Central Cholinergic Mechanisms and Adaptive Dysfunctions

Central Cholinergic Mechanisms and Adaptive Dysfunctions

Edited by

Man Mohan Singh

Southern Illinois University School of Medicine
Springfield, Illinois

David M. Warburton

University of Reading
Reading, United Kingdom

and

Harbans Lal

Texas College of Osteopathic Medicine
Fort Worth, Texas

assisted by

Barbara Mason

Southern Illinois University School of Medicine
Springfield, Illinois

Plenum Press • *New York and London*

Library of Congress Cataloging in Publication Data

Main entry under title:

Central cholinergic mechanisms and adaptive dysfunctions.

Includes bibliographies and index.
1. Mental illness — Physiological aspects. 2. Mental illness — Etiology. 3. Acetylcholine.
4. Psychopharmacology. I. Singh, Man Mohan. II. Warburton, David M. III. Lal,
Harbans. [DNLM: 1. Mental Disorders — etiology. 2. Psychopharmacology. 3. Recep-
tors, Cholinergic — psychopathology. WL 102.8 C397 1984]
RC455.4.B5C46   1984   616.89′071   84-18126
ISBN-13: 978-1-4684-1220-8   e-ISBN-13: 978-1-4684-1218-5
DOI: 10.1007/978-1-4684-1218-5

© 1985 Plenum Press, New York
Softcover reprint of the hardcover 1st edition 1985

A Division of Plenum Publishing Corporation
233 Spring Street, New York, N.Y. 10013

Dedicated to the mentally ill,
who will some day teach us to understand
the workings of the brain's minds

PREFACE

Although serious interest in studying the role of central cholinergic processes in psychopathology is just beginning to emerge, experimental literature on the part played by cholinergic mechanisms in brain behavior relations is quite extensive. During the past thirty years, cholinergic research has contributed significantly to the characterization and differentiation of adaptive mechanisms involved in input selection, perception, cortical, autonomic and behavioral activation, learning, memory, and inhibitory control of behavioral outputs. To say that dysfunction of one or more of these mechanisms may be at the root of neuropsychiatric illnesses such as schizophrenia would be stating the obvious.

This book examines the part cholinergic processes might play in dysfunctions of the adaptive processes involved in higher brain functions and their significance for the pathogenesis, classification, etiology, and treatment of psychopathological conditions.

In a series of wide ranging reviews of the available information, the subject is discussed from a variety of perspectives, using data derived from both experimental and clinical research. The purpose is not so much to determine whether cholinergic excess or deficiency is causal in this or that neuropsychiatric syndrome, but rather to try to understand the disease mechanisms in terms of adaptive processes in which cholinergic systems seem to play an important part. An underlying agenda for this exercise is to begin to prepare the ground for scientific psychiatry, or what we would like to term clinical neuroscience, in which the experimental and clinical observations can be understood and developed within a single framework. Only the development of such a framework can permit us to formulate experimentally testable hypotheses concerning disease mechanisms in terms of specific neurophysiological and neuropsychological processes, and go beyond sweeping hypotheses in which complex and heterogenous conditions such as schizophrenia are viewed as being due to too much or too little activity of a certain neurotransmitter system. It may well transpire that a central cholinergic abnormality as such proves not to be a primary etiological factor in any psychiatric illness, but still the information provided by cholinergic manipulations may help

us to understand the nature of abnormal mental functions because the
mechanisms involved include, or are affected by, cholinergic neurons.
Such information would, no doubt, be valuable.

The book starts with a historical overview of research on cholinergic systems and behavior. This is followed by a chapter on the
functional anatomy of the cholinergic pathways in the brain. Several
chapters are then devoted to reviewing the animal data concerning the
role of cholinergic mechanisms in orienting, habituation, learning,
memory, operant behavior, motor control, aggression, and electrophysiology. This sets the stage for chapters which review experimental
and clinical data in humans related to schizophrenia, affective disorders and dementia. The final chapter attempts a synthesis of the
foregoing information in the framework of a functional anatomical
brain model and speculates on a perspective for future research.

All the chapters went through a review and revision process which
was designed to decrease the unevenness of quality and style of a
multi-authored work and to avoid unnecessary duplication of information. A table of contents before every chapter should provide ready
reference to the information in that chapter, while the organization
of the book has been designed to allow for progression of ideas from
the laboratory to the clinic.

It is essentially a research monograph which should be of the
greatest appeal to both the clinical and laboratory researchers and
to those who may be described as neurotheoreticians. However, there
is much in it of interest for advanced level students of psychiatry,
psychology, psychopharmacology, and neuroscience. Parts of it would
undoubtedly also be of value to psychobiologically-oriented psychiatrists.

Contributing to a work of this kind is essentially a labor of
love in which the main reward for the long hours spent is the satis-
faction of sharing knowledge with others. We are most grateful to
all the authors and their assistants who have helped to bring this
project to fruition, and to Rosemary McCall, Ruth McLemore and Betty
Jo Taylor for the final typing. Also, we would like to thank those
involved at Plenum Publishing Corporation for their faith, patience
and helpfulness.

Man Mohan Singh

David M. Warburton

Harbans Lal

CONTENTS

Chapter 1

HISTORICAL OVERVIEW OF RESEARCH ON CHOLINERGIC SYSTEMS AND BEHAVIOR

David M. Warburton and Keith Wesnes

Department of Psychology
Reading University
Reading, RG6 2A1, U.K.

1.   INTRODUCTION

     This chapter will trace some of the history of work on the rela-
tion between cholinergic systems in the brain and behavior. The
problem of such a task is that work proceeded in parallel in several
laboratories and there was cross-fertilization of ideas between the
various research groups so that common themes evolved. However, a
chapter must of necessity be serial and so the reader should bear in
mind this interrelatedness of ideas between research groups. For the
purposes of exposition, the chapter is divided into four parts: Part
I covers the period from 1950 to 1970 and the development of a set of
competing hypotheses from human and animal research on cholinergic
systems and behavior; Part II describes the resolution of some of the
controversies of the previous 20 years during the early 1970's and the
development of a more comprehensive psychopharmacological hypothesis;
and in Part III the neuropharmacological work on the cholinergic
system from 1950 to 1980 is described and shown to be completely consonant with the behavioral research so that a neurochemical hypothesis
of cholinergic systems and behavior could be proposed. The final
Part IV describes the human research after 1975 which has confirmed
and extended the neurochemical theorizing.

2.   PART I: 1950–1970 EMERGENCE OF ACETYLCHOLINE–BEHAVIOR HYPOTHESES

     Some of the first interest in cholinergic systems and behavior
stemmed from the action of the anticholinesterase nerve gases which
were investigated extensively for chemical warfare. These agents are
organophosphorous esters and were first developed in Germany as insecticides at the end of the 1930's. The major agents developed were
Tabun (known as GA in the United States) and Sarin (GB). Soman (GE)
was also developed in Germany, but was not manufactured because its
toxicity was only comparable to Sarin. Since 1950, a new range of
anticholinesterase agents, the V compounds, were developed that were
more effective, because they could be absorbed through the skin due
to their low volatility. One of the first signs of poisoning by all
these anticholinesterases is muscular impairment. High doses of an
anticholinesterase are lethal but it was obviously interesting to discover the effects of sub-lethal doses on behavior and the counterac-
tive effects of cholinolytic antagonists to the compounds.

     From this military research and work stimulated by the initial
results, three rather different concepts of the involvement of the
cholinergic system in behavior developed in parallel. These were an
involvement in adaptive behavior, in mediating focus of attention and
in controlling behavioral inhibition.

2.1.   Acetylcholine and Adaptive Behavior

     Research in this area has followed two strategies: concomitant variation (experimental manipulation of the cholinergic system and measuring behavior) and correlated variation (relating individual differences in behavior to individual differences in cholinergic neurochemistry, Russell, 1969).

2.1.1. Concomitant Variations of Cholinergic Systems and Behavior

The pioneering experiments on changing the cholinergic system and testing animal behavior experimentally (Russell, 1954, 1958) were directed towards a search for general empirical relations between cholinesterase activity and behavior. Cholinesterase activity was reduced by administration of a potent organophosphorus agent, Systox (OO-diethyl-S-ethylmercaptoethanol thiophosphate). Since there were no clues about how behavior might be affected besides motor impairment, a wide variety of standardized behavior patterns were used in order to evaluate the behavioral changes resulting from manipulations of the cholinergic system. Initial results indicated that, although the acquisition of new response patterns appeared not to be affected by the reduction in enzyme activity, the extinction of responses was slower for the animals drugged with an anticholinesterase than for control animals. There was no evidence that other aspects of behavior were affected.

Further investigations (Russell et al., 1961) confirmed the differential effects of cholinesterase inhibition on conditioning and extinction when the same operant response was involved. Dose-response functions showed that the relation between cholinesterase activity and extinction was non-linear, but that there was a "critical level" between 40 and 50 percent of normal cholinesterase activity below which speed of extinction was inversely related to cholinesterase activity. A consistent tendency was found for the efficiency of performance to increase at levels of cholinesterase activity between this critical level and normal, but the effect was not statistically significant. In other experiments (Banks and Russell, 1967), the effect of chronic reductions of cholinesterase activity below the critical level of 40 to 50 percent was to increase errors in serial problem solving when new problems were presented.

These results were extended in a series of studies by Glow and his collaborators (Glow and Rose, 1966; Glow, Richardson and Rose, 1966), using several different behavioral tests. Glow and Rose confirmed by bioassay that there were "out of control" increases in acetylcholine after cholinesterase reduction to below 40 percent of normal. Slower extinction occurred when cholinesterase activity was reduced below 40 to 45 percent of normal. They also provided further evidence that the resistance to extinction could not be explained in terms of motivational or non-specific performance factors.

This biphasic action relates to the results of research on relations between cholinesterase activity and other psychobiological variables. Metz (1958) had described a cross-over from potentiation to decline in a respiratory reflex at about 40 percent of normal brain cholinesterase activity. This critical level is in the range where Aprison (1962) had reported that cholinesterase loses control of its substrate so that acetylcholine content in brain began increasing rapidly below this level and cholinergic nerve function was impaired (Wilson and Cohen, 1953).

Russell (1958) interpreted his work in terms of adjustment to the environment. Any adaptive behavior requires extinction of previous behavior patterns and the speed of extinction will determine the rate of adaptive behavior changes. If a cholinergic system in the brain is a part of this mechanism, then more efficient cholinergic transmission will produce more rapid extinction while cholinergic blockade will impair adjustment.

A line of research which ran in parallel with the work of Russell was that of Feldberg and Sherwood (1954b) who reported stereotyped behavior - an extreme form of maladaptive behavior - after blockade of the cholinergic system. They injected cats intraventricularly with either di-isopropylfluorophosphate (DFP) or physostigmine, two powerful anticholinesterase agents. A catatonic-like stupor was a dramatic feature of the response to these drugs (Feldberg and Sherwood, 1954a). For example, when placed in an erect posture with its front paws on the upper rung of a stool or when placed across two stools, the cat remained in these positions for many minutes. Nevertheless, its movements were not impaired because it jumped in a well-coordinated manner when pushed.

Signs of catatonia were also observed when large doses of acetylcholine were injected intraventricularly and so it is highly likely that these actions of DFP were an effect of unhydrolyzed acetylcholine, which was not exciting the neurons, but paralyzing them. It is known that, in the presence of an anticholinesterase, the main effect of stimulating a motor nerve, after an initial augmentation of contraction, is neuromuscular block. Thus Feldberg (1963) argued that unmetabolized acetylcholine may have a similar paralyzing action on synaptic transmission in central cholinergic neurons.

Stupor and catatonia occur in some forms of schizophrenia and it is interesting to note that other symptoms of this illness have been described in response to anticholinesterases. When DFP was used in the treatment of myasthenia gravis, patients experienced nightmares, confusion and hallucinations (Grob et al, 1947) and DFP given to schizophrenics caused reactivation of the psychosis (Rowntree et al., 1950). Feldberg (1964) claimed "In our cats, we also observed behavioral changes which suggested that the cats had hallucinations." (p430). If acetylcholine acts by blocking central synaptic transmission, it would explain why hallucinations can also be produced by cholinolytics. Atropine and scopolamine poisoning produce dramatic hallucinations (Warburton, 1979). If excessive acetylcholine acts by

blocking central synaptic transmission then it should have the same
effect as the central synaptic block produced by an antagonist.

Consequently, Feldberg (1964) argued that the hallucinations and
the catatonia seen after DFP are due to an effect of undestroyed acetylcholine, which produced a blockade of cholinergic function. However, when these symptoms occur in schizophrenic patients without
treatment with DFP, it cannot be concluded that they result from an
excess of acetylcholine. The most conservative conclusion is that
these failures of adaptation are due to impaired function of a system
which involves cholinergic neurons. These data suggest that treatment
with cholinergic drugs should be effective in the treatment of schizophrenia, as a diagnostic entity. Consequently, a number of investigators have tried cholinergic therapy with schizophrenics but have
obtained mixed results. However, important evidence suggests that
these differences of outcome are the result of choice of patient for
cholinergic therapy and not the total lack of efficacy of cholinergic
treatment per se.

Support for this conclusion has come more recently from the thorough, systematic studies of the countertherapeutic effects of cholino-
linolytics on neuroleptic medication in the schizophrenias, which have
been carried out by Singh and Smith (1973a,b) and Singh and Kay (1975,
1978, 1979). The studies were carried out using a longitudinal design
in which a neuroleptic alone was given before and after a period
during which a cholinolytic drug was also given with the neuroleptic.
All the patients were actively psychotic and drug-free when included
in the study, and particular emphasis was placed on differentiating
them diagnostically. Measures of psychopathology and social functioning were obtained at different points during the course of each study.

Analyses showed significant countertherapeutic effects of the
cholinolytic on the beneficial effects of neuroleptics in terms of
thought disorder, uncooperativeness and disorientation. The signs and
symptoms involved were clearly those considered characteristic of the
schizophrenias. Crow et al. (1981) have found support for the observations of Singh and his co-workers in terms of the action of cholinolytics on psychotic symptoms. When the changes were considered longi-
tudinally, the countertherapeutic cholinolytic effects were most evident in social measures when it was introduced early on in therapy,
whereas later on it was increasingly evident in the cognitive function
(Singh and Kay, 1975, 1979).

In addition, Singh and Kay (1978) made a very interesting set of
analyses on the treatment of diagnostic subtypes, which were most susceptible to the countertherapeutic effects of cholinolytics. It
seemed that the effects were most evident in the good prognosis, nonparanoid, mostly catatonic, type of schizophrenia and much less in the
hebephrenic and undifferentiated types, while paranoid schizophrenia
seems to be rather different neurochemically.

Thus there could be three biological subgroups of schizophrenia in terms of the cholinergic system function. The first group might be characterized as suffering from reversible deficit of cholinergic systems which still remain responsive, and so cholinergic stimulation can produce clinical improvement. The patients in this class would tend to belong to clinical types diagnosed as catatonic, acute, schizophreniform or good prognosis schizophrenia (Singh and Kay, 1978). The second group might be characterized as suffering from an under-activity in addition to an under-reactivity of cholinergic mechanisms. Patients of this type would tend to fall into the poor prognosis, or nuclear, nonparanoid categories such as hebephrenia and chronic undifferentiated schizophrenia. Patients with paranoid schizophrenia would be within normal limits cholinergically. Unfortunately, as Singh and Kay (Chapter 9) point out, these conclusions do not suggest any break-through in the treatment of schizophrenia. Most of the drugs which increase cholinergic activity tend to be too toxic and susceptible to the development of tolerance to be useful therapeutically. In addition, the cholinergic systems in chronic, nonparanoid schizophrenics, who represent a major part of the therapy-resistant schizophrenia population, seem to be more or less unresponsive to cholinergic agents. For this group, the search would have to be for the means of under-standing and reversing some sort of cholinergic receptor impairment. This digression has been included in order to show how the work of Russell and of Feldberg and Sherwood on "adaptive behavior" has been followed up and is producing fruitful hypotheses for the treatment of the schizophrenias.

2.1.2. The Correlative Approach to Cholinergic Systems and Behavior

A different method for trying to elucidate the relationships between cholinergic systems and adaptive behavior has been the correlative neurochemical approach. This research was begun in 1953 at the University of California at Berkeley by Krech, Rosenzweig, and Bennett, but had strong conceptual links with the work of Russell. This work was focused on the inactivating enzyme for acetylcholine, acetylcholinesterase, because of the ease of assay for this enzyme in the 1950's and the absence of a reliable biochemical assay technique for acetylcholine.

Krech and his colleagues regarded acetylcholinesterase activity per gram of neural tissue as a measure of cholinergic synaptic activity due to its localization at the membranes of nerve endings. This activity increases rapidly in the young rat to a maximum value at about 80 days. Similarly, cholinesterase activity per gram, was presumed to be related to glial function and was known to increase rapidly to peak at 40 days of age. In one set of experiments Rosenzweig et al., (1968) compared the cholinergic chemistry of the brains of a set of rats raised in a deprived environment with that of their littermates raised in an enriched environment. In the enriched condition, groups of animals lived in a large cage which contained ladders, tunnels, and levers, and were regularly put in mazes, discrimination boxes and other new environments. In the deprived environment each rat was isolated in a bare cage.

After this treatment, there was an increase in the cortical weight which was largest in the visual cortex, intermediate in the dorsal and ventral cortices and least in the somesthetic cortex. The cholinergic differences between the two experimental groups were found nearly as consistently as the weight differences. Enzyme activity can be expressed in terms of activity per unit weight (specific activity) or in terms of total activity for the samples. The activity of acetylcholinesterase increases in the cortex less rapidly than weight, since part of the cortical weight increase was made up of noncholinergic parts, such as glial cells and blood vessels. Thus, for the enriched rat there was an increase in total acetylcholinesterase in the cortex but a decrease in acetylcholinesterase per unit weight of cortical material. As a consequence, although total activity increases, the specific activity (the ability to hydrolyze acetylcholine) decreases slightly. In addition, the enriched brain had a considerably lower cortical to subcortical ratio of acetylcholinesterase per unit weight. If acetylcholinesterase is an inverse index of synaptic activity these results suggest that the cortex of an "environmentally enriched" brain has a small increase in functional ability at the cholinergic nerve endings due to the enriching experience.

In conjunction with, and consistent with, the histological observation of an increase in the glial cells of the enriched cortex, there was the increase in cortical cholinesterase, an enzyme found primarily in the glial cells. In addition, there was a greater cortical to subcortical ratio of cholinesterase activity in the deprived animals. Finally, if we can consider the ratio of cholinesterase to acetylcholinesterase reflects the ratio of glial to neuron cells, then we have a neurochemical index which indicates that the enriched rat has more glial cells serving each neuron than deprived rats.

The next step in the Krech, Rosenzweig and Bennett research program was to try and link these differences to problem-solving ability. Accurate measures of rat "intelligence" or problem-solving ability are complex, but Krech and his co-workers found significant correlations of performance in a reversal discrimination test with both the cortical to subcortical weight ratio and the cortical to subcortical ratio of acetylcholinesterase activity in those animals raised in different environments.

In a complementary set of genetic studies (Krech, 1968; Bennett and Rosenzweig, 1968), they tested ten different strains of rats (each of which had a characteristically different cholinergic-anatomical brain pattern) on problem-solving ability, and looked for relations between their cholinergic system and problem-solving performance. Prior to testing, these animals all received a brief period of enriched experience in order to give them optimum brain characteristics

prior to testing and to minimize further brain changes during the
reversal discrimination testing procedure. For each experiment they
determined the brightest and dullest strains and then compared the
anatomical and cholinergic, cortical to subcortical ratios of the
strains in order to see whether they differed in their cholinergic
neurochemistry.

They found that the brightest strains had a higher cortical to
subcortical weight ratio, a slightly lower acetylcholinesterase ratio
in these regions, a considerably higher cholinesterase ratio and an
equally higher cholinesterase to acetylcholinesterase ratio than the
dullest strains. When this profile was compared with the profile of
differences between the brains of enriched and deprived rats from a
single strain, the profile of similarities showed that animals of
different strains raised in the same environment but differing in
problem-solving ability, had brain differences similar to those of
animals from the same strain but raised in different environments.

In addition, they determined for the 299 rats in 22 groups, four
within-stock correlations: (1) the cortical to subcortical weight
ratio versus the error score; (2) the cortical, subcortical acetylcholinesterase ratio versus errors; (3) the cortical to subcortical
cholinesterase ratio versus errors; and (4) the combination of the
acetylcholinesterase and cholinesterase measures. Consistently, both
within-strain and between-strain correlational analyses supported the
hypothesis that anatomical and cholinergic measures are related to
problem-solving ability. Thus a good "adaptive" brain had a relatively high cortical to subcortical weight ratio, along with low acetylcholinesterase, high cholinesterase, and high cholinesterase to acetylcholinesterase ratios (i.e., more functional acetylcholine per unit
neuron) irrespective of whether the differences resulted from genes or
the environment.

In summary, the work of Russell and his co-workers, Feldberg and
Sherwood, the Berkeley group, and more recently Singh, Kay and Smith,
has suggested a relation between adaptive behavior and the functional
acetylcholine in the brain. The latter studies give some evidence for
the importance of cortical acetylcholine. The precise way in which
cholinergic systems are involved with adaptive behavior is not clear
from the work of these groups.

2.2. Acetylcholine and Learning

In 1966, Deutsch and his co-workers (Deutsch et al., 1966) presented some interesting data based on the earlier work on adaptive
behavior. Although Russell had found no changes in learning after
anticholinesterases, Deutsch wondered if there might be some relation
between the adaptive behavior changes and memory systems. He argued
that if learning involved increases in the effectiveness of cholinergic synapses, then it should be possible to strengthen or weaken

memory by cholinergic drugs. He tested this hypothesis using DFP (disopropylfluorophosphate), physostigmine and scopolamine. As physostigmine and DFP prolong the effects of ACh by inhibiting acetylcholinesterase, then these drugs should strengthen weak memories, but weaken strong memories because there will be excessive acetylcholine which will result in a depolarization block. Scopolamine would markedly impair weak memories but would have a much smaller effect on strong memories.

Rats were trained to escape shock in a simple Y maze. After training, some rats were given a delay of seven days before testing, while others waited 18 days. After the delay, the animals received either a placebo or a dose of drug before their memory was assessed. The predictions were strikingly confirmed and these experiments by Deutsch and others (see review by Deutsch, 1973) would seem to indicate that learning involves increased efficiency of cholinergic synapses.

There is also some evidence for the involvement of cholinergic processes in human learning. Drachman and Leavitt (1974) injected young adult volunteers with scopolamine or physostigmine. While immediate memory was spared, storage of new information was significantly impaired by scopolamine, both for ordered recall of digits and for free recall of word lists. Retrieval by category, a test presumed to depend on intactness of both the retrieval mechanisms and long-term memory stores, showed mild impairment. Interpretation of this test was made difficult, however, by the distractibility of the subjects, who would often retrieve items from other categories in the midst of an otherwise adequate performance. No subjects exhibited an alteration of the sensory input of sufficient degree to explain the impaired memory or cognitive performance, except for the effect of variation of the subjects' attention on the retrieval tests.

Physostigmine failed to produce any significant memory or cognitive effects although some performed marginally better. Drachmann and Leavitt speculated that in normal young adults there is sufficient acetylcholine present for cognitive functioning, and a slight increase in acetylcholine neither improves nor impairs function. However, it is just as likely that the tests used were not sensitive enough to detect improvements.

The findings of this study support and extend the observations of previous studies of human memory and cholinergic drugs (e.g., Safer and Allen, 1971). Several of these workers have noted that the performance of the scopolamine subjects was similar in many ways to that of undrugged senile people. Accordingly, they have hypothesized that the memory problems of Alzheimer's disease may be due to an acetylcholine deficiency. However, although memory is affected in Alzheimer's disease and after cholinolytics the behavioral process which results in impairment could be due to an alteration in the memory processing, it is possible that performance deficits with cholinolytics result from impairment of information input at the time of acquisition or retrieval.

2.3. Acetylcholine and Focus of Attention

The military used atropine in order to protect against, and provide an antidote for, nerve gas poisoning. Consequently, they were concerned about the more subtle psychological and neurological changes in soldiers who were given atropine and other cholinolytics and thus conducted and sponsored a whole series of human studies on the possible behavioral effects of these compounds.

It was found that soldiers who were given atropine could answer simple questions (Ostfeld et al., 1960) but could not understand complex conversations and carry out instructions (White et al., 1956; Ketchum et al., 1973). Their attention could not be attracted and they appeared to be daydreaming (Ketchum et al., 1973). Some of them felt a sense of detachment from reality (Callaway and Band, 1958). Usually, they reported loss of awareness or alertness, a difficulty in concentrating and a shortened attention span (White et al., 1956; Michelson, 1961; Ostfeld et al., 1960; Crowell and Ketchum, 1967; Ketchum et al., 1973).

In experimental tests, there were increased errors on the Stroop Test following drug administration (Callaway and Band, 1958; Ostfeld and Aruguete, 1962) which were the result of the subjects being distracted by the semantic information (e.g., the word "red" printed in blue), while naming the print color of a word. Subjects that had been injected with atropine also experienced difficulty in filtering out irrelevant parts of the design in the Gottschalk Embedded Figures Test in which they had to find a figure which is embedded within a larger design (Callaway and Band, 1958). In contrast, in the Luchins Test, which consists of a series of problems of how to obtain a given volume of water with three different measures, atropine improved performance when the mode of solution was changed. Thus, drugged subjects discovered the new, short method of solving the problems faster than the control group. Atropine also improved performance in a disjunctive reaction time experiment in which the subjects pressed one of two keys if they detected a light or heard a buzzer (Miles, 1955). These findings were the first to lead to the hypothesis that atropine and cholinolytics in general disrupt the attention of the subjects.

In two papers, Callaway (Callaway and Dembo, 1958; Callaway and Band, 1958) proposed that the impairment after a dose of atropine resulted from "broadened attention." Broadened attention was defined as an increase in the influence of peripheral factors such as relatively current environmental events which are removed from the central focus of attention by space, time, or by differences of meaning (Callaway and Dembo, 1958). The improved performance could also be explained in terms of cholinolytics broadening attention if one must use a broader focus of attention to respond to two modalities. Callaway and Band (1958) claimed that atropine improved performance by broadening attention, so that the subject attended to aspects of the task which were not essential for the original test but helped in discovering the simpler method by attending to peripheral factors. It was not explicitly stated but it was implied that atropine was acting on the focus of attention via some cholinergic system in the brain.

2.4. Acetylcholine and Behavioral Inhibition

A variety of closely related response inhibition hypotheses has been proposed, and will be considered in this section.

2.4.1. Pavlovian Internal Inhibition

At the beginning of the 1960's, Michelson (1961) summarized research in the Soviet Union which pointed to the idea that there was a cholinergic system in the brain mediating the process of conditioned internal inhibition. He reviewed studies which showed that anticholinesterases intensified cholinergic activity in the body and enhanced differential and extinctive inhibition while muscarinic cholinolytics weakened both forms of internal inhibition. Inhibition as a psychological concept was derived by Pavlov from physiology in which the term refers to arrest of the function of one neural structure by the activity of another, but the ability to execute that function is not abolished and can be manifested when the activity of the inhibiting structure is reduced (Brunton, 1883). Michelson concluded that these changes in behavioral inhibition were the result of action of drugs on cholinergic systems of the cerebral cortex and of the reticular formation.

2.4.2. Inhibition of Non-Reinforced Responses

Soon after this proposal, Carlton (1963) suggested a more adventurous and comprehensive theory. He speculated that there was a catecholamine system controlling behavioral excitation and an antagonistic cholinergic system producing inhibition of non-reinforced responses. The cholinergic system antagonized the diffuse effects of catecholaminergic activation and provided a basis for selective effects of activation on responses to the extent that these responses were correlated with non-reinforcement. The level of activation controlled the probability of occurrence for all responses while the cholinergic system acted to antagonize this activation of non-reinforced responses. The outcome of this interaction would be that a change in activation would only alter the probability of occurrence of a subset of responses, i.e., those that were reinforced (Carlton, 1963). Carlton's conception of inhibition is very close to the traditional physiological use of the term inhibition in which there is arrest of the function of one system by the activity of another.

     The relations between extinction and the effects of anticholin-
esterases on the cholinergic system were reinterpreted in terms of
inhibitory control over "competing responses" (Russell, 1966). Observation of behavior under even the most restricted environmental circumstances shows that an array of different responses are initially
available to the organism, the majority of which soon cease to appear
as they fail to be reinforced. That the latter have not been abolished from the organism's repertoire can be demonstrated by altering
some feature of the situation and they are reinstated wholly or partially, suggesting that, during exposure to the situation, competing
responses had merely been suppressed. If reduction in cholinesterase
activity were to enhance their suppression, competing responses would
not be as readily available to interfere with the dominant, reinforced
behavior and hence, the latter would be more resistant to extinction.

2.4.3. Inhibition of Stimulus-Response Associations

     Another type of response inhibition was suggested by Douglas
(1967). This was inhibition of learned responses, i.e., associations
between stimuli and responses. One version of this hypothesis
(Warburton, 1967; Russell and Warburton, 1973) proposed that a cholinergic system was important in the inhibitory control of all competing and dominant learned responses. A blockage of central neural
function by anticholinergics and high doses of anticholinesterases
would result in a disinhibition of all responses, but with lower
probability, competing responses increasing proportionally more than
the higher probability, dominant responses, especially if these higher
probability responses were already at their response ceiling. The
locus of this inhibitory control was thought to be in the hippocampus
(Douglas, 1967; Warburton, 1967).

2.4.4. Inhibition of Response Sets

     The remaining version of a behavioral inhibition mechanism has
been proposed by Mishkin (1964). This mechanism was said to involve
a system involving the frontal cortex and produced suppression of competing response sets. A particular mode of response might be appropriate in one situation but inappropriate in another and a correct
choice would depend on inhibition of the initial set. Damage to the
system would result in perseveration of a central "set" or mode of
responding rather than in perseveration of a specific response. This
perseveration would even produce lowered responding if the original
set had a strong "no go" tendency. This hypothesis was adopted by
Bignami and Rosic (1972) to explain the performance deficits caused
by cholinolytics and they suggested that there is a cholinergic system
which acts on the "motor" side of the stimulus-response chain to suppress competing response sets.

3.   PART II: 1970-1975 A PSYCHOPHARMACOLOGICAL HYPOTHESIS OF
     STIMULUS SELECTION

Many of the studies of the late 1960's and early 1970's were
devoted to obtaining evidence consistent with behavioral inhibition
ideas and not towards testing between the different hypotheses. It
is clear that there was a strong divergence of opinion about the behavioral mode of action of cholinergic drugs. In man, there was some
evidence which suggested that attentional processes were affected by
cholinergic drugs while in animals the research findings had been interpreted to indicate that cholinergic drugs were involved in response
control and so the stage was set for tests of the competing focus of
attention, memory and behavioral inhibition hypotheses at the beginning of the 1970's.

3.1. Tests of the Competing Hypotheses

In order to resolve this apparent disparity in hypotheses, a
series of animal experiments was performed to test directly the attention and behavioral inhibition hypotheses (Brown and Warburton, 1971;
Warburton and Brown, 1971; Warburton, 1972). In particular, they
examined extensively the hypothesis of a generalized loss of stimulus
control. In order to do this, several sorts of discrimination performance were analyzed using the theory of signal detectability. It was
predicted that a loss of response inhibition would result in an up-
wards shift in the response criterion. However, a loss of stimulus
sensitivity would produce equal conditional probabilities in all intervals whereas improved signal sensitivity would be reflected in a
decreased conditional probability of a response before the signal onset and an increased probability after the signal.

Application of the analysis was made to the effects of scopolamine on performance controlled by a temporal, i.e., internal, stimulus
in differential reinforcement of low rate (Brown and Warburton, 1971),
to performance controlled by an external stimulus in light-dark discrimination (Warburton, 1972; Warburton and Brown, 1974) and to performance controlled by a paired internal-external cue consisting of a
temporal discrimination with added external cue (Warburton and Brown,
1971). It was found that there were changes in stimulus sensitivity
which were not accompanied by any lowering of the animals' response
criterion. These results demonstrated unequivocally that cholinergic
blockade modified behavior by impairing the stimulus input but not by
changing the response output i.e., contradicting the loss of response
inhibition hypothesis.

In fact, evidence which could have been used to contradict the
response inhibition hypothesis had been obtained earlier by Carlton
himself in a study of habituation, but the data were not interpreted
in these terms. Carlton and Vogel (1965) had put some animals into a
novel chamber whereas others were not given this experience. Half of

the subjects in each group were injected with scopolamine prior to
exposure, while half received saline. Three days later, the animals
were water deprived and then placed in the chamber with water.
Animals who had been put in the chamber would be expected to have a
shorter drinking latency than animals who had not been given this
habituation experience. The two saline injected groups had shorter
latencies than before, but the scopolamine injected rats behaved as
if they had never been exposed.

    A crucial aspect of this study is that the animals were trained
under the influence of scopolamine but tested after an injection of
saline. If scopolamine acts on a behavioral inhibition system, it
should have no effect in terms of responding during the test session.
However, if the scopolamine had interfered with some stimulus input
mechanisms, then the amount of habituation would be less and the
effect would carry over to the test session. The group trained under
scopolamine, but tested without the drug did show marked impairment.
Obviously, this result cannot be explained in terms of scopolamine
impairing a cholinergic response output mechanism, but must have
affected a stimulus input system.

    A direct way of testing the stimulus selection hypothesis was to
compare the performance of animals on a double stimulus discrimination
with their performance when only a single exteroceptive stimulus was
presented. It would be predicted that double-cued discriminations
would be less sensitive to cholinolytics, because two cues would be
available if the animal switched modalities. A successive discrimination was used with either a light, a tone, or a light plus a tone as
the relevant stimuli (Warburton, 1974). After training, all animals
were tested for stimulus equivalence by presenting each animal with a
set of transfer trials, which were signaled by either one or other of
the two discriminative cues. Following the transfer test, the rats
were tested with scopolamine. The results showed that there was significantly more impairment produced by scopolamine in the group
trained with only one stimulus. In addition, individuals within the
double stimulus groups that responded mainly to one cue were more
affected by the drug than subjects who pressed almost equally in
response to both cues.

    This result was supported by a two-trial study by Heise (1975).
During the first trial, a stimulus was presented which set the occasion for a go or a no-go response on the second trial. One group has
to discriminate between two tones which determined the response on the
second trial. A second group had to respond on the first trial, and
the presence or absence of reinforcement was the cue for the second
trial responding. The third group discriminated between the two tones
and responded for reinforcement on the first trial, and the stimulus
for responding on the second trial was the double stimulus of the tone
together with the presence or absence of reinforcement on the first
trial. Scopolamine had the least effect on subjects in the third

group who had multiple cues for responding. These studies confirm that the number of stimuli can determine the magnitude of cholinergic blocking effects, which again indicates the involvement of a cholinergic system with stimulus processing rather than response output processes like response inhibition.

A comparison between single and multiple cues and between internal and external cues in the same subject was made by Warburton and Heise (1972). They trained rats in spatial double-alternation responding. Responding on different components of the sequence was controlled by a different set of internal and external stimuli. The first left response of the double-alternation sequence was controlled by a single "external" cue. The second left and first right were controlled by two internal cues, while the second right was under the control of a single internal cue. Scopolamine increased the total number of errors. The mean number of errors for each dose was divided up into switching errors, i.e., changing levers on successive trials and perseveration errors, which would be expected to reflect the amount of response inhibition. The number of errors in each category increased as the total number of errors increased, and the proportions of perseverative and switching errors changed very little with increasing doses of the drug, until at the higher doses the probabilities of both switching and perseveration were nearly equal. It seems that perseveration and switching errors were being made because animals did not discriminate the cues for responding correctly. However, there does not appear to be any strong stimulus specificity in the action of scopolamine on internal as opposed to external cues, which suggests that the drug results in a general loss of stimulus control. In addition, since the "internal" cue was a remembered one, there was no evidence of a specific effect on memory. However, the drug effects on multi-cued discriminations were less than on the single-cued performance, which once again gave evidence for a stimulus input process being affected.

In summary, these tests have given no evidence for a cholinergic mechanism which could be involved in response inhibition. The impairment of performance was independent of memory, although it cannot be concluded that a change in cholinergic systems would not impair memory. Instead, the evidence points to an effect on a stimulus input process.

3.2. Stimulus Selection Hypothesis

From this sort of evidence, it was hypothesized that a cholinergic system is involved in a mechanism which is responsible for selecting the relevant stimuli from the environment. These stimuli are the information which leads to the performance of relevent responses and the inhibition of irrelevant behavior. Organisms have many sorts of stimuli which could potentially influence their behavior in any situation. From the external environment, stimuli impinge on the exteroceptors, while after a response there are outcome stimuli. In

addition, responses are influenced by internal stimuli, including
response-produced cues and previous "remembered" stimuli. These two
classes of stimuli may be relevant, irrelevant or partially relevant
for behavior. Responses will be determined by selection by a cholinergic mechanism of a subset of stimuli from these various sources.

     If cholinergic drugs were affecting a mechanism of this sort, it
might be predicted that impairment would be increased in discrimination acquisition when irrelevent cues were present, or when multiple
relevant cues were available. This was demonstrated by Whitehouse
(1967) when be trained rats on a simultaneous discrimination with
relevant visual cues of black or white arms of the maze. The introduction of tactile and auditory irrelevant cues slowed acquisition
rate. Injections of atropine slowed acquisition, and there were a
larger number of trials to a criterion. In a successive discrimination, where the relevent visual cue was color and the irrelevant cues
were tactual and auditory, atropine again retarded the acquisition of
the discrimination. In a series of experiments with multiple relevant
stimuli, Whitehouse (1967) trained rats with visual, auditory, and
tactile cues as relevant. The control animals learned the multi-cued
discrimination faster and with fewer errors than the rats that were
trained with a single cue. Atropine had little effect on the single-
cued discrimination, but acquisition was much slower than control in
the multi-cued discrimination.

     In another set of studies on stimulus control and cholinergic
function (Warburton, 1977), rats were trained for four days on a discrimination with two relevant cues. The rats were injected with doses
of scopolamine prior to session. After training, subjects were given
a transfer test which was preceded by an injection of the dose of drug
given during training, in order to determine the amount that they had
learned about the two cues. Acquisition performance showed that scopolamine impaired the acquisition of the discrimination. The drug
also slowed up the decrease in intertrial-interval responses, another
measure of discrimination learning. A stimulus selection explanation
of this impairment is that the scopolamine-injected animals were
switching cues more frequently than control animals and showing slower
learning. This prediction was examined in the transfer tests which
showed that animals who learned with two relevant cues did learn something about both cues but that the more a subject learned about one
cue the less he learned about the other. An interesting difference
was found between the transfer scores of the scopolamine and placebo
subjects. Most placebo subjects learned more about one cue than the
other, but animals injected with scopolamine tended to respond almost
equally in terms of both cues.

     These studies show clearly that cholinergic drugs are modifying
some cholinergic mechanism which is controlling the input of information. The latter studies give evidence for a cholinergic mechanism
which is involved in the processes of stimulus selection (Warburton,
1972) or "attention" as proposed by Callaway and Band (1958). Further

support for this involvement in stimulus processing can be derived
from a consideration of the anatomical distribution of the cholinergic
systems and their role in the control of electrocortical activity.

4.   PART III: 1950-1980 NEUROPHARMACOLOGICAL STUDIES OF CHOLINERGIC
     SYSTEMS

     In the 1950's and early 1960's we had very superficial knowledge
about the neurochemistry of the brain and, certainly, little information about the organization of the central nervous system. Biochemical content analysis had demonstrated that the brain contained some
of the peripheral nervous system transmitters and revealed that there
were very marked differences in concentration from region to region.
However, content analysis gave only a general idea of the regional
variation. Acetylcholine was identified in many places in the brain
but research in the 1960's showed that it was the only compound that
fitted the most stringent criteria for a central nervous system transmitter, i.e., evidence of release and identity of action.

     The criterion of demonstrating that the transmitter is released
from neurons in the central nervous system is one of the hardest to
satisfy. However, the presence of acetylcholine at the cortex was
discovered when cups were placed on the cortex and push-pull cannulae
were used to perfuse cortical areas. The cortical acetylcholine is
known to have been released from presynaptic terminals at the cortex
because the amount that is collected can be reduced by the removal of
calcium ions which are necessary for transmitter release at peripheral
cholinergic synapses (see Phillis, 1970).

     The origin of the fibers which initiated acetylcholine release
was outside the cortex because release was not observed when the
cortex was undercut and deprived of its afferent input (Mitchell,
1963). Cortical acetylcholine release was enchanced by sensory stimulation (Mitchell, 1963) but was not restricted to the cortical area
which corresponded to the modality of stimulation (Phillis, 1970).
This evidence points to release from a non-sensory pathway which projects to most areas of the cortex. The origin of this pathway seems
to be in the mesencephalic region of the brain stem; unilateral destruction of this region produced cortical synchronization and reduced
acetylcholine release in comparison with release from the cortex on
the intact side. In a second study, stimulation of the mesencephalic
reticular formation produced electrocortical arousal and increased
acetylcholine release from the cortex (Celesia and Jasper, 1966).
Thus release was independent of specific sensory input but was a
result of activity in a diffusely projecting pathway from the brain
stem.

     Important additional evidence for acetylcholine being a trans-
mitter in the central nervous system was establishing the presence of
synthesizing and inactivating enzymes for it. The terminals from

which the acetylcholine was collected were not in the sensory layer but in the deeper layers (Phillis, 1970). These deep layers are a region of pyramidal cells and have been shown to contain choline acetyltransferase, which is the synthesizing enzyme for acetylcholine. Acetylcholinesterase, the inactivating enzyme for acetylcholine, is present in neurons which are located in these regions (Krnjevic and Silver, 1965), and the origin of these acetylcholinesterase-containing fibers is the ventral tegmental area of the mesencephalic reticular formation (Shute and Lewis, 1967).

The second major criterion for acetylcholine being a central nervous system transmitter is evidence that it excites neuronal cells. Studies with iontophoretically applied acetylcholine have revealed that this transmitter excites neurons in many regions of the brain (Phillis, 1970), including the medullary and mesencephalic reticular formation, lateral and medial geniculate, caudate nucleus, ventrobasal complex of the thalamus, hippocampus, cerebellum, inferior colliculus and the Betz cells of the deep pyramidal layer of the cerebral cortex. Direct application of acetylcholine to the deep pyramidal layer of cortical cells, which appear to be the origin of the released acetylcholine, consistently produced prolonged excitation with slow onset (Krnjevic and Phillis, 1963) and also prolonged the evoked potentials to sensory stimulation (Krnjevic et al., 1971). Although acetylcholine has not been applied directly to the cortex and cortical activity measured, injections of acetylcholine into the carotid artery which supplies blood to the cortex produced electrocortical arousal (Bremer and Chatonnet, 1949).

In summary, the major criterion of collectability of transmitters had been satisfied together with evidence for the presence of synthesizing and inactivating enzymes in association with a diffuse pathway from the ventral tegmental area to the cortex. Microinjection studies have shown that acetylcholine acts as an excitatory transmitter in many parts of the brain. Acetylcholine has been collected as a consesequence of stimulating the ventral tegmental region. Transmitter release at the terminals of the pathway increase the excitation of nonsensory cells at the cortex and potentiate existing cortical excitation (Krnjevic and Phillis, 1963; Krnjevic et al., 1971). Electrophysiologically, the cortical excitation is manifested as increased electrocortical arousal and enhancement of sensory evoked potentials.

Histochemical techniques have been used to trace fiber pathways of acetylcholine. These studies revealed in considerable detail the unique patterns of distribution of acetylcholine pathways and the organizational complexity of them which content analysis had not indicated. The cholinergic pathways which have their origin in the brain stem have been analyzed thoroughly by Shute and Lewis over the last ten years and their work is summarized in the chapter by Robinson in this book. From their studies it can be seen there are at least three main systems - two ascending systems to the cortex and a hippocampal system. The ascending reticular systems are the dorsal and ventral tegmental pathways. The dorsal tegmental system projects to the thalamic regions including some, at least, of the primary sensory pathways and the ventral tegmental system projects to the neocortex and to diencephalic nuclei. The hippocampal cholinergic system ascends from the ventral tegmental area via the lateral preoptic, the diagonal band and medial septal nuclei to the hippocampus. This latter system could be the neurochemical substrate for stimulus selection.

4.1. A Hippocampal Mechanism for Stimulus Selection

Although there is little evidence for the involvement of the lateral preoptic nuclei in stimulus selection, there is some support for the involvement of the medial septal nuclei and hippocampal formation. Douglas and Pribram (1966) proposed a hippocampal system which gates out irrelevant aspects of the environment by inhibiting the input along the primary sensory pathways. Douglas and Pribram postulated that the probability of attention to a stimulus was increased by virtue of its association with reinforcement and other significant events in the environment. In a similar theory, Kimble (1968, 1969) has also emphasized the importance of hippocampal function for inhibition during habituation, extinction and discrimination. Novel stimuli would elicit cortical arousal via activity in the nonspecific sensory systems of the midbrain and thalamus. An organism would remain attentive to stimuli associated with reinforcement. Repeated presentation of the stimulus in the absence of reinforcement would result in the hippocampus inhibiting the non-specific arousal systems. The organism can switch its attention from that stimulus to new or more important environmental events. Several workers noted that the effects of lesions in the septal area and the hippocampal formation closely parallel the changes obtained after impairment of cholinergic function with cholinolytics (Meyers and Domino, 1964; Douglas and Isaacson, 1966).

In a test of the idea that the cholinergic hippocampal system was mediating stimulus selection, Warburton and Russell (1969) examined the effects on single alternation discrimination performance of atropine and carbachol injected into the ventral portion of the hippocampal formation. Atropine increased both no-go and inter-trial responding while carbachol reduced both which is consistent with the hypothesis of a hippocampal locus for selection. The hippocampal formation has cholinergic pathways which are projecting from the medial septal nuclei (Shute and Lewis, 1967). Cholinergic stimulation of these nuclei produced increased theta activity in the hippocampal formation analogous to that produced by sensory stimulation (Stumpf, 1965). Stimulation of the septal nuclei with carbachol with 0.5 to 5.0 micrograms produced a decrease in incorrect lever pressing in a discrimination test, while similar doses of atropine sulfate increased the error rate (Grossman, 1964) in the same way as intraperitoneally injected atropine. These two sets of data are consistent with information processing being mediated by a cholinergic, septo-hippocampal system.

The origin of the septo-hippocampal system is the tegmental
nuclei of the mesencephalic reticular formation. Carbachol, a cholinomimetic, and atropine methylbromide, were injected bilaterally
close to the ventral tegmental nuclei. The effects of these compounds
were examined using alternation discrimination performance (Warburton,
1972). The effects of atropine were clear; there was an increase in
both the internally-cued responding and the externally-cued responding
at all doses. The effects of carbachol were opposite at low "physiological" doses and all animals showed a decrease in errors, i.e., improved discrimination. This finding, together with the previous two
pieces of evidence, suggests that a cholinergic tegmental-septo-
hippocampal system may be involved in information processing.

However, these hippocampal and tegmental studies indicate that
the hippocampal circuit is not a simple negative feedback loop
(Warburton, 1975). If it were, it would have been expected that
blockade of the pathway with atropine would have produced effects
opposite to those resulting from cholinergic blockade of the ventral
tegmental nuclei. Evidence supporting this idea comes from a study of
Endroczi et al. (1963) in which they found that injections of acetylcholine directly into the dorsal hippocampus of the cat, which is
equivalent to the ventral hippocampus of the rat, did not induce theta
activity, but did produce transient desynchronization at the cortex.
Injections into the dorsal and ventral tegmental areas resulted in
neocortical desynchronization for up to an hour, and also gave rise
to marked hippocampal theta activity for five to ten minutes. These
qualitatively similar results showed a relationship between hippocampus and the ventral tegmental region in the control of information
processing, but the last data show that selection could be mediated
by a cholinergic pathway to the cortex.

4.2. A Cortical Selection Mechanism

In some of the earliest work on cholinergic drugs, cortical activity and behavior, Wikler (1952) reported an "EEG behavioral dissociation." Dogs that had been given a large dose of atropine exhibited EEGs characterized by continuous high voltage slow activity,
irrespective of whether they were quiet and dozing or whether they
were barking and struggling. On the basis of this failure of cortical
activity to change consistently in the direction of desynchronization
when the animals were alert, Wikler concluded that the cholinergic
mechanisms that desynchronize or synchronize the spontaneous electrical activity of the cortex are distinct from those systems that control alertness, thinking, level of awareness and sensation i.e., information processing. This very early speculation has proved to be
incorrect as we shall see.

4.2.1. Electrocortical Activity and Attention

The first step in the disproof came from studies of attention and electrocortical arousal. By the mid-1960's, it was clear that behavioral efficiency was highly correlated with desynchronization in the electrical activity of the cortex (Thompson, 1967). When a person wakes and becomes alert, the waves increase in amplitude and increase in frequency through theta waves (4 to 7 Hz), alpha waves (8 to 12 Hz) to beta waves (13 to 50 Hz). A high proportion of beta activity, cortical desynchronization, is correlated with a state of full alertness and concentration in the person while a high proportion of alpha activity is correlated with relaxed wakefulness. The alpha rhythm of the resting person is blocked by sudden stimulation and replaced by low voltage high frequency waves (Adrian, 1944). Lindsley (1952) has reviewed much of the literature and has listed the electrocortical correlates of various states of awareness and behavioral efficiency. In an awake organism, as behavioral efficiency varies from an uncoordinated state lacking in sequential timing to an efficient, selective state with fast reactions and well organized movements - so the electrical activity at the cortex increases both in frequency and in the amount of low amplitude activity.

Using sophisticated frequency analyses of EEG recordings, Groll (1966) studied the relationship between EEG frequencies and the performance of a 90 minute sequential brightness discrimination. The results showed parallel decreases in the percentage of correct detections and the average EEG frequency over the session. Most interesting were the analyses of the average frequencies during the one second interval preceding the targets. Groll discovered that the average frequency immediately before a missed target was slower than before a detected target. Furthermore, the latency of responses for detected targets was significantly negatively correlated with the EEG frequencies in the one second intervals preceding the targets. In a simulated radar task, O'Hanlon and Beatty (1977) found that the number of sweeps to detect the targets was directly related to the amount of energy in the theta band and inversely to the amount of energy in the alpha and beta bands. Thus, slower detections were accompanied by lower electrocortical arousal. In both cases, increased desynchronization was correlated with better performance. Altogether, these studies and others like them provide evidence that the efficiency of attentional performance is directly related to electrocortical arousal.

Further evidence interlinking electrocortical activity and attention has come from studies of Event-related Potentials. Event-related Potentials, sometimes known as Averaged Evoked Potentials, are the complex electrical changes recorded at the same time as an external or internal event and reflect the activity of groups of neurons in the brain. With repetitive stimulation, the post-stimulus waveform between 0 and 2.50 milliseconds consists of components which are essentially constant in amplitude, latency and scalp site distribution for a given stimulus. These exogenous components occur whether the subjects are attending or not attending, are awake or asleep, aroused or relaxed. Further support for the cortical selection theory comes from

studies which have related the size of Event-related Potentials to
attentional performance.

For example, in a study of Schwent and Hillyard (1975) subjects
were presented with randomized trains of stimuli concurrently to both
ears, but were asked to attend to one ear at a time. Tones which were
presented to the attended ear produced evoked potentials with larger
N1 components than the tones presented to the unattended ear. This
method of presentation controlled for non-specific influences and a
multi-channel technique controlled for any peripheral factors such as
middle ear contractions which could have contributed to the observed
effects. These experiments have demonstrated that the magnitude of
evoked potentials is related to both the efficiency and direction of
attention.

In order to locate those levels at which different stimulus selection processes take place, Picton and Hillyard (1974) examined the
evoked potentials recorded concurrently from all levels of the auditory system. They found that when attention was directed towards
auditory stimuli in order to perform a difficult loudness discrimination, no changes were found in the Event-related Potentials prior to
the N1-P2 components. Since the N1-P2 waves are believed to be cor-
tically generated, Picton and Hillyard concluded that the absence of
effect was evidence that the selection mechanism was operating at the
cortex. These results supplement an earlier finding that cochlear
nerve potentials were unchanged during an identical attention task
(Picton et al., 1971). These data give a clear indication of a mechanism which enhances evoked discharges at the cortex. Evidence reviewed above suggests that acetylcholine facilitates sensory evoked
discharges at the cortex (Krnjevic et al., 1971; Spehlmann, 1969) and
so we will now consider in detail some of the evidence interrelating
acetylcholine release and electrocortical activity.

4.2.2. Acetylcholine and Electrocortical Activity

The next step in the argument is the mass of evidence that electrocortical arousal is controlled by cholinergic pathways from the
reticular formation. The first suggestion that a cholinergic system
was mediating electrocortical desynchronization was made by Funderbunk
and Case, 1951.

From the initial attempts to establish the role of acetylcholine
release in behavior it seemed that the rate of release was associated
with the sleep-waking cycle. Celesia and Jasper (1966) observed high
rates of acetylcholine liberation (three to four nanograms per square
centimeter) in the intact alert animal with electrocortical arousal
(desynchronization) which was halved during sleep with a synchronized
pattern of cortical electrical activity. This finding was confirmed
by Jasper and Tessier (1971) but they also showed that there was
marked release during paradoxical sleep when the cortex was desynchronized but the animal was not behaviorally aroused. Clearly, the

cortical acetylcholine release was related to electrocortical arousal rather than behavioral arousal. Domino et al. (1968) have reviewed twenty-two studies of the effects of cholinergic drugs upon electro-cortical activity and have concluded that there is strong support for the involvement of cholinergic mechanisms in electrocortical arousal.

A number of studies have attempted to determine the precise loca-tion of cholinergic pathways which are controlling electrocortical arousal. Rinaldi and Himwich (1955a) infused acetylcholine into the carotid and found that this produced electrocortical arousal. How-ever, no effects were observed in an isolated cortex preparation in-dicating that the arousal was dependent upon subcortical structures. Other studies revealed that physostigmine does not induce cortical desynchronization in isolated hemisphere preparations, thus confirming the importance of subcortical structures in cholinergic-induced arous-al (Rinaldi and Himwich, 1955b). Kawamura and Domino (1969) have dem-onstrated that the electrocortical arousal produced by nicotine is blocked both by midbrain reticular lesions and by rostral midbrain transections, but not by caudal midbrain transections. The authors concluded that the midbrain reticular formation was an indispensible structure for the activation of electrocortical activity by nicotine. Further evidence that the ascending reticular cholinergic pathways are involved in electrocortical activation comes from a study in which acetylcholine, when applied directly to the reticular formation, pro-duced electrocortical desynchronization (Hernandez-Peon, 1963). On the basis of their studies of the distribution of cholinergic pathways in the central nervous system, Shute and Lewis (1967) proposed that cholinergic pathways form the anatomical basis of the electrocortical arousal system.

While these studies strongly suggested that the ascending reticu-lar cholinergic system is the origin of the control of electrocortical activity, cholinergic neurons in the cortex appear to form the basis of the electrocortical activity recorded at the surface of the brain or the scalp. Electrical stimulation of the midbrain reticular for-mation produces electrocortical desynchronization which is accompanied by a marked release of acetylcholine at the cortex (Celesia and Jasper 1966; Kanai and Szerb, 1965). Furthermore, cholinolytics applied to the cortex block the electrocortical arousal produced by physostigmine, by peripheral stimulation and by electrical stimulation of the reticu-lar formation (Cuculic et al., 1968). Microelectrophoresis studies indicate that between 15 and 25 percent of cortical cells, mainly in the sensory cortices, are excited by acetylcholine (Krnjevic and Phillis, 1963a and b). This excitatory action of acetylcholine upon cortical neurons has been confirmed by intracellular recording (Krnjevic et al., 1971). Krnjevic et al. concluded that acetylcholine lowers the membrane resting conductance of cortical neurons so that the excitatory action of other inputs is increased and sensory evoked discharges are prolonged. This hypothesis is supported by a study in which acetylcholine was applied directly to the visual cortex and

prolonged both the neural discharges produced by mesencephalic reticular stimulation and the after-discharge of stimulating the visual
afferent pathways (Spehlmann, 1969). Atropine had the opposite effects upon the evoked potential discharge. In addition, the threshold
for the facilitation of cortical discharges that are produced by stimulation of the midbrain reticular formation was raised by cholinolytics (Il'yutchenok and Gilinskii, 1969).

Thus, there is strong support for a cholinergic involvement in
electrocortical activity. The evidence presented so far strongly im-
plicates the ascending reticular cholinergic pathways in the control
of electrocortical activation and attention.

4.3. A Neurochemical Hypothesis of Attention

On the basis of the animal behavior research of Part II and the
neuropharmacological evidence of Part III, Warburton (1972) concluded
that there was a cholinergic pathway ascending from the reticular formation to the cortex that was important in the selection of information for responding. As we saw in previous sections, the selection
mechanism seems to be correlated with changes in electrocortical
arousal. From the evidence, it seems possible that, with a low level
of reticular activation, the slightly increased cortical activity will
enhance small evoked potentials while a higher level of increased cortical activity would occlude the sensory input by masking the smaller
potentials with cortical "noise" (Bremer, 1961). The largest potentials will be a function of not only the activity in the cortex but
also the modulation that has occurred at successive sites along the
primary sensory pathway by the corticofugal fibers, for example. Such
findings led to the proposal that cholinergic pathways were mediating
the selection of stimuli from the environment by controlling the
degree of electrocortical arousal. The release of acetylcholine at
the cortex, which accompanied cholinergic activation, increased the
size of the potentials and thus improved the probability of their
being distinguished from the background cortical activity. On the
other hand, cholinergic blockade, by reducing the size of the evoked
potentials, increased the likelihood that irrelevant stimuli would be
detected and become part of the subset controlling behavior. In subsequent restatements of this position, Warburton (1975, 1977, 1981)
has proposed that electrocortical arousal has the effect of masking
smaller Event-related Potentials, and thus increasing the probability
of larger potentials initiating responses.

Thus the ascending cholinergic system makes the final selection
of inputs by masking the smaller potentials by increasing the background noise and so determining the response emitted. Increased
activity in this system will usually produce better performance by
reducing irrelevant sensory inputs. However, very high levels of
activity could result in disrupted performance if the relevant stimuli
are also masked. When activity in the cholinergic arousal pathways

is low, normally less intense stimuli are not eliminated and become part of the stimulus subset controlling behavior so that irrelevant responses will occur.

In summary, the evidence in the previous sections supports the hypothesis that cholinergic pathways are involved in the processes controlling stimulus selection. From neurophysiological studies, there appears to be a generalized arousal mechanism operating on all modalities at the cortex. This mechanism is a separate system from that maintaining behavioral arousal and although they are usually co-ordinated, only electrocortical arousal is modified by cholinergic agents such as anticholinesterases and cholinolytics.

5.   PART IV: 1975-1983 ACETYLCHOLINE AND HUMAN INFORMATION
      PROCESSING

It is clear from the mass of evidence considered in the preceding sections that there is much support from animal experimentation that cholinergic pathways exert control over stimulus selection as a result of their involvement in electrocortical activity. There was also some suggestion that similar mechanisms are operating in man, which came from human studies with cholinolytics (Callaway and Band, 1958) and from studies showing a cholinergic involvement in pathologies which exhibit attentional dysfunction, such as certain forms of schizophrenia (Singh and Kay, Chapter 9). In order to consolidate and extend these findings we have carried out an extensive series of studies of the effects of cholinergic drugs on human information processing.

In our laboratory we have studied the effects of nicotine and scopolamine on the performance of tests of sustained mental efficiency. In animals nicotine increases the release of acetylcholine at the cortex and increases cortical desynchronization (Armitage et al., 1969). Nicotine produces this effect by acting at the midbrain reticular formation (Il'yutchenok and Ostrovskaya, 1962; Kawamura and Domino, 1969), and this effect can be blocked by both muscarinic and nicotinic cholinergic blockade, but not by adrenergic blockade. On the other hand, scopolamine blocks acetylcholine receptor sites. In man, nicotine injections also produce an increase in electrocortical arousal (Kenig and Murphree, 1973), whereas scopolamine decreases electrocortical arousal (Ostfeld and Aruguette, 1962).

In a study of smoking and vigilance (Wesnes and Warburton, 1978), a signal detection analysis was used to examine the effects of the nicotine, which was delivered in the cigarette smoke, on the perform-ance of a prolonged visual vigilance task. Groups of deprived and smoking smokers, as well as non-smokers were tested. Over the 80 minute task both the non-smokers and deprived smokers showed a marked vigilance decrement, whereas the smoking group maintained their ini-tial level of concentration over the session. In a similar experiment with nicotine tablets (Wesnes et al., 1983), nicotine tablets helped reduce the vigilance decrement in non-smokers, light smokers and heavy smokers. For all three types of smokers, nicotine significantly counteracted the decrement in stimulus sensitivity which occurred over time in the placebo condition, while having no effect on response bias, giving no evidence for a change in any response output systems. Smokers and non-smokers were also similarly improved by nicotine tablets in a study using the Stroop Test (Wesnes and Warburton, 1978).

In a second set of experiments (Wesnes and Warburton, 1983b), we investigated the effects of smoking on the performance of a rapid visual information processing task. The task involves the detection of sequences of three consecutive odd or even digits from a series of digits presented visually at the rate of 100 per minute. In the first experiment, smoking improved both the speed and accuracy of performance above rested baseline levels, the greatest improvement occurring with the highest nicotine delivery cigarette. In the second experiment, smoking again improved the speed and accuracy of performance above baseline levels, while performance deteriorated over time after not smoking as well as after smoking a nicotine-free cigarette. These findings demonstrate that nicotine from smoking produces absolute improvements in performance. Thus, nicotine from cigarettes does not simply restore information processing performance to pre-smoking levels, but actually improves this performance above such levels.

This finding has been substantiated by further studies of the effects of cigarettes having a range of covarying nicotine and tar yields on the performance of a rapid information processing task. Smokers were tested on different days with each of the cigarettes and in a non-smoking control condition. Not only did smoking help to prevent the decrease in speed and accuracy which occurred over time in the non-smoking condition, but it actually improved performance over baseline levels. Furthermore, the greatest improvements were found with the high nicotine yielding cigarettes (Wesnes and Warburton, in preparation).

In animals, it had been demonstrated that cholinolytics impair the selection of environmental stimuli, while having little involvement in response control (see review in Warburton, 1977). Signal detection analysis was also used to examine the effects of scopolamine on the visual vigilance tasks (Wesnes and Warburton, 1983a). Non-smokers performed the 60 minute task on three separate occasions, receiving a different dose of scopolamine each time. Scopolamine significantly lowered stimulus sensitivity and did not increase response bias. Methscopolamine had no effect on either stimulus sensitivity or response bias, showing that peripheral cholinergic blockade was not involved in the effects of scopolamine. Thus, central cholinergic blockade disrupted vigilance performance by lowering stimulus sensitivity as it had in animal studies with an equivalent visual discrimination and a signal detection data analysis.

The purpose of a second scopolamine experiment was to determine the effects of cholinergic blockade on the efficiency of rapid visual information processing performance which was used in the nicotine studies (Wesnes and Warburton, 1983b). In order to control for the peripheral actions of scopolamine, the effects of methscopolamine were also measured. On the basis of the reduction in stimulus sensitivity produced by scopolamine in a vigilance task (Wesnes and Warburton, 1983a), we predicted that the drug would lower the efficiency of task performance. Following scopolamine, correct detections were significantly lower over the 20 minute period whereas no decrement was observed in the other three conditions. In the second experiment a similar design was used to study the effects of nicotine tablets except that post-drug testing was carried out 10 minutes after baseline due to the faster absorption of nicotine. Nicotine helped prevent both the decline in detections and the increase in reaction time which occurred over time in the placebo condition. These findings indicate that compounds with opposite effects on central cholinergic pathways produce opposite effects on performance.

An extension of the previous work determined whether these two drugs have mutually antagonistic effects on the efficiency of the performance of the rapid visual information processing task (Wesnes, Revell and Warburton, unpublished data). In a pilot study, subjects received single and combined doses of scopolamine and nicotine, and there was some evidence of antagonism. In another experiment, subjects received the same doses but testing was carried out over a longer time period and the Stroop Test was introduced at the end of the 2.5 hour session. In this study, nicotine completely counteracted the decrement in performance produced by scopolamine on both the rapid information processing task and the Stroop Test. These results provide further support for the theory that central cholinergic pathways play a major role in human information processing.

These experiments, therefore, provide evidence that cholinergic pathways are involved in human information processing. The cholinergic stimulation produced by nicotine increased efficiency while the cholinergic blockade produced by scopolamine decreased efficiency. Further studies have provided evidence that the behavioral changes, resulting from increased cholinergic function in man, are paralleled by changes in electrocortical activity.

Many human studies have shown that smoking increases the amount of cortical desynchronization in the form of an upward shift in dominant alpha frequency i.e., more 10 to 12 Hz (e.g., Hauser et al., 1958), less total alpha activity and more beta activity (e.g., Knott, 1979). In a study correlating performance with electrocortical activity, Warburton and Wesnes (1979) found that both cigarettes and nicotine tablets increased the dominant alpha frequencey (11.5 to 13.5 Hz) and beta activity (13.5 to 20 Hz) and these changes were correlated with more efficient performance in the rapid visual information processing task described earlier.

     In a further study we recorded the Event-related Potentials pro-
duced by the target stimuli in the rapid information processing task.
As in previous studies, smoking increased both the number of correctly
detected targets and the speed of detection. We were particularly
interested in the so-called endogenous or late components of Event-
related Potentials which are emitted or elicited, often in the absence
of stimulation. Their characteristics are partially independent of
the physical aspects of stimuli. The major endogenous component which
has been identified is the P3 or P300 whose latency ranges from 275 to
600 milliseconds. The P300 is particularly sensitive to the subject's
prior experience, intentions and decisions and varies according to the
task requirements and experimental instructions. In the present study
smoking significantly decreased the latency of this component of the
Event-related Potentials to targets which were correctly detected.
This is particularly relevant because McCarthy and Donchin (1981) have
shown that the latency of the P300 component "..is sensitive to the
duration of stimulus evaluation processes and relatively insensitive
to response selection processes" (p.79). This finding indicates that
improvements in information processing resulting from cholinergic
stimulation are paralleled by changes in electrocortical activity
which are indicative of enhanced stimulus evaluation as opposed to
changes in response control.

6.   SUMMARY

     In this chapter, we have traced out some of the strands of re-
search that have contributed to our knowledge of the relationships
between brain cholinergic systems and behavior. Systematic behavioral
information began to be collected in the early 1950's, at a time when
it was only a working hypothesis that acetylcholine was a neurotransmitter in the central nervous system, but major lines of theorizing
were developing by the middle of the decade. From careful experimental analyses of the behavioral mode of action of anticholinesterases
in animals, a hypothesis of a relation between cholinergic systems and
adaptive behavior was formulated.

     However, human studies with cholinolytic compounds suggested a
rather different view of the function of cholinergic systems in behavior. This hypothesis was that cholinergic drugs act on a mechanism
for focusing attention, i.e., a stimulus input control mechanism. In
contrast, behavioral studies of animals given cholinolytics resulted
in a completely different hypothesized mode of action for these drugs.
Interpretations of the animal data by various workers resulted in a
set of hypotheses whose common theme was that a brain cholinergic system was controlling the inhibition of responses.

     Clearly, the adaptive behavior, attentional focusing and response
inhibition hypotheses were in conflict. These issues could not be
resolved by merely accumulating data by performing experiments which

were similar to those carried out previously. Rejection of this approach by applying the method of "strong inference" (i.e., comparing hypotheses rather than testing only one) resulted in a resolution of the conflict in favor of the idea of a cholinergic system mediating stimulus selection processes, at least in animals. Previous studies which were thought to demonstrate a response inhibition mechanism could be reinterpreted in stimulus selection terms. Studies with direct stimulation of the brain by cholinergic drugs associated this stimulus selection system with the ascending cholinergic pathways from the mesencephalic reticular formation to the cortex.

In people, stimulus selection is termed attention and human tests of the stimulus selection hypothesis showed that a similar cholinergic system was important in human attention. More recent evidence suggests that this system seems to be important in the control of the efficiency of information processing, in general. Combined behavioral testing and electrophysiological measurements have shown that the cholinergically-induced improvements in behavioral efficiency could be related to changes in electrocortical activity. These findings place behavioral cholinergic research among the more general theories that have related behavioral efficiency with electrocortical activity controlled from the reticular formation.

Future behavioral work (some of which is hinted at in this volume) will indicate the particular components of information processing that involve the cholinergic system. From the recent exciting developments in cholinergic neurochemistry, we will understand better the relation of the cholinergic systems to other transmitter systems and the role of these interacting systems in behavioral dysfunction. The cholinergic system has had a brief, but vigorous, history and a bright and exciting future lies ahead.

REFERENCES

Adrian, E. D., 1944, Brain rhythms, Nature 153:360-362.
Aprison, M. H., 1962, On a proposed theory of the mechanism of action of serotonin in the brain, Rec. Adv. Biol. Psychiat. 4:133-146.
Armitage, A. K., Hall, G. M., and Sellers, C. M., 1969, Effects of nicotine on electrocortical activity and acetylcholine release from the cat cerebral cortex, Br. J. Pharmacol. 35:152-160.
Banks, A., and Russell, R. W., 1967, Effects of chronic reductions in acetylcholinesterase activity on serial problem solving behavior, J. Comp. Physiol. Psychol. 64:262-267.
Bartus, R. T., 1979, Physostigmine and recent memory: Effects in young and aged nonhuman primates, Science 206:1087-1089.
Bennett, L. E., and Rosenzweig, M. R., 1968, Brain chemistry and anatomy: implications for theories of learning and memory, in "Mind as Tissue," C. Rupp ed., Harper and Row, New York.

Bignami, G., and Rosic, N., 1970, The nature of disinhibitory phenom-
    ena caused by central cholinergic (muscarinic) blockade, in "Proc.
    of VIIth Int. Congr. Coll. Int. Neuropsycholog." pp. 270–273,
    Pergamon, Oxford.
Bremer, F., 1961, Neurophysiological mechanisms in cerebral arousal,
    in "The Nature of Sleep," G. E. W. Wolstenholme and M. O'Connor
    eds., pp. 30–56, Little, Brown, Boston.
Bremer, F., and Chatonnet, J., 1949, Acetylcholine et cortex cerebral,
    Arch. Int. Physiol. 57:106–109.
Brown, K., and Warburton, D. M., 1971, Attenuation of stimulus sensi-
    tivity by scopolamine, Psychon. Sci. 22:297–298.
Brunton, T. L., 1883, On the nature of inhibition and the action of
    drugs upon it, Nature 27:419–422.
Callaway, E., and Band, I., 1958, Some psychopharmacological effects
    of atropine, Arch. Neurol. 79:91–102.
Callaway, E., and Dembo, D., 1958, Narrowed attention: A psychologi-
    cal phenomenon that accompanies a certain physiological change,
    J. Neurol. Psychiatry 79:74–90.
Carlton, P. L., 1963, Cholinergic mechanisms in the control of behav-
    ior by the brain, Psychol. Rev. 70:19–39.
Carlton, P. L., and Vogel, J. R., 1965, Studies of the amnesic prop-
    erties of scopolamine, Psychonomic Sci. 3:261–262.
Celesia, G. G., and Jasper, H. H., 1966, Acetylcholine released from
    cerebral cortex in relation to state of excitation, Neurology
    16:1053–1064.
Crow, T. J., Frith, C. D., Johnstone, E. C., and Owens, D. G. C.,
    1981, The influence of anticholinergic medication on the extra-
    pyramidal and antipsychotic effects of neurological drugs in the
    treatment of acute schizophrenia, in "Proc. IIIrd World Biol.
    Cong. Psychiat." Elsevier-North Holland Press, Amsterdam.
Crowell, E. B., and Ketchum, J. S., 1967, The treatment of
    scopolamine-induced delirium with physostigmine, Clin. Pharmacol.
    Ther. 8:409–414.
Cuculic, Z., Bost, K., and Himwich, H. E., 1968, An examination of a
    possible cortical cholinergic link in the EEG arousal reaction,
    Prog. Brain Res. 28:27–39.
Deutsch, J. A., 1973, The cholinergic synapse and the site of memory,
    in "The Physiological Basis of Memory," J. Deutsch, ed., pp. 13–16,
    Academic Press, New York.
Deutsch, J. A., Hamburg, M. D., and Dahl, H., 1966, Anticholinesterase
    induced amnesia and its temporal aspects, Science 151:221–223.
Domino, E. F., Yamamoto, K., and Dren, A. T., 1968, Role of cholin-
    ergic mechanisms in states of wakefulness and sleep, Prog. Brain
    Res. 28:113–133.
Douglas, R. J., 1967, The hippocampus and behavior, Psychol. Bull.
    67:416–442.
Douglas, R. J., and Isaacson, R. L., 1966, Spontaneous alternation
    and scopolamine, Psychon. Sci. 4:283–284.
Douglas, R. J., and Pribram, K. H., 1966, Learning and limbic lesions,
    Neuropsychologia 4:197–220.

Drachman, D. A., and Leavitt, J., 1974, Human memory and the cholin-
    ergic system, Arch. Neurol. 30:113-121.
Endroczi, E., Hartmann, G., and Lissak, K., 1963, Effect of intra-
    cerebrally administered cholinergic and adrenergic drugs on neo-
    cortical and archicortical activity, Acta. Physiol. Acad. Sci.
    Hung. 24:200-209.
Feldberg, W., 1963, "A Pharmacological Approach to the Brain from its
    Inner and Outer Surface," p. 430, Williams and Wilkins, Baltimore.
Feldberg, W., 1964, Discussion on extrapolation from animals to man:
    catatonia, in "Animal Behavior and Drug Action," H. Steinberg, ed.
    pp. 429-439, Churchill, London.
Feldberg, W., and Sherwood, S. L., 1954b, Behavior of cats after
    intraventricular injections of eserine and DFP, J. Physiol.
    125:488-500.
Feldberg, W., and Sherwood, S. L., 1954a, Injection of drugs into the
    lateral ventral of the cat, J. Physiol. 123:148-167.
Ferris, S. H., Sathananthan, G., Reisman, B., and Gershon, S., 1979,
    Long-term choline treatment of memory-impaired elderly patients,
    Science 205:1039-1040.
Funderbunk, W. H., and Case, T. J., 1951, The effect of atropine on
    cortical potentials, Electroencephalogr. Clin. Neurophysiol.
    3:213-223.
Glow, P. H., and Rose, S., 1966, Cholinesterase levels and operant
    extinction, J. Comp. Physiol. Psychol. 61:165-172.
Glow, P. H., Richardson, A., and Rose S., 1966, Effects of acute and
    chronic inhibition of cholinesterase upon body weight, food in-
    take, and water intake in the rat, J. Comp. Physiol. Psychol.
    61:295-298.
Grob, D., Lilienthal, J. D., Jr., Harvey, A. M., and Jones, B. F.,
    1947, The administration of diisopropylfluorophosphate (DFP) to
    man. 1, Effect on cholinesterase and systemic effects, Johns
    Hopkins Hospital Bull. 81:217-244.
Groll, E., 1966, (Central nervous system and peripheral activation
    variables during vigilance performance), Z. Exp. Angew. Psychol.
    13:248-264.
Grossman, S. P., 1964, Effects of chemical stimulation of the septal
    nuclei on motivation, J. Comp. Physiol. Psychol. 58:194-200.
Hauser, H., Schwartz, B. E., Roth, G., and Bickford, R. G., 1958,
    Electroencephalographic changes related to smoking, Electroen-
    cephalogr. Clin. Neurophysiol. 10:567.
Heise, G. A., 1975, Discrete trial analysis of drug action, Fed.
    Proc. 34:1898-1903.
Hernández-Peón, R., 1963, Sleep induced by localized electrical or
    chemical stimulation of the forebrain, Electroencephalogr. Clin.
    Neurophysiol. Suppl. 24:188-198.
Hillyard, S. A., Hink, R. F., Schwendt, V. L., and Picton, T. W.,
    1973, Electrical signs of selective attention in the human brain,
    Science 182:177-180.
Il'yutchenok, R. Yu., and Gilinskii, M. A., 1969, Deistvie kholino-
    liticheskikh veschestv na spontannuyu i vyzannuyu akitivnost,
    karkovykh neironov, Farmakol. Toksikol. 32:515-519.

Il'yutchenok, R. Yu, and Ostrovskaya, R. U., 1962, The role of mesen-
    cephalic cholinergic systems in the mechanism of nicotine activa-
    tion of the electroencephalogram, Expt. Biol. Med. 54:753-757.
Jasper, H. H., and Tessier, J., 1971, Acetylcholine released from the
    cortex in relation to its state of activation, Science 172:601-
    602.
Kanai, T., and Szerb, J. C., 1965, The mesencephalic reticular acti-
    vating system and cortical acetylcholine output, Nature 205:81-
    82.
Kawamura, M., and Domino, E. F., 1969, Differential actions of m and n
    cholinergic agonists on the brain stem activating system, Int. J.
    Neuropharmacol. 8:105-115.
Kenig, L., and Murphree, M. B., 1973, Effects of intravenous nicotine
    in smokers and non-smokers, Fed. Proc. 32:805.
Ketchum, J. S., Sidell, F. R., Crowell, E. B., Aghajanian, G. K., and
    Haines, A. H., 1973, Atropine, scopolamine and ditran: compara-
    tive pharmacology and antagonists in man, Psychopharmacologia
    28:121-145.
Kimble, D. P., 1968, Hippocampus and internal inhibition, Psychol.
    Bull. 70:285-295.
Kimble, D. P., 1969, Possible inhibitory functions of the hippo-
    campus, Neuropsychologia 7:235-244.
Knott, V. J., 1979, Psychophysical correlates of smokers and non-
    smokers: studies on cortical, autonomic and behavioral respon-
    sivity, in "Electrophysiological Effects of Nicotine," A. Remond
    and C. Izard, eds., Elsevier, Amsterdam.
Krech, D., 1968, Brain chemistry and anatomy: Implications for behav-
    ior therapy, in "Mind as Tissue," C. Rupp, ed., pp. 39-54, Hoeber
    Medical Division, Harper and Row, New York.
Krnjevic, K., Pumain, R., and Renaud, L., 1971, The mechanisms of
    excitation by acetylcholine in the cerebral cortex, J. Physiol.
    (Lond.) 215:247-268.
Krnjevic, K., and Phillis, J. W., 1963a, Acetylcholine-sensitive
    cells in the cerebral cortex, J. Physiol. (Lond.) 166:296-327.
Krnjevic, K., and Phillis, J. W., 1963b, Pharmacological properties
    of acetylcholine-sensitive cells in the cerebral cortex, J.
    Physiol. (Lond.) 166:328-350.
Krnjevic, K., and Silver, A., 1965, A histochemical study of cholin-
    ergic fibers in cerebral cortex, J. Anat. 99:711-759.
Lindsley, D. B., 1952, Psychological phenomenon and the electroen-
    cephalogram, Electroencephalogr. Clin. Neurophysiol. 4:443-446.
McCarthy, G., and Donchin, E., 1981, A metric for thought: a compari-
    son of P300 latency and reaction time, Science 211:77-80.
Metz, B., 1958, Brain cholinestersase and the respiratory reflex, Am.
    J. Physiol. 192:101-105.
Michelson, M. J., 1961, Pharmacological evidences of the role of ace-
    tylcholine in the higher nervous activity of man and animals,
    Act. Nerv. Super. (Praha) 3:140-147.
Miles, S., 1955, "Some Effects of Injection of Atropine Sulphate in
    Healthy Young Men," U.K. Ministry of Defense Unpublished Report.

Mishkin, M., 1964, Preservation of central sets after frontal lesions in monkeys, in "The Frontal Granular Cortex and Behavior," J. M. Warren and K. Akert, eds., pp. 219-241, McGraw-Hill, New York.

Mitchell, J. F., 1963, The spontaneous and evoked release of acetylcholine from the cerebral cortex, J. Physiol. (Lond.) 165:98-116.

Myers, B., and Domino, E. F., 1964, The effect of cholinergic blocking drugs on spontaneous alternation in rats, Arch. Int. Pharmacodynam. Therap. 150:525-529.

O'Hanlon, J. F., and Beatty, J., 1977, Concurrence of electroencephalographic and performance changes during a simulated radar watch and some implications for the arousal theory of vigilance, in "Vigilance: Theory: Operational Performance and Physiological Correlates," G. Mackie, ed., pp. 189-201, Plenum Press, London.

Ostfeld, A. M., and Araguette, A., 1962, Central nervous system effects of hyoscine in man, J. Pharmacol. Exp. Ther. 137:133-139.

Ostfeld, A. M., Machne, X., and Unna, K. R., 1960, The effects of atropine on the electroencephalogram and behavior in man, J. Pharmacol. Exp. Ther. 128:265-272.

Phillis, J. W., 1970, "The Pharmacology of Synapses," Pergamon Press, Oxford.

Picton, T. W., and Hillyard, S. A., 1974, Human auditory evoked potentials II. Effects of attention, Electroencephalogr. Clin. Neurophysiol. 36:191-200.

Picton, T. W., Hillyard, S. A., Galambos, R., and Schiff, M., 1971, Human auditory attention: a central or peripheral process? Science 173:351-353.

Rinaldi, F., and Himwich, H. E., 1955a, Altering responses and actions of atropine and cholinergic drugs, AMA Arch. Neurol. Psychiatry 73:387-395.

Rinaldi, F., and Himwich, H. E., 1955b, Cholinergic mechanisms involved in function of mesodiencephalic activating system, AMA Arch. neurol. Psychiatry 73:396-402.

Rosenzweig, M. R., Krech, D., Bennett, E. L., and Diamond, M. C., 1968, Modifying brain chemistry and anatomy by enrichment or impoverishment of experience, in "Early Experience and Behavior," G. Newton and S. Levine, eds. pp. 258-298, C. C. Thomas, Springfield, Illinois.

Rowntree, D. W., Nevin, S., and Wilson, A., 1950, The effects of diisopropylfluorophosphate in schizophrenia and manic depressive psychosis, J. Neurol. Neurosurg. Psychiatry 13:47-62.

Russell, R. W., 1969, Behavioral aspects of cholinergic transmission, Fed. Proc. 28:121-131.

Russell, R. W., 1966, Biochemical substrates of behavior, in "Frontiers in Physiological Psychology," R. W. Russell, ed., pp. 185-246, Academic Press, New York.

Russell, R. W., 1958, Effects of "biochemical lesions" on behavior, Acta Psychol. 14:281-294.

Russell, R. W., 1954, Effects of reduced brain cholinesterase on behavior, Bull. Brit. Psychol. Soc. 23:6-7.

Russell, R. W., and Warburton, D. M., 1973, Biochemical bases of behavior, in "Handbook of General Psychology," B. B. Wolman, ed., Prentice-Hall, New Jersey.

Russell, R. W., Watson, R. H. J., and Frankenhaeuser, M., 1961, Effects of chronic reductions in brain cholinesterase on the acquisition and extinction of a conditioned avoidance response, Scand. J. Psychol. 2:21-29.

Safer, D. J., and Allen, R. P., 1971, The central effects of scopolamine in man, Biol. Psychiatry 3:347-355.

Schwent, V. L., and Hillyard, S. A., 1975, Evoked potential correlates of selective attention with multi-channel auditory inputs, Electroencephalogr. Clin. Neurophysiol. 38:131-138.

Shute, C. C. D., and Lewis, P. R., 1967, The ascending cholinergic reticular system: neocortical, olfactory and subcortical projections, Brain 90:497-520.

Singh, M. M., and Kay, S. R., 1978, Nosological and prognostic distinctions in schizophrenia: Pharmacological validation in terms of therapeutic antagonism between anticholinergic anti-Parkinsonism drugs and neuroleptics, Neuropsychobiology 4:288-304

Singh, M. M., and Kay, S. R., 1979, Therapeutic antagonism between anticholinergic anti-Parkinsonism agents and neuroleptics in schizophrenia: Implications for a neuropharmacological model, Neuropsychobiology 5:74-86.

Singh, M. M., and Kay, S. R., 1975, Therapeutic reversal with benztropine in schizophrenia, J. Nerv. Ment. Dis. 160:258-266.

Singh, M. M., and Smith, J. M., 1971, Reversal of some therapeutic effects of haloperidol in schizophrenia by anti-Parkinsonism drugs, Pharmacologist 13:207.

Singh, M. M., and Smith, J. M., 1973a, Kinetics and dynamics of response to haloperidol in acute schizophrenics: A longitudinal study of the therapeutic process. Compr. Psychiatry 14:393-414.

Singh, M. M., and Smith, J. M., 1973b, Reversal of some therapeutic effects of antipsychotic agent by an anti-Parkinsonism drug, J. Nerv. Ment. Dis. 157:50-58.

Spehlmann, R., 1969, Acetylcholine facilitation and atropine block of synaptic excitation of cortical neurons, Science 165:404-405.

Stumph, C., 1965, Drug action on the electrical activity of the hippocampus, Int. J. Neurobiol. 8:77-138

Thompson, R. F., 1967, "Foundations of Physiological Psychology," Harper and Row, New York.

Warburton, D. M., 1975, "Brain, Behavior and Drugs," Wiley, London.

Warburton, D. M., 1979, Neurochemical bases of consciousness, in "Chemical Influences on Behavior," K. Brown and S. J. Cooper, eds., Academic Press, London.

Warburton, D.M., 1981, Neurochemical bases of behavior, Br. Med. Bull. 37:121-125.

Warburton, D. M., 1967, Some behavioral effects of central hippocampal stimulation with special reference to the hippocampus, Unpublished Doctoral Thesis of Indiana University.

Warburton, D. M., 1977, Stimulus selection and behavioral inhibition, in "Handbook of Psychopharmacology, Vol. 8," L. L. Iversen, S. D. Iversen and S. H. Snyder, eds., pp. 385-431, Plenum Press, London.

Warburton, D. M., 1972, The cholinergic control on internal inhibition, in "Inhibition and Learning," R. Boakes and M. S. Halliday eds., pp. 431-460, Academic Press, London.

Warburton, D. M., 1974, The effect of scopolamine on a two-cue discrimination, Q. J. Exp. Psychol. 26:395-404.

Warburton, D. M., and Brown, K., 1974, Effects of scopolamine on a double stimulus discrimination, Neuropharmacology 15:659-663.

Warburton, D. M., and Brown, K., 1971, Scopolamine-induced attentuation of stimulus sensitivity, Nature 230:126-127.

Warburton, D. M., and Brown, K., 1972, The facilitation of discrimination performance by physostigmine sulphate, Psychopharmacologia 27:275-284.

Warburton, D. M., and Heise, G. A., 1972, The effects of scopolamine on spatial double alternation in rats, J. Comp. Physiol. Psychol. 81:523-532.

Warburton, D. M., and Russell, R. W., 1969, Some behavioral effects of cholinergic stimulation of the hippocampus, Life Sci. 8:617-627.

Warburton, D. M., and Wesnes, K., 1979, The role of electrocortical arousal in the smoking habit, in "Electrophysiological Effects of Nicotine," A. Remond and C. Izard, eds., pp. 183-200, Elsevier North Holland Biomedical Press, Amsterdam.

Wesnes, K., and Warburton, D. M., 1978, The effects of cigarette smoking and nicotine habits on human attention, in "Smoking Behaviour Physiological and Psychological Influences," R. E. Thornton, ed., pp. 131-147, Churchill-Livingston, London.

Wesnes, K., and Warburton, D. M., 1983a, Effects of scopolamine on stimulus sensitivity and response bias in a visual vigilance task, Neuropsychobiology 9:154-157.

Wesnes, K., and Warburton, D. M., 1983b, Effects of smoking on rapid visual information processing performance, Neuropsychobiology 9:223-229.

Wesnes, K., Warburton, D. M., and Matz, B., 1983, Effects of nicotine on stimulus sensitivity and response bias in a visual vigilance task, Neuropsychobiology 9:41-44.

White, R. P., Rinaldi, F., and Himwich, H. E., 1956, Central and peripheral nervous system effects of atropine sulfate and mepiperphenidol bromide (Darstine) on human subjects, J. Appl. Psychol. 8:635-642.

Whitehouse, J. M., 1967, Cholinergic Mechanisms in discrimination learning as a function of stimuli, J. Comp. Physiol. Psychol. 63:448-451.

Wikler, A., 1952, Pharmacologic dissociation of behavior and E.E.G. "sleep patterns" in dogs: Morphine, N-allylnormorphine and atrophine, Proc. Soc. Exp. Biol. Med. 79:261-264.

Wilson, I. B., and Cohen, M., 1953, The essentiality of acetylcholinesterase in conduction, Biochem, Biophys. Acta, 11:147-156.

Chapter 2

CHOLINERGIC PATHWAYS IN THE BRAIN

Susan E. Robinson

Department of Pharmacology and Toxicology
Medical College of Virginia
Richmond, Virginia 23298, U.S.A.

---

1. INTRODUCTION

Although acetylcholine (ACh) was the first neurotransmitter to be discovered, in many ways less is known about central cholinergic pathways than about many other neurotransmitters discovered much later. Reliable histochemical techniques for identifying cholinergic neurons have been slow to develop. Although excellent histochemical methods for locating acetylcholinesterase (AChE) exist, this enzyme is only a necessary, but not sufficient, means of identifying cholinergic neurons. However, with improved methods for measuring ACh, choline acetyltransferase (ChAT), high affinity choline uptake, muscarinic and nicotinic receptors, and ACh turnover, more is being learned about central cholinergic pathways. In addition, the development of a possible cholinergic specific neurotoxin, ethylcholine mustard aziridinium (AF64A) holds promise for expediting the mapping of cholinergic pathways in the brain (Fisher et al., 1982).

The purpose of this chapter is to describe central cholinergic pathways which are relevant to behavioral mechanisms or to the actions

of centrally acting drugs. Evidence for the existence of these pathways is given, as well as evidence for the interaction of these pathways with other neurotransmitters.

2.   SEPTAL - HIPPOCAMPAL PATHWAY

One of the best-described cholinergic pathways in the brain is
the septal-hippocampal cholinergic pathway (Fig. 1). Cholinergic cell
bodies located in the medial septum and the nucleus of the diagonal
band send projections through the fimbria to the hippocampus where
they form axodendritic synapses with the pyramidal and granular cells
(Storm-Mathisen, 1970). A great deal of information, electrophysiological, biochemical and histochemical in nature, has been gathered
concerning this pathway.

Stimulation of the septal area activates neurons in the hippocampus (Gogolak et al., 1968), increases the release of ACh from the
hippocampus (Smith, 1984; Dudar, 1975), and decreases hippocampal ACh
content (Rommelspacher and Kuhar, 1974). Furthermore, microelectro-
phoretic application of ACh results in the activation of pyramidal and
granular cells in the hippocampus (Steiner, 1968; Bland et al., 1974).
Benardo and Prince (1980) have recently carried out studies in an in
vitro preparation of guinea pig hippocampal slices that suggest that
ACh serves as an excitatory neuromodulator in the hippocampus. Lesion
of the septum has been found to cause supersensitivity of ACh in the
pyramidal cells of the hippocampus, most likely due to loss of AChE
activity (Bird and Aghajanian, 1975).

The septal-hippocampal pathway has been well-described histologically in the rat, using degeneration techniques, as well as histochemically, with techniques staining for AChE (Lewis and Shute, 1967;
Storm-Mathisen, 1970; Mellgren and Srebro, 1973) and techniques for
ChAT (Lewis et al., 1967). Both nicotinic and muscarinic receptors
have been described in the hippocampus. Using autoradiographic binding studies with quinuclidinyl benzilate (QNB), Kuhar and Yamamura
(1976) have demonstrated muscarinic receptors in many of the same
areas of the hippocampus and dentate gyrus that contain AChE. Binding
studies with radiolabeled nicotine and radiolabeled ACh have demonstrated the existence of nicotinic receptors in the hippocampus (Marks
and Collins, 1982; Schwartz et al., 1982).

Acute and chronic lesions of the medial septum in the rat have
been found to decrease ACh in the hippocampus, as well as to decrease
the activity of ChAT and choline uptake in this area (Kuhar et al.,
1973; Sethy et al., 1973). Section of the fimbria, through which the
cholinergic neurons pass, has a similar effect (Pepeu et al., 1973).
Moroni et al. (1978b) demonstrated in the rat that electrical stimulation of the medial septum increases the turnover of ACh in the hippocampus, whereas acute section of the fimbria reduces the turnover.

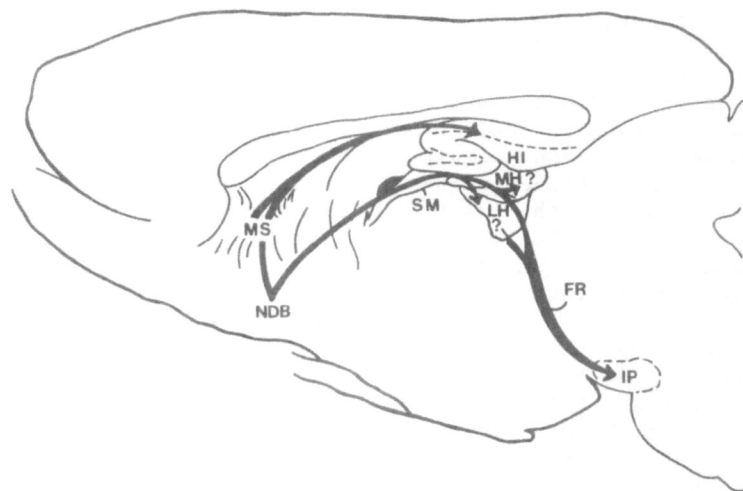

Fig. 1.   Cholinergic Projections to Hippocampus and Medially-located
          Structures. FR, fasciculus retroflexus; HI, hippocampus;
          IP, interpenduncular nucleus; LH, lateral habenular nucleus;
          MH, medial habenular nucleus; MS, medial septum; NDB, nucleus
          of the diagonal band; SM, stria medullaris.

        In addition to being well-described in the adult animal, the
ontogeny of the cholinergic septal-hippocampal pathway also has been
extensively studied. The cholinergic innervation of the hippocampus
is rather late in developing, as shown in studies measuring the activity of AChE and ChAT, as well as by AChE histochemistry (Matthews
et al., 1974; Nadler et al., 1974). AChE activity does not appear in
the medial septum or the nucleus of the diagonal band until the second
day postnatally and does not appear in the hippocampal formation until
the fourth day postnatally. Activity of cholinergic enzymes throughout the entire hippocampus does not reach adult levels until eleven
days after birth. This development is blocked by septal lesion
(Ben-Barak and Dudai, 1980). On the other hand, development of hippocampal innervation by certain other neurotransmitters begins much
earlier and may even serve as a trophic signal for later-arriving
innervation. Noradrenergic input from the locus coeruleus first
arrives at the septal end of the hippocampus on the eighteenth day of
gestation and gradually moves temporally until fluorescence is apparent over the entire hippocampal formation by postnatal day ten (Loy
and Moore, 1979). Likewise, serotonergic innervation of the hippocampus begins prenatally (Lauder and Krebs, 1978).

        The septal-hippocampal cholinergic pathway may be of great func-
tional importance. This pathway is thought to be involved in the generation of the theta rhythm in the hippocampus, and Steiner (1968) has

reported a cholinergic involvement in hippocampal activation during photic stimulation. Vanderwolf and Robinson (1981) have written an extensive review concerning two inputs from the reticular activating system to the hippocampus and the cortex: one of which is atropine-sensitive and presumably cholinergic in nature and the other of which is urethane-sensitive and postulated to involve an unknown type of monoamine receptor. Although the effect of these inputs on the EEG has been well studied, the exact behavioral and anatomical significance of these two systems is unknown. Singh (1981) has suggested that irregularities in the hippocampal cholinergic circuitry may be important in certain forms of schizophrenia.

Cholinergic neurons have been postulated to play an important role in learning and memory (Deutsch, 1971). Therefore, it is extremely interesting that a neuronal pathway extending from the medial septal nucleus to the dentate granule cells has been reported to be involved in sensory discrimination learning (Deadwyler et al., 1981) and that the hippocampus is required for nonspatial working memory (Olton and Feustle, 1981). In Alzheimer's disease, a condition characterized by progressive dementia and memory loss, there is a reduction in cholinergic markers (ChAT, AChE) in the hippocampus (Davies and Maloney, 1976; Rossor et al., 1982; Coyle et al., 1983). All this suggests that the septal-hippocampal cholinergic projection is important in learning and memory.

The septum occupies a pivotal position in the brain, connecting lower centers of the CNS with the limbic areas. Many pathways projecting from these lower centers to the septum have been identified. Dopaminergic neurons project to the lateral septum from the cell body group A10 in the ventral medial tegmentum (Lindvall, 1975; Assaf and Miller, 1977). This dopaminergic pathway has been found to exert an inhibitory influence on the septal hippocampal cholinergic pathway. The directly-acting dopaminergic agonist apomorphine has been found to decrease the turnover rate of ACh (TR_{ACh}) in the hippocampus. Furthermore, local injection of the dopamine antagonist, haloperidol, or depletion of septal dopamine by local injection of 6-hydroxydopamine into the septum or area A10 results in an increase in hippocampal TR_{ACh} (Robinson et al., 1979). However, since the dopaminergic nerve terminals are located in the lateral septum and the cholinergic cell bodies are located in the medial septum, an interneuron must be involved to connect the two. A most likely candidate for this neurotransmitter is GABA. Intraseptal injection of the GABA agonist muscimol, like apomorphine, decreases TR_{ACh} in the hippocampus. Furthermore, intraseptal injection of the GABA antagonist bicuculline blocks the decrease in the TR_{ACh} seen after apomorphine (Cheney et al., 1978).

The septum, as well as the hippocampus itself, also receives projections from the brain stem noradrenergic cell groups (Fuxe, 1965). It appears that norepinephrine exerts an excitatory effect on TR_{ACh} in the hippocampus, and that the septum is the site of this action. Amphetamine increases TR_{ACh} in the hippocampus: this action is not due to dopamine, since dopaminergic neurons have been found to decrease TR_{ACh} in the hippocampus (Robinson et al., 1979). The excitatory effect of amphetamine on hippocampal TR_{ACh} appears to involve a noradrenergic receptor in the septum, as intraseptal injection of the irreversible α-adrenergic antagonist phenoxybenzamine blocks the amphetamine-induced increase in TR_{ACh} (Robinson et al., 1978).

The medial septum receives serotonergic input from both the dorsal and median raphe nuclei (Kuhar et al., 1972; Conrad et al., 1974; Segal and Landis, 1974), and the hippocampus also receives direct serotonergic input largely from the median raphe nucleus (Bobillier et al., 1979). Despite the large input of serotonergic neurons from the median raphe nucleus to the hippocampus, lesion of the median raphe by local injection of 5,7-dihydroxytryptamine does not affect TR_{ACh} in the hippocampus (Robinson, 1983). This would suggest that hippocampal cholinergic neurons do not interact with these serotonergic neurons, or, at least, are not under tonic control of these neurons. On the other hand, lesion of the dorsal raphe nucleus, which projects to the medial septum with only a slight input to the hippocampus, results in an increase in hippocampal TR_{ACh}, as reflected in an increased rate of decline of ACh levels after administration of hemicholinium-3. This would suggest that the dorsal raphe nucleus tonically inhibits cholinergic neurons terminating in the hippocampus (Robinson, 1983).

Morphine has been found to decrease TR_{ACh} in the hippocampus (Zsilla et al., 1977). This action is most likely due to an inhibitory effect in the septum, as intraseptal injection of β-endorphin also decreases hippocampal TR_{ACh}, and this decrease is blocked by naltrexone (Moroni et al., 1978a). Interestingly, β-endorphin, like dopamine, may be exerting its inhibitory action through a GABA interneuron, as intraseptally-injected bicuculline blocks the β-endorphin-induced decrease in hippocampal TR_{ACh} (Cheney et al., 1978). Furthermore, Wood and Stotland (1980) have evidence that the opiate receptors involved in the inhibition of the septal-hippocampal cholinergic neurons are μ- but not κ-receptors.

Septal-hippocampal cholinergic neurons may also be regulated by peptidergic neurons. Substance P, which has been found in substantial amounts in the septum, has been reported to significantly decrease hippocampal TR_{ACh} when injected intraseptally (Malthe-Sorenssen et al., 1978a). On the other hand, the pituitary polypeptides alpha-MSH and ACTH have been found to increase TR_{ACh} in the hippocampus when given intraventricularly (Wood et al, 1978). The site where these polypeptides act to increase hippocampal TR_{ACh} remains to be established. Finally, the peptides thyrotropin-releasing hormone (TRH), somatostatin, neurotensin, and angiotensin II have all been

found to have no effect on hippocampal TR$_{ACh}$ (Malthe-Sorenssen
et al., 1978b).

3.   CORTICAL CHOLINERGIC NEURONS

Another group of cholinergic neurons are those terminating in the
cortex (Fig. 2). AChE and ChAT have been demonstrated histochemically
in the cerebral cortex of the rat, cat, and monkey (Hebb et al.,1963;
Krnjevic and Silver, 1965; Kimura et al., 1980); levels of these enzymes are greatly reduced after cortical undercutting experiments,
suggesting that the cell bodies are located outside of the cortex.
However, recent studies by Johnston et al., (1981) using kainic acid
lesions of the cortex suggest the presence of intrinsic cortical cholinergic neurons. Binding studies have shown that the cortex contains
both nicotinic and muscarinic cholinergic receptors (Kuhar and
Yamamura, 1976; Schwartz et al., 1982; Marks and Collins, 1982). As
in the hippocampus, ACh has been found to act as an excitatory muscarinic agent in the cortex (Krnjevic et al., 1971).

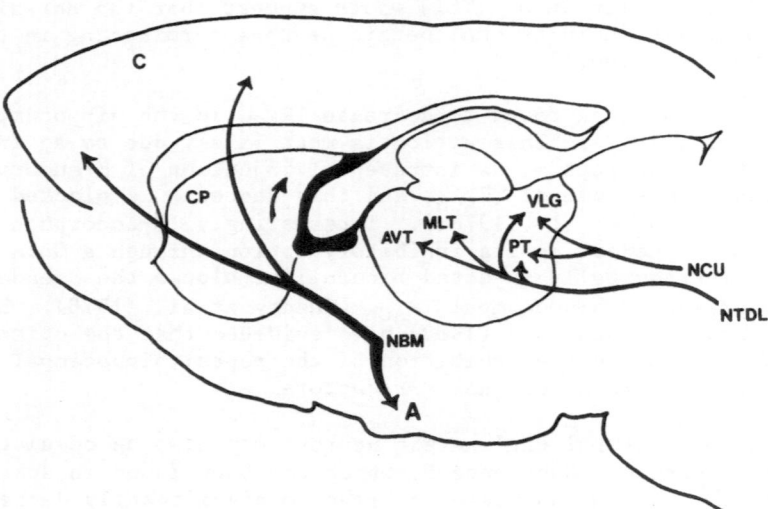

Fig. 2.   Cholinergic Projections to Laterally-located Structures.
          A, amygdala; AVT, anteroventral thalamic nucleus; C, cortex;
          CP, caudate putamen; MLT, medial thalamic nucleus pars lat-
          eralis; NBM, nucleus basalis magnocellularis; NCU, nucleus
          cuneiformis; NTDL, nucleus tegmentalis dorsalis lateralis;
          PT, posterior thalamic nucleus; VLG, ventral lateral genicu-
          late body.

Much evidence exists that the main source of the cholinergic terminals located in the cerebral cortex is a group of cell bodies located near the septal area. Szerb (1967) has demonstrated in the cat that stimulation of septal nuclei increases the release of ACh from the cortex. Septal lesions in the rat have been demonstrated to reduce the level of ACh in the frontal cortex as well as to reduce ChAT activity and choline uptake in the cortex (Pepeu et al., 1973; Kuhar et al., 1973). Also, medial septum lesions have been found to block the amphetamine-induced increase in release of ACh from the cerebral cortex in the cat and rat (Nistri et al., 1972; Mulas et al., 1974).

It is now apparent that the above studies most likely included lesions that extended outside of the medial septal nucleus or perhaps included fibers of passage, because the most recent studies have indicated that a source of cholinergic neurons projecting to the cerebral cortex is a group of neurons that are located in the ventromedial extremity of the globus pallidus and extend caudally from the septum, the nucleus basalis magnocellularis. Histochemical studies using horseradish peroxidase and AChE staining techniques have identified this projection in the rat (Johnston et al., 1979; Lehmann et al., 1980). From the histochemistry, it appears that the nucleus basalis is a large source of cholinergic neurons in the cortex. Specific decreases in cholinergic markers (ChAT, ACh, and choline uptake) in the cortex after kainic acid lesion of the nucleus basalis further support the existence of this projection (Johnston et al., 1979).

Using electrolytic lesions of the basal forebrain and following changes in ChAT and AChE activity in various cortical areas, Wenk et al. (1980) suggested that cholinergic neurons in the basal forebrain project to cortical areas in a widespread, but specific topographical fashion. By the use of a pharmacohistochemical method for AChE determination coupled with fluorescent retrograde tracing techniques, the location of putative cholinergic neurons projecting to the ipsilateral frontal, parietal, temporal, and visual cortices has been identified in the rat. Projections to medial neocortical structures have been found to be innervated by more rostral structures and projections to the more laterally-oriented neocortical structures have been found to be innervated by more caudally-located cells (Bigl et al., 1982).

Horseradish peroxidase injections indicate that neither the medial septum nor the nucleus of the diagonal band project to the cortex (Lehmann et al., 1980). A thalamocortical cholinergic pathway and a cortical cholinergic projection from a site caudal to the nucleus basalis have also been ruled out (Johnston et al., 1979; Lehmann et al., 1980). The neurons in the nucleus basalis, which in the rat is a homologue of the substantia innominata, are clearly different from pallidal neurons. However, it is uncertain whether they are functionally part of a system intermediate between the limbic and extrapyramidal systems or are a rostral extension of the reticular

formation. This pathway could be considered part of the ventral tegmental pathway proposed by Shute and Lewis (1967).

ACh may play an important functional role in the cortex. An
atropine-sensitive pathway projects from the reticular activating
system to the cortex and is associated with specific types of behavior
and EEG activity (Vanderwolf and Robinson, 1981). Montplaisir (1975)
has suggested that cholinergic mechanisms may be involved in cortical
activation during arousal in the cat. In the rabbit, Collier and
Mitchell (1966) found that stimulation of the visual pathway increased
the release of cortical ACh. Most importantly, the basal forebrain
cholinergic projection to the cortex is very likely involved in cognitive behavior. Specific degeneration of cholinergic cell bodies that
project from the basal forebrain to the cortex has been described in
Alzheimer's disease (Coyle et al., 1983). A major symptom of
Alzheimer's disease is dementia, a severe impairment in cognitive
function. Autopsies of victims of Alzheimer's disease indicate a
reduction in ChAT and AChE activity and ACh content in the cerebral
cortex (Davies, 1979; Richter et al., 1980; Rossor et al., 1982).

Although the function of cortical cholinergic neurons is not
completely understood, they are known to be affected by a number of
drugs with powerful behavioral effects. Amphetamine is known to increase the release of ACh from the cortex and to increase TR_{ACh} in
the cortex (Nistri et al., 1972; Mulas et al., 1974; Robinson et al.,
1978). It is most likely that this effect is due to the action of
amphetamine on noradrenergic neurons, for the dopamine agonist apomorphine has no significant effect on TR_{ACh} in the cortex (Robinson
et al., 1978). Since injection of the α-blocker phenoxybenzamine
directly into the septal area significantly reduces the amphetamine-
induced increase in cortical TR_{ACh}, it is likely that the excitatory
action is taking place at an α-adrenergic synapse in this region
(Robinson et al., 1978).

Both the cortex and the septal area receive serotonergic projections from the dorsal and the median raphe nuclei (Kuhar et al., 1972;
Conrad et al., 1974; Segal and Landis, 1974; Descarries et al., 1975);
therefore, the possibility exists for an interaction between these
serotonergic neurons and cortical cholinergic neurons. Specific
lesioning of the median raphe nucleus and of the dorsal raphe nucleus
with the neurotoxin 5,7-dihydroxytryptamine has been found to significantly increase the turnover of ACh in the cortex, as evidenced by
an increased rate of decline of ACh after intraventricular injection
of hemicholinium-3 (Robinson, 1983). Therefore, it appears that serotonergic neurons arising in the median raphe and dorsal raphe nuclei
may exert a chronic inhibitory effect on cortical cholinergic neurons.

As is the case in the hippocampus, morphine has been found to
decrease the turnover of ACh in the cortex, an effect which can be
blocked by naltrexone (Zsilla et al., 1977). Wood and Stotland (1980)

substantiated and extended these findings with several narcotic agonists and partial agonists in the parietal cortex, but found no effect
on TR_{ACh} in the frontal cortex. Thus, it appears that cholinergic
neurons in the parietal, but not in the frontal, cortex possess or are
regulated by neurons with μ or κ receptors. Unlike the hippocampus,
TR_{ACh} in the cortex is not decreased after intraseptal injection of
β-endorphin, although intraventricular injection of β-endorphin does
result in a decrease in cortical TR_{ACh} (Moroni et al., 1978a). Thus,
the action of opiates on cortical cholinergic neurons does not take
place directly in the septal area. It is unlikely, too, that the interaction occurs directly in the cortex, because the distribution of
enkephalins and opiate receptors in that area is rather light (Atweh
and Kuhar, 1977; Simantov et al., 1977). Experiments by Jhamandas and
Sutak (1976) point to the medial thalamus as a likely site for the
action of opiates on cortical ACh, although the actual neuronal circuitry involved remains unclear.

The basal forebrain cholinergic projection to the cortex is also
regulated by a phasically active GABAergic mechanism. Local injection
of the GABA agonist muscimol into the "substantia innominata" decreases TR_{ACh} in the parietal and frontal cortices; this action is
blocked by picrotoxin. Picrotoxin by itself has no effect on TR_{ACh} in
the cortex (Wood and Richard, 1982). The source of the GABAergic
input to the "substantia innominata" remains uncertain.

TRH has been found to significantly increase TR_{ACh} in the
parietal cortex (Malthe-Sorenssen et al., 1978b). Yarbrough (1976)
has also reported that TRH potentiates the excitatory effect of ACh on
cortical neurons. Since TRH reduces barbiturate sleeping time, and
barbiturates are known to decrease cortical TR_{ACh} (Trabucchi et al.,
1975a), it is possible that the interaction between TRH and cholinergic neurons is involved in maintaining a state of consciousness. On
the other hand, although the peptides somatostatin, neurotensin and
angiotensin II lower the ACh content of the parietal cortex, they do
not affect TR_{ACh} in the parietal or the frontal cortex (Malthe-
Sorenssen et al., 1978b; Wood et al., 1978). Neither ACTH, alpha-
MSH, nor substance P affect TR_{ACh} in the cortex (Malthe-Sorenssen
et al., 1978a; Wood et al., 1978).

4.   STRIATAL CHOLINERGIC NEURONS

The caudate-putamen (striatum) contains one of the highest concentrations of ACh and its related enzymes in the brain (Cheney et al.
1975). Furthermore, muscarinic and nicotinic receptors have been
reported in the striatum (Kobayashi et al., 1978; Schwartz et al.,
1982; Marks and Collins, 1982). The nicotinic receptors appear to be
located on serotonergic and catecholaminergic terminals (Schwartz and
Kellar, 1983). It is most likely that the cholinergic neurons are
intrinsic to the striatum (Fig. 2). Deafferentation of this structure

does not reduce the level of AChE, ChAT or ACh in the striatum (McGeer et al., 1971; Butcher and Butcher, 1974).

Cholinergic neurons within the striatum are thought to play an important role in the extrapyramidal system and to be involved in the generation of tremors in Parkinson's disease. It is well-known that the muscarinic agonist oxotremorine induces tremors in experimental animals. Anticholinergic drugs are known to be very useful in the milder stages of Parkinson's disease.

Parkinsonism reflects a deficiency of dopamine in the striatum. One of the best-known pathways in the CNS is the dopaminergic nigro-striatal pathway, which projects from the zona compacta of the sub-stantia nigra to the caudate-putamen. ACh is known to interact in a reciprocal manner with dopamine in the striatum, although the exact pathway involved is not certain. Dopamine inhibits neuronal discharge in the striatum (Bloom et al., 1965), and dopaminergic agonists in-crease the striatal content of ACh, presumably due to a decrease in release (Consolo et al., 1974). Treatment with dopamine agonists such as L-DOPA, apomorphine, and amphetamine all reduce striatal TR_{ACh} (Trabucchi et al., 1975b). Conversely, dopamine blockers, such as chlorpromazine, increase striatal TR_{ACh} (Trabucchi et al., 1974) and increase the release of ACh from the striatum (Stadler et al., 1973). After interruption of dopaminergic impulse flow by acute lesion of the nigrostriatal pathway, levels of ACh are reduced in the striatum; this is reversed by administration of apomorphine (Rommelspacher and Kuhar, 1975). There seems to be an important feedback loop involved, for atropine reduces dopamine turnover in the striatum (Bowers and Roth, 1972).

The interaction between ACh and dopamine in the striatum may also include a GABAergic link. A large projection of GABA neurons extends from the striatum to the substantia nigra via the globus pallidus (Fonnum et al., 1974). Ladinsky et al., (1976) have suggested that a GABAergic (inhibitory)-dopaminergic (inhibitory)-cholinergic (inhibi-tory) feedback loop exists between the striatum and substantia nigra. This concept is supported by their findings that the GABA antagonist picrotoxin increases striatal ACh, presumably due to decreased firing of striatal cholinergic neurons, which is blocked by depletion of dop-amine by alpha-methylparatyrosine. This particular circuit may not be a complete explanation for the interactions between ACh, dopamine, and GABA in the striatum. However, as supported by data from Ferkany and Enna (1980), it is apparent that these three neurotransmitters inter-act quite closely in the striatum, as atropine blocks the increased striatal dopamine receptor binding resulting from treatment with GABA transaminase inhibitor.

Another projection to the striatum which appears to regulate striatal cholinergic neurons is the corticostriatal pathway, which most likely uses the excitatory neurotransmitter, glutamate (Spencer,

1976; McGeer et al., 1977). Scatton and Bartholini (1979, 1980) have
reported that GABA-mimetic agents increase striatal ACh levels, sup-
posedly reflecting a decrease in cholinergic neuronal firing, by a
mechamism involving the corticostriatal neurons and independent of
nigrostriatal dopaminergic neurons. Interestingly, Mitchell (1980)
has presented evidence for facilitation of glutamate release from
corticostriatal terminals by a GABA receptor. However, the results
of Mitchell (1980) would predict an increase in ACh release by GABA-
mimetic agents, unless an inhibitory interneuron is located between
the ACh and the glutamate neurons.

    The striatum receives serotonergic input from the dorsal raphe
nucleus (Lorens and Guldberg, 1974). Furthermore, the dorsal and the
median raphe nuclei send serotonergic projections to the substantia
nigra where it is possible for these neurons to interact indirectly
with striatal cholinergic neurons (Dray et al., 1976; Vander Kooy and
Hattori, 1980). Several groups of researchers have found evidence
for interaction between these serotonergic neurons and dopaminergic
neurons in the nigrostriatal system (Giambalvo and Snodgrass, 1978;
Nicolaou et al., 1979).

    There is evidence for an interaction between serotonergic neurons
and striatal cholinergic neurons. Fenfluramine, which releases and
blocks the reuptake of serotonin, has been found to increase the content of ACh in the striatum (Consolo et al., 1979). This was suggest-
sted to indicate a reduction in the activity of striatal cholinergic
neurons, and a possible inhibitory action of serotonin on these neurons. However, changes in levels of ACh do not always represent
changes in turnover of the neurotransmitter. Specific lesion of
either the dorsal or the median raphe nucleus with 5,7-dihydroxytryp-
tamine does not change the rate of decline of ACh seen after intraventricular administration of hemicholinium-3 (Robinson, 1983). On
the other hand, these results do not rule out a phasic regulation of
striatal cholinergic neurons by these serotonergic neurons. However,
studies by Butcher et al. (1976) have found that $^2H_9$-ACh synthesis
is decreased in rats with lesions in the dorsal raphe area or the
median raphe area and which have been treated with ammonium chloride
intravenously. This would instead suggest a tonic excitatory influence of these areas on striatal cholinergic neurons. However, radio-
frequency lesions were made in this study and this does not rule out
lesion of non-serotonergic neurons or fibers of passage. Therefore,
the interaction of serotonergic neurons with striatal cholinergic
neurons remains unsettled.

    Despite a substantial distribution of opiate receptors and en-
kephalins in the striatum (Atweh and Kuhar, 1977; Simantov et al.,
1977), it appears that the striatal cholinergic neurons are unaffected
by opiates. Neither morphine, β-endorphin, partial opiate agonists,
nor enkephalin analogues modify striatal ACh or TR_{ACh} (Zsilla et al.,
1977; Moroni et al., 1978a; Wood and Stotland, 1980). Only the potent

μ-receptor agonist etorphine depresses striatal TR$_{ACh}$, but very large
doses of naloxone are required to reverse this response (Wood and
Scotland, 1980). The following peptides also do not affect ACh content or TR$_{ACh}$ in the striatum: alpha-MSH, ACTH, angiotensin II,
somatostatin, substance P, and TRH (Malthe-Sorenssen et al., 1978a,
1978b; Wood et al., 1978). Although neurotensin does not change
striatal TR$_{ACh}$, it was observed to increase the ACh content of the
striatum (Malthe-Sorenssen et al., 1978b).

5.   CHOLINERGIC PROJECTIONS TO THE INTERPEDUNCULAR NUCLEUS

     Despite its small size, the interpeduncular nucleus has the dis-
tinction of having the highest ChAT activity of any brain part studied
(Kataoka et al., 1973; Cheney et al., 1975). The interpenduncular
nucleus also exhibits a very high synaptosomal choline uptake activity
(Sorimachi et al., 1974). Lake (1973) reported that neurons within
the interpeduncular nucleus were excited by microiontophoresis of ACh.
Also, muscarinic receptors have been located in the lateral aspect of
the interpeduncular nucleus (Rotter et al., 1979). Thus it is obvious
that the interpeduncular nucleus receives a cholinergic projection.

     Historically, the cholinergic innervation of the interpeduncular
nucleus has been thought to arise in the habenula, an epithalamic
nucleus with input from both the extrapyramidal and limbic systems.
Histochemical studies staining for AChE have described a projection
from the habenula to the interpeduncular nucleus via the fasciculus
retroflexus (Shute and Lewis, 1963; Krnjevic and Silver, 1965; Lewis
and Shute, 1967) (Fig. 1). Léranth et al. (1975) have described a
similar pathway using histochemical techniques for ChAT. Furthermore,
lesions of the habenula in the rat result in a decrease in the activity of AChE, ChAT and choline uptake (Kataoka et al., 1973; Kuhar et
al., 1975; Emson et al., 1977). It has also been reported that electrical stimulation of the lateral habenula increases the release of
ACh from the interpeduncular nucleus (Sastry et al., 1979).

     However, it appears that only part of the cholinergic cell
bodies that project to the interpeduncular nucleus are located in the
habenula. The rest of the cholinergic innervation of the interpeduncular nucleus probably occurs as fibers of passage through the habenula (Fig. 1). Gottesfeld and Jacobowitz (1978) have found that extensive septal lesions, including the vertical limb of the nucleus of the
diagonal band, result in an approximately 50 percent reduction in ChAT
activity in the interpeduncular nucleus. Also, more specific lesions
of the nucleus of the diagonal band, which is known to contain cholinergic cell bodies, also result in an approximately 50 percent reduction of ChAT activity in the interpenduncular nucleus. This extra-
habenular source of cholinergic neurons has been confirmed by McGreer
et al. (1979). Injection of kainic acid, which has been suggested to
spare fibers of passage, into the habenula destroys most of the cell

bodies in the habenula, but only reduces interpeduncular ChAT activity
by about one-half. On the other hand, cutting the fasciculus retroflexus reduces the ChAT activity to less than 20 percent of control.
This suggests that half of the cholinergic neurons terminating in the
interpeduncular nucleus arise elsewhere, but pass through the habenula.
Further supporting an extra-habenular source of interpeduncular cholinergic neurons are the results of Lehmann and Fibiger (1981). Using
AChE histochemistry in combination with difluophosphate, they have
reported a probable cholinergic projection from the horizontal limb
of the nucleus of the diagonal band to the interpeduncular nucleus
(Fig. 1).

In addition to the nucleus diagonal band-interpeduncular cholinergic projection, Gottesfeld and Jacobowitz (1979) also report a
differential projection from the septal-diagonal band area to the
median and lateral habenular nuclei (Fig. 1).

6.   CHOLINERGIC INNERVATION OF THE AMYGDALA

A good amount of evidence exists for cholinergic innervation of
the amygdala. ACh and its synthetic enzyme, ChAT, are found in substantial amounts in the various amygdalar nuclei (Cheney et al., 1975;
Ben-Ari et al., 1977). Most studies indicate that the highest ChAT
activity is located in the lateral amygdalar nuclei (posterolateral
> anterolateral > basolateral) and the lowest activity in the medial
nuclei. AChE activity correlates fairly well with the distribution
of ChAT activity. One source of the cholinergic innervation of the
amygdala is believed to be the basal forebrain (Fig. 2). ChAT and
AChE-containing neurons project from the lateral preoptic area and
ventral pallidum to the basolateral and corticomedial nuclei of the
amygdala (Emson et al., 1979). These projections have been confirmed
by combined fluorescent retrograde tracer-AChE analysis (Woolf and
Butcher, 1982). Injection of kainic acid into the amygdala has been
found to reduce ChAT activity and muscarinic and nicotinic binding
sites in the amygdala. If it is assumed that kainic acid spares
fibers of passage and terminals, this can be taken to suggest that
much of the cholinergic innervation of the amygdala not from the nucleus basalis magnocellularis is intrinsic to the amygdala (McCaughran
et al., 1980).

The cholinergic innervation of the amygdala may have behavioral
importance, for local injection of carbachol into the amygdala results
in a rage reaction (Hernández-Peón et al., 1967). Furthermore, the
amygdala is an area of the brain which exhibits a loss of cholinergic
markers in Alzheimer's disease and senile dementia of Alzheimer's type
(Rossor et al., 1982). There is evidence that the amygdala is involved in emotional and motivational behavior (Gloor, 1972). Therefore,
the loss of initiative observed in Alzheimer's disease may result from
deficits in cholinergic innervation of the amygdala.

7.   OTHER CHOLINERGIC PATHWAYS

There are varying amounts of evidence for the existence of other cholinergic pathways, although the anatomy or the possible functional importance of these pathways is not as well known.

ACh seems to have a role in the visual system. There is a good deal of evidence that ACh is a neurotransmitter in the retina (for a review, see Neal, 1976). Furthermore, there is evidence for cholinergic innervation of other parts of the visual system: the lateral geniculate body, the superior colliculus, and the visual cortex. A substantial amount of AChE and ChAT activity is found in the lateral geniculate body and superior colliculus (Domino et al., 1973). ACh in these areas appears to have functional importance. Stimulation of the retina by light and direct electrical stimulation of the lateral geniculate body produces a large increase in ACh release from the primary visual cortex in the rabbit (Collier and Mitchell, 1966). ChAT activity is reduced in the lateral geniculate body and the superior colliculus, but not in the visual cortex, of rats deprived of light from birth (Maletta and Timiras, 1968). However, little change is found in AChE activity in the lateral geniculate body and superior colliculus of the rat or in the optic tectum of the pigeon after enucleation (Henke and Fonnum, 1976; Urano, 1977).

The lateral geniculate body is not the only thalamic nucleus to receive cholinergic innervation. On the basis of AChE histochemistry, Shute and Lewis (1967) proposed a cholinergic projection through the dorsal tegmental pathway from the nucleus cuneiformis (midbrain reticular formation) to the thalamus (Fig. 2). Hoover and Jacobowitz (1979) expanded these findings in the rat by measuring ChAT activity in thalamic nuclei after electrolytic lesion of the nucleus cuneiformis. An ipsilateral projection was found to the anterior thalamic nuclei, the medial thalamic nucleus pars lateralis, pretectal nucleus, parafascicular nucleus, posterior thalamic nucleus, and superior colliculus, as well as possible bilateral innervation of the reticular nucelus of the thalamus and the lateral geniculate body. More recent studies from the same laboratory now suggest that part of the decrease in ChAT activity in thalamic nuclei following lesion of the nucleus cuneiformis in the rat is actually due to destruction of fibers of passage. Cholinergic neurons located in the nucleus tegmentalis dorsalis lateralis and passing through the nucleus cuneiformis terminate in the anteroventral thalamic nucleus, posterior thalamic nucleus, medial thalamic nucleus pars lateralis, and the ventral lateral geniculate body (Rotter and Jacobowitz, 1981) (Fig. 2). Studies with combined horseradish peroxidase-AChE histochemistry suggest that the nucleus tegmentalis dorsalis lateralis is the actual source of cholinergic innervation of the anteroventral thalamic nucleus (Hoover and

Baisden, 1980). However, it was also reported that the posterior thalamic nucleus and ventrolateral geniculate body receive additional cholinergic innervation from neurons located in the nucleus cuneiformis (Rotter and Jacobowitz, 1981). The dorsal tegmental cholinergic pathway may serve to interconnect the limbic midbrain and the limbic forebrain. Therefore, it is an exciting area to study with reference to emotional behavior.

The hypothalamus receives cholinergic innervation, although the exact anatomy of the connections is not clear. ACh, AChE, and ChAT are all found in the hypothalamus as well as moderate muscarinic and nicotinic receptor binding (Shute and Lewis, 1966; Yamamura et al., 1974; Cheney et al., 1975; Schwartz et al., 1982; Marks and Collins, 1982). Since surgical deafferentation reduces ChAT activity in certain hypothalamic nuclei, it is evident that the source of part of the cholinergic innervation of the hypothalamus is extrinsic (Brownstein et al., 1976). Because of the large limbic input into the hypothalamus and the important role that the hypothalamus plays in autonomic control, this area of the brain could be involved in the influence of emotion on homeostatic mechanisms. For example, cholinergic mechanisms in the hypothalamus have been found to influence blood pressure. Since the hypothalamus receives substantial innervation from brain stem neurons, the possibility for interaction between these systems and hypothalamic cholinergic neurons exists. Specific lesion of serotonergic neurons originating in the median raphe nucleus results in a decrease in ACh turnover in the hypothalamus (Robinson, 1982). This would suggest a tonic excitatory influence of serotonergic neurons on cholinergic neurons in the hypothalamus.

The last cholinergic projection to be discussed is one terminating on the locus coeruleus. This small brain stem structure, a major source of noradrenergic innervation throughout the CNS, contains cell bodies which are positive for both AChE and norepinephrine (Albanese and Butcher, 1980). Cheney et al. (1975) have reported ACh and ChAT activity in the locus coeruleus and concluded that cholinergic neurons terminate on this structure. It has been suggested that noradrenergic neurons in the locus coeruleus receive functional cholinergic input from the parabrachial nucleus or the nucleus tegmentalis dorsalis lateralis (Kimura and Maeda, 1982). It appears that cholinergic neurons may play a functional role in the locus coeruleus because iontophoretic ACh increases the firing rate of the locus coeruleus, and this effect is potentiated by physostigmine (Kuhar et al., 1978). However, the source of this cholinergic innervation is unknown, and electron microscopic studies by Lewis and Schon (1975) detecting no AChE in synaptic clefts or on presynaptic membranes even suggest that functional innervation is not present in the locus coeruleus.

Table 1. Proposed Action of Neurotransmitters on Cholinergic Activity
          in Specific Brain Areas[a]

NEUROTRANSMITTER	BRAIN AREA		
	Hippocampus	Cortex	Striatum
Dopamine	↓	↔	↓
Norepinephrine	↑	↑	
Serotonin	↔, ↓	↔, ↓	↑, ↔, ↓
Opiates	↓	↓	↔
Substance P	↓	↔	↔
ACTH	↑	↔	↔
Alpha-MSH	↑	↔	↔
TRH	↔	↑	↔
Somatostatin	↔	↔	↔
Neurotensin	↔	↔	↔
Angiotensin II	↔	↔	↔

[a]See Text for references

8.   CONCLUSION

In this chapter a number of cholinergic projections and the
actions of other neurotransmitters on these pathways have been described. This information has been summarized in Table 1. One must
be cautioned, however, that brain cholinergic pathways do not exist
in a vacuum. Although a drug may act on a specific neurotransmitter
controlling cholinergic neurons, it may also act at a point distal to
the cholinergic neuron, negating that effect. Thus, one cannot make
definitive predictions concerning the actions of a drug until the complete organization of the brain is known. Since the balance between
cholinergic neurons and other neurotransmitters is thought to be important in many diseases, such as Parkinson's disease, Alzheimer's
disease, and schizophrenia, it is important that the exact relationship between cholinergic and other neurotransmiters be understood.

ACKNOWLEDGEMENTS

    The author wishes to thank Ms. Debbie Maljarik, Ms. Kathy Weight
and Ms. Delaine Harris for their assistance in preparing this
manuscript. Part of the work reported therein was supported by
National Institute of Mental Health Grant MH-37450, American Heart
Association Grant-in-Aid #80684 with funds contributed in part by
AHA, Texas Affiliate, Inc. and an American Parkinson Disease
Association Grant.

REFERENCES

Albanese, A., and Butcher, L. L., 1980, Acetylcholinesterase and cate-
    cholamine distribution in the locus coeruleus of the rat, Brain
    Res. Bull. 5:127-134.
Assaf, S. Y., and Miller, J. J., 1977, Excitatory action of the meso-
    limbic dopamine system on septal neurons, Brain Res. 129:353-360.
Atweh, S. F., and Kuhar, M. J., 1977, Autoradiographic localization
    of opiate receptors in rat brain III. The telencephalon, Brain
    Res. 134:393-405.
Benardo, L. S., and Prince, D. A., 1980, Acetylcholine induced modu-
    lation of hippocampal pyramidal neurons, Brain Res. 211:227-234.
Ben-Ari, Y., Zigmond, R. E., Shute, C. C. D., and Lewis, P. R., 1977,
    Regional distribution of choline acetyltransferase and acetylcho-
    linesterase in the amygdaloid complex and stria terminalis system,
    Brain Res. 120:435-445.
Ben-Barak, J., and Dudai, Y., 1980, Early septal lesion: effect on
    the development of the cholinergic system in rat hippocampus,
    Brain Res. 185:323-334.
Bigl, V., Woolf, N. J., and Butcher, L. L., 1982, Cholinergic projec-
    tions from the basal forebrain to frontal parietal, temporal,
    occipital, and cingulate cortices: a combined fluorescent tracer
    and acetylcholinesterase analysis, Brain Research Bull. 8:727-749.
Bird, S. J., and Aghajanian, G. K., 1975, Denervation supersensitiv-
    ity in the cholinergic septohippocampal pathway: A microionto-
    phoretic study, Brain Res. 100:355-370.
Bland, B. H., Kostropoulos, G. K., and Phillis, J. W., 1974, Actyl-
    choline sensitivity of hippocampal formation neurons, Can. J.
    Physiol. Pharmacol. 52:966-971.
Bloom, F. E., Costa, E., and Salmoiraghi, G. C., 1965, Anethesia and
    the responsiveness of individual neurons of the caudate nucleus
    of the cat to acetylcholine, norepinephrine and dopamine admin-
    istered by microelectrophoresis, J. Pharmacol. Exp. Ther.
    150:244-252.
Bobillier, P., Seguin, S., Degueurce, A., Lewis, B. D., and Pujol, J.
    F., 1979, The efferent connections of the nucleus raphe centralis
    superior in the rat as revealed by radioautography, Brain Res.
    166:1-8.

Bowers, M. B., Jr., and Roth, R. H., 1972, Interaction of atropine-like drugs with dopamine-containing neurons in rat brain, Br. J. Pharmacol. 44:301-306.

Brownstein, M. J., Palkovits, M., Tappaz, M. L., Saavedra, J. M., and Kizer, J. S., 1976, Effect of surgical isolation of the hypothalamus on its neurotransmitter content, Brain Res. 117:287-295.

Butcher, S. G., and Butcher, L. L., 1974, Origin and modulation of acetylcholine activity in the neostriatum, Brain Res. 71:167-171.

Butcher, S. G., Butcher, L. L., and Cho, A. K., 1976, Modulation of neostriatal acetylcholine in the rat by dopamine and 5-hydroxytryptamine afferents, Life Sci. 18:733-744.

Cheney, D. L., LeFevre, H. F., and Racagni, G., 1975, Choline acetyltransferase activity and mass fragmentographic measurement of acetylcholine in specific nuclei and tracts of rat brain, Neuropharmacology 14:801-809.

Cheney, D. L., Robinson, S. E., Malthe-Sorenssen, D., Wood, P. L., Commissiong, J. W., and Costa, E., 1978, Regulation of the cholinergic septal-hippocampal pathway: role of dopaminergic septal afferents, in "Advances in Pharmacology and Therapeutics," Vol. 5 C. Dumont, ed., pp. 241-250, Pergamon Press, New York.

Collier, B., and Mitchell, J. F., 1966, The central release of acetylcholine during stimulation of the visual pathway, J. Physiol. (Lond.) 84:239-254.

Conrad, L. C. A., Leonard, C. M., and Pfaff, D. W., 1974, Connections of the median and dorsal raphe nuclei in the rat: an autoradiographic and degeneration study, J. Comp. Neurol. 156:179-206.

Consolo, S., Ladinsky, H., and Garattini, S., 1974, Effect of several dopaminergic parameters in the rat striatum, J. Pharm. Pharmacol. 26:275-277.

Consolo, S., Ladinsky, H., Tirelli, A. S., Crunelli, V., Samanin, R., and Garattini, S., 1979, Increase in rat striatal acetylcholine content by d-fenfluramine, a serotonin releaser, Life Sci. 25:1975-1981.

Coyle, J. T., Prince, D. L., and DeLong, M. R., 1983, Alzheimer's disease: a disorder of cortical cholinergic innervation. Science 219:1184-1190.

Davies, P., 1979, Neurotransmitter-related enzymes in senile dementia of the Alzheimer type, Brain Res. 171:319-327.

Davies, P., and Maloney, A. J. R., 1976, Selective loss of central cholinergic neurons in Alzheimer's disease, Lancet 2:1403.

Deadwyler, S. A., West, M. O., and Robinson, J. H., 1981, Entorhinal and septal inputs differentially control sensory-evoked responses in the rat dentate gyrus, Science 211:1181.

Descarries, L., Beaudet, A., and Watkins, K. C., 1975, Serotonin nerve terminals in adult rat neocortex, Brain Res. 100:563-588.

Deutsch, J. A., 1971, The cholinergic synapse and the site of memory, Science 174:788-794.

Domino, E. F., Krause, R. R., and Bowers, J., 1973, Regional distribution of some enzymes involved with putative neurotransmitters in the human visual system, Brain Res. 58:79-189.

Dray, A., Gonye, T. J., Oakley, N. R., and Tanner, T., 1976, Evidence
    for the existence of a raphe projection to the substantia nigra
    in rat, Brain 133:45-57.
Dudar, J. D., 1975, The effect of septal nuclei stimulation on the
    release of acetylcholine from the rabbit hippocampus, Brain Res.
    83:123-133.
Emson, P. C., Cuello, A. C., Paxinos, G., Jessell, T., and Iversen,
    L. L., 1977, The origin of substance P and acetylcholine projec-
    tions to the ventral tegmental area and interpeduncular nucleus
    in the rat, Acta Physiol. Scand., Suppl. 452:43-46.
Emson, P. C., Paxinos, G., Le Gal La Salle, G., Ben-Ari, Y., and
    Silver, A., 1979, Choline acetyltransferase and acetylcholines-
    terase containing projections from the basal forebrain to the
    amygdaloid complex of the rat, Brain Res. 165:271-282.
Ferkany, J. W., and Enna, S. J., 1980, Interaction between GABA-
    agonists and the cholinergic muscarinic system in rat corpus
    striatum, Life Sci. 27:143-149.
Fisher, A., Mantione, C. R., Abraham, D. J., and Hanin, I., 1982,
    Long-term central cholinergic hypofunction induced in mice by
    ethylcholine aziridinium ion (AF 64A) in vivo, J. Pharmacol. Exp.
    Ther. 222:140-145.
Fonnum, F., Grofova, I., Rinvik, E., Storm-Mathisen, J., and Walberg,
    F., 1974, Origin and distribution of glutamate decarboxylase in
    substantia nigra of the cat, Brain Res. 71:77-92.
Fuxe, K., 1965, Distribution of monoamine nerve terminals in central
    nervous system, Acta Physiol. Scand., 64 (Suppl. 247):41-85.
Giambalvo, C. T., and Snodgrass, S. R., 1978, Biochemical and behav-
    ioral effects of serotonin neurotoxins on the nigrostriatal dopa-
    mine system: comparison of injection sites, Brain Res.
    152:555-566.
Gloor, P., 1972, Temporal lobe epilepsy: its possible contribution to
    the understanding of the functional significance of the amygdala
    and of its interaction with neocortical-temporal mechanisms, in
    "The Neurobiology of the Amygdala," B. E. Eleftheriou, ed.,
    pp. 423-457, Plenum Press, New York.
Gogolak, G., Stumpf, C. H., Petske, H., and Sterc, J., 1968, The
    firing pattern of septal neurons and the form of the hippocampal
    theta wave, Brain Res. 7:201-207.
Gottesfeld, Z., and Jacobowitz, D. M., 1978, Cholinergic projection of
    the diagonal band to the interpeduncular nucleus of the rat brain,
    Brain Res. 156:329-332.
Gottesfeld, Z., and Jacobowitz, D. M., 1979, Cholinergic projections
    from the septal-diagonal band area to the habenular nuclei, Brain
    Res. 176:391-394.
Hebb, C. O., Krnjevic, K., and Silver, A., 1963, Effect of undercut-
    ting on the acetylcholinesterase and choline acetyltransferase
    activity in the cat's cerebral cortex, Nature 198:692.
Henke, H., and Fonnum, F., 1976, Topographical and subcellular distri-
    bution and choline acetyltransferase and glutamate decarboxylase
    in pigeon optic tectum, J. Neurochem. 27:387-391.

Hernández-Peón, R., O'Flaherty, J. J., and Mazzuchelli-O'Flaherty, A.
    L., 1967, Sleep and other behavioral effects induced by acetyl
    cholinic stimulation of basal temporal cortex and striate struc-
    ture, Brain Res. 4:243-267.
Hoover, D. B., and Baisden, R. H., 1980, Localization of putative cho-
    linergic neurons innervating the anteroventral thalamus, Brain
    Res. Bull. 5:519-524.
Hoover, D. B., and Jacobowitz, D. M., 1979, Neurochemical and histo-
    chemical studies of the effect of a lesion of the nucleus cunei-
    formis on the cholinergic innervation of discrete areas of the rat
    brain, Brain Res. 170:113-122.
Jhamandas, K., and Sutak, M., 1976, Morphine-naloxone interaction in
    the central cholinergic system: the influence of subcortical le-
    sioning and electrical stimulation, Br. J. Pharmacol. 58:101-107.
Johnston, M. V., McKinney, M., and Coyle, J. T., 1979, Evidence for a
    cholinergic projection to neocortex from neurons in basal fore-
    brain, Proc. Natl. Acad. Sci. USA 76:5392-5396.
Johnston, M. V., McKinney, M., and Coyle, J. T., 1981, Neocortical-
    cholinergic innervation: a description of extrinsic and intrinsic
    components in the rat, Exp. Brain Research 43:159-172.
Kataoka, K., Nakemura, Y., and Hassler, R., 1973, Habenulo-interpe-
    duncular tract: a possible cholinergic neuron in rat brain,
    Brain Res. 63:264-267.
Kimura, H., and Maeda, T., 1982, Aminergic and cholinergic systems in
    the dorsolateral pontine tegmentum, Brain Research Bull.
    9:493-499.
Kimura, H., McGeer, P. L., Peng, F., and McGeer, E. G., 1980, Choline
    acetyltransferase-containing neurons in rodent brain demonstrated
    by immunohistochemistry, Science 208:1057-1059.
Kobayashi, R. M., Palkovits, M., Hruska, R. E., Rothschild, R., and
    Yamamura, H. I., 1978, Regional distribution of muscarinic cholin-
    ergic receptors in rat brain, Brain Res. 154:13-23.
Krnjevic, K., Pumain, R., and Renaud, L., 1971, The mechanism of
    excitation by acetylcholine in the cerebral cortex, J. Physiol.
    (Lond.) 215:247-268.
Krnjevic, K., and Silver, A., 1965, A histochemical study of choliner-
    gic fibers in the cerebral cortex, J. Anat. 99:711-759.
Kuhar, M. J., Aghajanian, G. K., and Roth, R. H., 1972, Tryptophan
    hydroxylase activity and synaptosomal uptake of serotonin in dis-
    crete brain regions after midbrain raphe lesion: correlations
    with serotonin levels and histochemical fluorescence, Brain Res.
    44:165-176.
Kuhar, M. J., Atweh, S. F., and Bird, S. J., 1978, Studies of cholin-
    ergic-monoaminergic interactions in rat brain, in "Cholinergic-
    monoaminergic Interactions in the Brain," L. L. Butcher, eds.,
    pp. 211-227, Academic Press, New York.
Kuhar, M. J., Dehaven, R. N., Yamamura, H. I., Rommelspacher, H., and
    Simon, J. R., 1975, Further evidence for cholinergic habenulo-
    interpeduncular neurons: pharmacologic and functional character-
    istics, Brain Res. 97:265-275.

Kuhar, M. J., Sethy, V. H., Roth, R. H., and Aghajanian, G. K., 1973, Choline: Selective accumulation by central cholinergic neurons, J. Neurochem. 20:581-593.

Kuhar, M. J., and Yamamura, H. I., 1976, Localization of cholinergic muscarinic receptors in rat brain by light microscopic radioautography, Brain Res. 110:229-243.

Lake, N., 1973, Studies of the habenulo-interpeduncular pathway in cats, Exp. Neurol. 41:113-132.

Landinsky, H., Consolo, S., Bianchi, S., and Jori, A., 1976, Increase in striatal acetylcholine by picrotoxin in the rat: evidence for a gabergic-dopaminergic-cholinergic line, Brain Res. 108:351-361.

Lauder, J. M., and Krebs, H., 1978, Serotonin as a differentiation signal in early neurogenesis, Dev. Neurosci. 1:15-30.

Lehmann, J., and Fibiger, H. C., 1981, Anatomical organization of some cholinergic systems in the mammalian forebrain, in "Cholinergic Mechanisms: Phylogenetic Aspects, Central and Peripheral Synapses, and Clinical Significance," G. Pepeu and H. Ladinsky, eds., Plenum Press, New York.

Lehmann, J., Nagy, J. I., Atmadja, S., and Fibiger, H. C., 1980, The nucleus basalis magnocellularis: The origin of a cholinergic projection to the neocortex of the rat, Neuroscience 5:1161-1174.

Leranth, C. S., Brownstein, M., Zaborszky, L., Jardanyi, Z. S., and Palkovits, M., 1975, Morphological and biochemical changes in the rat interpenduncular nucleus following the transection of the habenulo-interpeduncular tract, Brain Res. 99:124-128.

Lewis, P. R., and Schon, F. E. G., 1975, The localization of acetylcholinesterase in the locus coeruleus of the normal rat after 6-hydroxydopamine treatment, J. Anat. 120:373-385.

Lewis, P. R., and Shute, C. D., 1967, The cholinergic limbic system: projections to hippocampal formation, medial cortex, nuclei of the ascending cholinergic reticular system and the subfornical organ and supraoptic crest, Brain 90:521-539.

Lewis, P. R., Shute, C. C. D., and Silver, A., 1967, Confirmation from choline acetylase of a massive cholinergic innervation to the rat hippocampus, J. Physiol. (Lond.) 191:215-224.

Lindvall, O., 1975, Mesencephalic dopaminergic afferents to the lateral septal nucleus of the rat, Brain Res. 87:89-95.

Lorens, S. A., and Guldberg, H. C., 1974, Regional 5-hydroxytryptamine following selective midbrain raphe lesions in the rat, Brain Res. 78:45-56.

Loy, R., and Moore, R. Y., 1979, Ontogeny of the noradrenergic innervation of the rat hippocampal formation, Anat. Embryol. (Berl.) 157:243-253.

Maletta, G. J., and Timiras, P. S., 1968, Choline acetyltransferase activity and total protein content in selected optic areas of the rat after complete light-deprivation during CNS development, J. Neurochem. 15:787-793.

Malthe-Sorenssen, D., Cheney, D. L., and Costa, E., 1978a, Modulation of acetylcholine metabolism in the hippocampal cholinergic pathway by intraseptally injected substance P, J. Pharmacol. Exp. Ther 206:21-28.

Malthe-Sorenssen, D., Wood, P. L., Cheney, D. L., and Costa, E.;
    1978b, Modulation of the turnover rate of acetylcholine in rat
    brain by intraventricular injection of thyrotropin-releasing
    hormone, somatostatin, neurotensin and angiotensin II, J.
    Neurochem. 31:685-691.
Marks, M. J., and Collins, A. C., 1982, Characterization of nicotine
    binding in mouse brain and comparison with the binding of
    α-bungarotoxin and quinuclidinyl benzilate, Mol. Pharmacol.
    22:554-564.
Matthews, D. A., Nadler, J. V., Lynch, G. S., and Cotman, C. W., 1974,
    Development of cholinergic innervation in the hippocampal forma-
    tion of rat. I. Histochemical demonstration of acetylcholines-
    terase activity, Dev. Biol. 36:130-141.
McCaughran, J. A., Genovese, F. L., and Schechter, N., 1980, The
    effect of kainic acid on cholinergic enzymes and receptors in the
    amygdala complex of the rat, Brain Res. 199:127-133.
McGeer, P. L., McGeer, E. G., Fibiger, H. C., and Wickson, V., 1971,
    Neostriatal cholineacetylase and cholinesterase following selec-
    tive brain lesions, Brain Res. 35:308-314.
McGeer, P. L., McGeer, E. G., Sherer, U., and Singh, K., 1977, A
    glutaminergic corticostriatal path? Brain Res. 128:369-373.
McGeer, E. G., Scherer-Singler, U., and Singh, E. A., 1979, Confirma-
    tory data on habenular projections, Brain Res. 168:375-376.
Mellgren, S. I., and Srebro, B., 1973, Changes in acetylcholinesterase
    and distribution of degenerating fibers in the hippocampal region
    after septal lesions in the rat, Brain Res. 52:19-36.
Mitchell, R., 1980, A novel GABA receptor modulates stimulus-induced
    glutamate release from cortico-striatal terminals, Eur. J.
    Pharmacol. 67:119-122.
Montplaisir, J. Y., 1975, Cholinergic mechanisms involved in cortical
    activation arousal, Electroencephr. Clin. Neurophysiol.
    38:263-272.
Moroni, F., Cheney, D. L., and Costa, E., 1978a, The turnover rate of
    acetylcholine in brain nuclei of rats injected intraventricularly
    and intraseptally with alpha and beta-endorphin, Neuropharmacology
    17:191-196.
Moroni, F., Malthe-Sorenssen, D., Cheney, D. L., and Costa, E., 1978b,
    Modulation of ACh turnover in the septal-hippocampal pathway by
    electrical stimulation and lesioning, Brain Res. 150:333-341.
Mulas, A., Mulas, M. L., and Pepeu, G., 1974, Effect of limbic system
    lesions on acetylcholine release from the cerebral cortex of the
    rat, Psychopharmacologia 39:223-230.
Nadler, J. V., Matthews, D. A., Cotman, C. W., and Lynch, G. S., 1974,
    Development of cholinergic innervation in the hippocampal forma-
    tion of the rat. II. Quantitative changes in choline acetyltrans-
    ferase and acetylcholinesterase activities, Dev. Biol. 36:142-154.
Neal, M. J., 1976, Acetylcholine as a retinal transmitter substance,
    in "Transmitters in the Visual Process," S. L. Bonting, ed., pp.
    127-143, Pergamon Press, Oxford.

Nicolaou, N. M., Garcia-Munoz, M., Arbuthnott, G. W., and Eccleston, D., 1979, Interactions between serotonergic and dopaminergic systems in rat brain demonstrated by small unilateral lesions of the raphe nuclei, Eur. J. Pharmacol. 57:295-305.

Nistri, A., Bartolini, A., Deffenu, G., and Pepeu, G., 1972, Investigations into the release of acetylcholine from the cerebral cortex of the cat: effects of amphetamine, of scopolamine and of septal lesions, Neuropharmacology 11:665-674.

Olton, D. S., and Feustle, W. A., 1981, Hippocampal function required for nonspatial working memory, Exp. Brain Res. 41:380-389.

Pepeu, G., Mulas, A., and Mulas, M. L., 1973, Changes in the acetylcholine content in the rat brain after lesions of the septum, fimbria, and hippocampus, Brain Res. 57:153-164.

Richter, J. A., Perry, E. K., and Tomlinson, B. E., 1980, Acetylcholine and choline levels in post-mortem human brain tissue: preliminary observations in Alzheimer's disease, Life Sci. 26:1683-1689.

Robinson, S. E., 1982, Interaction of the median raphe nucleus and hypothalamic serotonin with cholinergic agents and pressor responses in the rat, J. Pharmacol. Exp. Ther. 223:662-668.

Robinson, S. E., 1983, Effect of specific serotonergic lesions on cholinergic neurons in the hippocampus, cortex and striatum, Life Sci. 32:345-353.

Robinson, S. E., Cheney, D. L., and Costa, E., 1978, Effect of nomifensine and other antidepressant drugs on acetylcholine turnover in various regions of rat brain, Naunyn Schmiedebergs Arch. Pharmacol. 304:263-269.

Robinson, S. E., Malthe-Sorenssen, D., Wood, P. L., and Commisssiong, J., 1979, Dopaminergic regulation of the cholinergic septal hippocampal pathway, J. Pharmacol. Exp. Ther. 208:476-479.

Rommelspacher, H., and Kuhar, M. J., 1974, Effects of electrical stimulation on the acetylcholine levels in central cholinergic nerve terminals, Brain Res. 81:243-251.

Rommelspacher, H., and Kuhar, M. J., 1975, Effects of dopaminergic drugs and acute medial forebrain bundle lesions on striatal acetylcholine levels, Life Sci. 16:65-70.

Rossor, M. N., Garrett, N. J., Johnson, A. L., Mountjoy, C. Q., Roth, M., and Iversen, L. L., 1982, A post-mortem study of the cholinergic and GABA systems in senile dementia, Brain 105:313-330.

Rotter, A., Birdsall, N. J. M., Burgen, A. S. V., Field, P. M., Hulme, E. C., and Raisman, G., 1979, Muscarinic receptors in the central nervous system of the rat. I. Technique for autoradiographic localization of the binding of [^{3}H]propylbenzilylcholine mustard and its distribution in the forebrain, Brain Research Rev. 1:141-165.

Rotter, A., and Jacobowitz, D. M., 1981, Neurochemical identification of cholinergic forebrain projection sites of the nucleus tegmentalis dorsalis lateralis, Brain Res. 6:525-529.

Sastry, B. R., Zialkowski, S. E., Hansen, L. M., Kavanagh, J. P., and Evoy, E. M., 1979, Acetylcholine release in interpeduncular nucleus following the stimulation of habenula, Brain Res. 164:334-337.

Scatton, B., and Bartholini, G., 1980, Increase in striatal acetylcho-
    line levels by GABA-ergic agents: dependence on corticostriatal
    neurons, Brain Res. 200:174-178.

Scatton, B., and Bartholini, G., 1979, Increase in striatal actylcho-
    line levels by GABA mimetic drugs: lack of involvement of the
    nigrostriatal dopaminergic neurons, Eur. J. Pharmacol. 56:181-182.

Schwartz, R. D., and Kellar, K. J., 1983, ^{3}H-Acetylcholine binding
    sites located on catecholamine and serotonin terminals in rat
    striatum, Fed. Proceed. 42:879.

Schwartz, R. D., McGee, R., and Kellar, K. J., 1982, Nicotinic cholin-
    ergic receptors labeled by [^{3}H]acetylcholine in rat brain, Mol.
    Pharmacol. 22:56-62.

Segal, M., and Landis, S. C., 1974, Afferents to the septal areas of
    the rat studied with the method of retrograde axonal transport of
    horseradish peroxidase, Brain Res. 82:263-268.

Sethy, V. H., Kuhar, M., Roth, H. R., Van Woert, M. H., and Aghajanian
    K. G., 1973, Cholinergic neurons: effect of acute septal lesion
    on acetylcholine and choline content of rat hippocampus, Brain
    Res. 55:481-484.

Shute, C. C. D., and Lewis, P. R., 1966, Cholinergic and monoaminergic
    pathways in the hypothalamus, Br. Med. Bull. 22:221-226.

Shute, C. C. D., and Lewis, P. R., 1963, Cholinesterase-containing
    systems of the brain of the rat, Nature 199:1160-1164.

Shute, C. C. D., and Lewis, P. R., 1967, The ascending cholinergic
    reticular system: neocortical, olfactory and subcortical projec-
    tions, Brain 90:467-520.

Simantov, R., Kuhar, M. J., Uhl, G. R., and Snyder, S. H., 1977,
    Opioid peptide enkephalin: immunohistochemical mapping in rat
    central nervous system, Proc. Natl. Acad. Sci. USA 74:2167-2171.

Singh, M. M., 1981, Cholinergic mechanisms and the psychobiology of
    schizophrenia, in "Biological Psychiatry 1981," C. Perris, G.
    Strüwe and B. Jansson, eds., pp. 793-800, Elsevier/North Holland,
    Amsterdam.

Smith, C. M., 1974, Acetylcholine release from the cholinergic septo-
    hippocampal pathway, Life Sci. 14:2159-2166.

Sorimachi, M., and Kataoka, K., 1974, Choline uptake by nerve termi-
    nals: a sensitive and a specific marker of cholinergic innerva-
    tion, Brain Res. 72:350-353.

Spencer, H. J., 1976, Antagonism of cortical excitation of striatal
    neurons by glutamic acid diethyl ester: evidence for glutamic
    acid as an excitatory transmitter in the rat striatum, Brain Res.
    102:91-101.

Stadler, H., Lloyd, K. G., Gadea-Ciria, M., and Bartholini, G., 1973,
    Enhanced striatal acetylcholine release by chlorpromazine and its
    reversal by apomorphine, Brain Res. 55:476-480.

Steiner, F., 1968, Influence of microelectrophoretically applied
    acetylcholine on the responsiveness of hippocampal and lateral
    geniculate neurons, Pfluegers Arch. 303:173-180.

Storm-Mathisen, J., 1970, Quantitative histochemistry of acetylcho-
    linesterase in rat hippocampal region correlated to histochemical
    staining, J. Neurochem. 17:739-750.

Szerb, J. C., 1967, Cortical acetylcholine release and electorencepha-
    lographic arousal, J. Physiol. 192:329-343.
Trabucchi, M., Cheney, D., Racagni, G., and Costa, E., 1974, Involve-
    ment of brain cholinergic mechanisms in the action of chlorprom-
    zine, Nature 249:664-666.
Trabucchi, M., Cheney, D. L., Racagni, G., and Costa, E., 1975a, Pen
    tobarbital and in vivo turnover rate of actylcholine in mouse
    brain and in regions of rat brain, Pharmacol. Res. Commun.
    1:81-94.
Trabucchi, M., Cheney, D. L., Racagni, G., and Costa, E., 1975b, In
    vivo inhibition of striatal acetylcholine turnover by L-DOPA,
    apomorphine and (+)-amphetamine, Brain Res. 85:130-134.
Urano, A., 1977, Effects of the eye enucleation on the activity of
    monoamine oxidase and acetylcholinesterase in the superior colli-
    culus of the rat, Cell Tissue Res. 179:331-345.
Vander Kooy, D., and Hattori, T., 1980, Dorsal raphe cells with col-
    lateral projections to the caudate-putamen and substantia nigra:
    A fluorescent retrograde double labeling study in the rat, Brain
    Res. 186:1-7.
Vanderwolf, C. H., and Robinson, T. E., 1981, Reticulo-cortical activ-
    ity and behavior: A critique of the arousal theory and a new syn-
    thesis, Behav. Brain Sciences 4:459-514.
Wenk, H., Bigl, V., and Meyer, V., 1980, Cholinergic projections from
    magnocellular nuclei of the basal forebrain to cortical areas in
    rats. Brain Research Rev. 2:295-316.
Wood, P.L., Malthe-Sorenssen, D., Cheney, D.L., and Costa, E., 1978,
    Increase of hippocampal acetylcholine turnover rate and the
    stretching-yawning syndrome elicited by alpha-MSH and ACTH, Life
    Sciences 22:673-678.
Wood, P. L., and Richard, J., 1982, GABAergic regulation of the sub-
    stantia innominata-cortical cholinergic pathway, Neuropharmacology
    21:969-972.
Wood, P. L., and Stotland, L. M., 1980, Actions of enkephalin, μ and
    partial agonist analgesics on acetylcholine turnover in rat brain,
    Neuropharmacology 19:975-982.
Woolf, N. J., and Butcher, L. L., 1982, Cholinergic projections to the
    basolateral amygdala: a combined Evans blue and acetylcholines-
    terase analysis, Brain Research Bull. 8:751-763.
Yamamura, H. I., Kuhar, M. J., and Snyder, S. H., 1974, In vivo iden-
    tification of muscarinic cholinergic receptor binding in rat
    brain, Brain Res. 80:170-176.
Yarbrough, G. G., 1976, TRH potentiates excitatory actions of actyl-
    choline on cerebral cortical neurons, Nature 263:523-524.
Zsilla, G., Racagni, G., Cheney, D. L., and Costa, E., 1977, Constant
    rate infusion of deuterated phosphorylcholine to measure the
    effects of morphine on acetylcholine turnover rate in specific
    nuclei of rat brain, Neuropharmacology 16:25-31.

Chapter 3

FUNCTIONS OF CENTRAL CHOLINERGIC SYSTEMS IN THE BRAIN-BEHAVIOR

Albert Wauquier and G.H.C. Clincke

Department of Neuropharmacology
Janssen Pharmaceutica
B-2340 Beerse
Belgium

---

1. INTRODUCTION

"Most impressive is the singular fact that acetylcholine is the

only substance that can influence every physiological and behavioral
response thus far examined." (Myers, 1974, pp. 759). The present
review deals with three levels of the relationship between brain and
behavior: input, integration and output, but obviously in a much more
restricted way than the citation would suggest.

The different parts of the review are separately described,
because of the methodologies employed. The first part (input) deals
with changes in brain electrical activity and the changes in sleep and
wakefulness, caused by acetylcholine itself and agonists-antagonists
of acetylcholine. The second part (integration) describes the cholinergic involvement in learning and memory mechanisms. The third part
(output) focuses on operant behavior, of which brain self-stimulation
was chosen as a representative example.

2.   BRAIN ELECTRICAL ACTIVITY: WAKEFULNESS AND SLEEP

The release of acetylcholine (ACh) from brain during wakefulness
and a decreased liberation during sleep, suggest cholinergic mechanisms are involved in waking. ACh itself and agonists or antagonists
modify electrical brain activity during the awake state and induce
arousal or sleep, further suggesting that cholinergic mechanisms might
be involved in sleep-wakefulness regulation. However, an apparent
dissociation between EEG and behavior, originally observed with atropine, deserves attention. This suggests that the behavioral changes
are not always reflected in changes in electrical brain activity in
the appropriate way. By summarizing the knowledge on the effects of
ACh and the effects of agonists and antagonists, it might be possible
to get a better insight into the role of ACh in sleep-wakefulness.

2.1. Acetylcholine

2.1.1. Release of Acetylcholine

Celesia and Jasper (1966) were the first to report ACh liberation
from the cerebral cortex in cats. Jasper and Tessier (1971) found
that the release of ACh at the cortical surface in cats was higher
during paradoxical sleep and wakefulness than during slow wave sleep.
In dogs, Haranath and Venkatakrishna-Bhatt (1973) found a diminished
ACh release from the cerebral ventricles during sleep. The release in
the ventricles paralleled that of the cerebral cortex. The increase
of ACh during REM sleep appeared consistent with the activity of the
brain, but it cannot be stated whether the release of ACh is initiated
by REM or vice versa. However, those studies suggested that the release of ACh is associated with brain activation. One would expect,
therefore, to observe brain EEG activation following ACh application.

2.1.2. Acetylcholine Application

Unless severe cardiovascular changes are induced, ACh given i.v.

does not cause major changes of the EEG (Longo, 1962; Nakao et al., 1956). Haranath et al. (1967) found that an acute injection of 1000 µg of ACh or an infusion of 30 µg/min of ACh into the internal carotid artery produced high voltage slow wave patterns as well as an 'activation pattern of sleep' (paradoxical sleep), associated with twitches of the eyelids, snout muscles and feet. These patterns started about 10 minutes after injection and lasted about one hour. A lower dose of 500 µg of ACh produced drowsiness for only about 30 minutes. Awakening occurred 10 minutes after stopping the infusion. An infusion of 3 to 10 µg/min of ACh did not produce sleep and an infusion of 300 µg/min elicited sleep interrupted by frequent awakening due to strong peripheral effects such as profuse salivation.

A similar state of drowsiness has been observed following i.cv. application of low doses of ACh ($\leq$ 1 µg) in cats, but higher doses > 10 µg) elicited seizure activity (Feldberg and Sherwood, 1954). Such EEG activation and seizure patterns were also observed following direct cortical application of small amounts of ACh in cats (Miller et al., 1940). Other cholinergic substances such as carbachol, were found to shift the cortical EEG to low voltage fast activity when applied into the mesencephalic brain stem in the rat (Grossman, 1968). ACh at the dose of 1 to 2 µg applied into the lateral ventricle of dogs (Haranath and Venkatakrishna-Bhatt, 1977) produced drowsiness after 10 to 15 minutes; subsequently, sleep period of 3 to 10 minutes occurred for about one hour: at 2 µg of ACh, sleep lasted longer and at 10 µg restlessness but no sleep was found.

The fact that both slow-wave and REM sleep are elicited through systemic application of ACh casts doubt on the validity of the generality of these findings. Direct brain application avoiding peripheral effects, appears to elicit fast EEG activity. However, other studies suggested a brain-site specificity and the presence of cholinoceptive hypnogenic areas.

Hernández-Peón et al. (1963) carried out an extensive study on the application of minute amounts of crystals of ACh through implanted cannulae in a large number of brain structures in the cat. When applied into Nauta's limbic-forebrain-limbic-midbrain circuit, extending from the preoptic region through the hypothalamus and into the midbrain and pons, the desynchronized EEG was replaced by spindles and high voltage slow waves which progressed towards a desynchronized pattern of sleep (paradoxical sleep). Sleep lasted for three to four hours. Nociceptive stimuli failed to awaken the cats, but strong electrical stimulation of the lateral mesencephalic reticular formation did.

Bilateral lesions of the medial forebrain bundle in posterior areas prevented the cholinergic-induced sleep, whereas cholinergic stimulation in points posterior to the lesions still evoked sleep. From these studies the authors concluded that the neocortex is not essential for the production of sleep and wakefulness, and that the

hypnogenic system directly inhibited the mesodiencephalic arousal
system.

In a later study Hernández-Peón et al. (1967) found behavioral
and electroencephalographic manifestations of two patterns of sleep
following ACh application in the prepyriform and peri-amygdaloid
cortex, olfactory tubercle and of extrapyramidal structures such as
the globus pallidus, putamen and caudate nucleus. These effects were
prevented by lesioning of the medial forebrain bundle, the ventral
anterior thalamus and the reticulogigantocellular nucleus. In extending this work, Mazzuchelli-O'Flaherty et al. (1967) found that sleep
was induced over a wide area of the limbic cortex, but not in the posterior parts of the mesial surface. These sleep-inducing effects were
prevented by preoptic lesions.

Thus, ACh application along the medial forebrain bundle extending into the cortex produces sleep. Since physostigmine produced
similar effects in these regions and atropine blocked the sleep
produced by electrical stimulation of sites into the orbitofrontal
cortex (Mazzuchelli-O'Flaherty et al., 1967), it was postulated that
the effects found after direct ACh application reflect the presence
of a physiological cholinergic limbic substrate involved in the production of sleep.

2.2. Ganglion Stimulation: Nicotine

Because of the prominent peripheral autonomic effects of nicotine, the central nervous system (CNS) effects of nicotine were not
fully appreciated for some time. It was initially thought that nicotine only produced a transient desynchronization of the EEG at low
doses in intact or brain stem transected animals, which were mainly
due to cardiovascular effects; whereas at higher doses seizure activity was produced.

The EEG desynchronization by nicotine (doses of about 0.01 mg/kg)
has been reported in intact rabbits (Longo et al., 1954) and cats
(Hudson, 1979), while in high doses (1 mg/kg, i.p.) it has been found
to reduce the EEG power in the genetically selected 'long-sleep' mice
(Ryan et al., 1979). EEG desynchronization has also been observed in
brain stem transected rabbits, cats, dogs and monkeys (Domino, 1967;
Knapp and Domino, 1963). A brain stem transection was applied because
of the necessity to have a preparation showing slow wave EEG activity.

Some species differences were, however, evident. Knapp and
Domino (1962, 1963) found that 10 to 20 µg/kg i.v. nicotine produced
EEG activation in midpontine (pretrigeminal section) rabbits, cats,
dogs and high pontine monkeys, and in prepontine rabbits and cats, but
not in the prepontine dog. High doses (> 0.05 mg/kg) produce seizure
in mesencephalic transected rabbits (Floris et al., 1962) and in
intact rats, guinea pigs and rabbits (Longo et al., 1967). Knapp and

Domino (1962, 1963) found that at subconvulsive doses (0.01 and 0.02 mg/kg, i.v.) the EEG desynchronization could not be ascribed to a peripheral action, because such activation was also obtained in completely de-afferented dogs (Domino, 1967; Knapp and Domino, 1962).

This biphasic action of nicotine; arousal followed by sedation, has been described in different species. Yamamoto and Domino (1967) gave a one minute infusion of 0.005 to 0.01 mg/kg in slow wave sleeping cats. An arousal reaction of about three minutes was then followed by slow wave sleep and activated sleep with the presence of cortical fast activity and a theta rhythm in the hippocampus 15 to 30 minutes later. Repeated injections of 0.005 mg/kg of nicotine at one hour intervals were also given. There is thus some confusion as to the interpretation of the EEG effects found by these authors. However, tachyphylaxis towards the peripheral effects of nicotine were observed. No seizure activity was seen, as has been reported by others (e.g., Floris et al., 1962), because low doses were used. Along with the findings of Dunlop et al. (1960) in rabbits, that the hippocampus had a low seizure threshold for nicotine, Yamamoto and Domino (1965) described the appearance of hippocampal theta and 35 to 45 Hz/sec burst discharges in the amygdala.

A biphasic action and an increase in the frequency as well as in the duration of the paradoxical sleep episodes following an i.v. injection of 10 μg/kg of nicotine was also found in rabbits by Goldstein et al. (1967). They also showed that nicotine produced a significant reversal of the effects of 3 mg/kg i.v. of pentobarbital which was confirmed by Hudson (1979) showing that pentobarbital-induced splindling in cats was suppressed.

Studying the cortical-subcortical relationship, Goldstein et al. (1967) described that nicotine diminished the mutual involvement of the cortex-hippocampus and of the cortex-reticular formation, suggesting a decreased inhibitory mechanism, thus lessening the control of the cortex over subcortical structures.

Bhattacharya and Goldstein (1970) found a somewhat longer-lasting biphasic effect in rabbits following a s.c. injection of 200 μg/kg in rabbits. In accordance with above, they found that the mean amplitude of the integrated EEG increased in the cortex and the reticular formation, decreased in the hippocampus and did not change in the amygdala and the hypothalamus. However, following repeated s.c administration of 200 μg/kg of nicotine (five times per day) over three weeks, nicotine did not change the cortical amplitude, but decreased the amplitude of the EEG in the reticular formation, hippocampus and amygdala. They concluded that nicotine administration produced a shift from the reticular to the 'limbic system arousal mechanism' and that this increased the incentive for nicotine intake.

Guha and Pradhan (1976) found that 12.5 μg/kg i.p. of nicotine

in cats, produced a biphasic effect, whereas 25, 50 or 100 μg/kg i.p.
or 10 μg i.cv. showed a typical depressive type of EEG pattern from
the beginning, characterized by an increase in the duration of low
and high amplitude alpha-bursts. The EEG synchronization resembled
the effects obtained with pentobarbital, confirming previously obtained data in rabbits by Goldstein et al. (1967).

Schaeppi (1967) gave nicotine intravertebrally in cats; the
threshold dose was 0.01 to 0.3 μg; at doses of 0.3 to 3 μg, an initial
arousal associated with an increase in blood pressure was followed by
relaxation of the animals and occasionally a late phase with enhanced
synchronization. Similar effects were obtained following an injection
of nicotine into the fourth ventricle, but with a longer onset and
occasionally leading to a prolonged phase of EEG synchronization. An
intracisternal injection of doses of nicotine exceeding 0.3 μg also
produced EEG desynchronization, without being followed by EEG synchronization.

Stadnicki and Schaeppi (1970) found that 10 μg of nicotine infused over one minute into the fourth ventricle of cats produced an
initial generalized arousal followed by a phase of inactivity and
cortical EEG hypersynchronization, which might be due to an action
upon the solitary tract nucleus. The same authors (Stadnicki and
Schaeppi, 1972) studied various i.v. doses of nicotine in cats:
1 μg/kg caused only temporary EEG desynchronization; at 10 μg/kg initial desynchronization was followed by cortical EEG hypersynchronization, hippocampal theta, and high frequency burst (40 Hz/sec) activity
in the amygdala. Thereafter, high voltage slow waves appeared in
subcortical structures along with episodes of slow-wave sleep and
paradoxical sleep. A dose of 30 to 100 μg/kg of nicotine caused
desynchronization of the EEG or flattening of the cortical EEG and
subsequently slow-wave activity throughout the cortex and subcortex;
at 100 μg/kg the cortical EEG flattened progressing to EEG silence,
but no seizure activity was found.

After i.cv. application of (-)-nicotine (1 to 10 μg) or the
(+)-isomer [1/100 of the dose of the (-)-isomer] in rats, behavioral
sedation was induced; in the hippocampus the amplitude and the number
of the 6-8 Hz discharges decreased; high doses produced seizure activity (Abood et al., 1979).

The EEG activation is ascribed to the ability of nicotine to
mimic or release ACh, which acts on the reticular formation, whereas
the second phase of EEG synchronization might be due to a noradrenergic preponderance. This later phase is blocked by the alpha-antagon-
ists phenoxybenzamine and phentolamine (Guha and Pradhan, 1976) and
nicotine itself decreased the noradrenaline concentration in whole rat
brain (Westfall, 1967).

Thus in general, nicotine produces an initial EEG activation lasting a few minutes, an action which is related to both a central and peripheral cholinergic action, but the EEG effects are predominantly due to a central action, probably via an action on the reticular formation. This is followed by EEG synchronization and periods of paradoxical sleep. The sleep increasing effects are probably not related to a direct nicotine action, but are due to an action on other transmitter systems, such as the noradrenergic systems.

2.3. Neuromuscular Blockers

A number of drugs which, by virtue of their peripheral ACh antagonism, interfere with transmission at the neuromuscular junction, are used to produce muscle relaxation and to immobilize animals. Nevertheless, some of the substances, such as d-tubocurarine, were tested for their possible central effects, on the one hand by direct brain application and on the other hand, following interventions which may disturb the blood brain barrier. Haranath et al. (1967) injected 500 μg of d-tubocurarine in the carotid artery of dogs. After a latency of about 20 minutes, dogs slept for periods of 5 to 10 minutes when they showed high voltage slow wave EEG patterns. Some of the periods were followed by an activated sleep pattern during which muscle twitches occurred.

In a further study, Haranath and Shyamalakumari (1973) injected or infused d-tubocurarine in the cerebral ventricles of dogs. Doses of 2 μg to 25 μg produced excitement and convulsions respectively. About 20 minutes after injecting 500 μg, sleep periods of varying durations were found and on some occasions REM sleep was observed. Low doses of 50 to 250 μg elicited sleep but after a latency of about 40 minutes. After perfusion of tubocurarine at the dose of 10 ng/min into the lateral ventricles, sleep was seen starting after 20 to 30 minutes and lasting either for 30 to 45 minutes continuously or for periods of 5 to 20 minutes. Haranath and Venkatakrishna-Bhatt (1977) described how doses of 10 to 20 ng of tubocurarine injected into the inferior horn of the lateral ventricle of dogs were sufficient to produce sleep. The authors stated that sleep was produced only when the dogs were left undisturbed. The long latencies and the lack of adequate controls caused doubt whether sleep was really induced or rather that spontaneous sleep was promoted, by virtue of the muscle relaxation.

In fact, in conscious cats, doses of 0.05 to 1 ng of tubocurarine given i.cv. induced desynchronization, characterized by a decrease in the 7 to 9 and 10 to 14 Hz waves, which was associated with behavioral arousal (Ashorobi et al., 1979), whereas Cohen et al. (1981) reported tonic-clonic seizure in rats.

Von Wild (1980) found that both pancuronium and succinylcholine given i.v. over a large dose range in cats under narcosis did not change the EEG. Using an encephale isole preparation, succinylcholine produced a desynchronization of the cortical EEG and a synchronization of the hippocampal EEG, starting 20 seconds after the injection and lasting for 40 to 120 seconds. In cats submitted to a series of electroshocks (20 to 93) which served to induce a pathophysiological model of a disturbed blood brain barrier and vasogenic edema, in a number of experiments with both succinylcholine and pancuronium, short-lasting arousal reactions were found.

Thus, in contrast to a postulated direct central effect séen by certain authors (e.g. Halpern et al., 1967) muscle relaxants did not cause EEG changes unless penetration of the drug into the brain was facilitated. Furthermore, these effects were very short-lasting and not seen in all experiments.

Pokorny and Sterc (1980) gave 0.5 mg/kg i.m. of tubocurarine in rats and found no noticeable effects on the frontal cortex, more slow waves of 1 to 2 Hz in the septum, rhythms of 2 to 3 and 5 Hz/sec in the hypothalamus and a peak at 2 Hz and 4 to 5 Hz in the hippocampus. The dose used is very unlikely to affect nerve cells. Immobilization itself may be the primary reason for the effects seen, leading to an activation of limbic structures due to stimulation from the periphery.

Using another muscle relaxant (gallamine triethiodide) in cats (Glenn et al., 1980) there was somewhat more wakefulness at the expense of non-REM sleep, but with a preservation of the sequence of sleep stages just like that found in freely moving animals.

Thus, it appears that muscle relaxants may slightly affect the EEG. This effect occurs especially when the blood brain barrier is disturbed. Alternatively, it may be due to immobilization and the resultant stress response.

2.4. Muscarinic Agonists: Pilocarpine and Arecoline

The muscarinic agonists arecoline and pilocarpine have seldom been investigated for their inherent effects on the EEG. The most extensive studies are those by Herz (1963) and Yamamoto and Domino (1967).

Herz (1963) gave different doses of arecoline in the rabbit. At 0.002 mg/kg arecoline caused a desynchronization of the cortex and had a synchronizing action in the hippocampus and thalamus; the effects were maximal at 1 to 2 minutes and lasted for about 5 minutes. Full arousal was observed at 20 to 40 µg/kg; there were no spike discharges and no tachyphylaxis was seen following repeated doses. An antagonism was found with a whole series of divergent substances, such as anticholinergics, chlorpromazine, imipramine and pentobarbital.

Yamamoto and Domino (1967) gave 0.04 mg/kg of arecoline i.v. in cats and found that it induced a short-lasting (12 minutes) EEG arousal in slow wave sleeping cats; at the same time a synchronization of

the hippocampus occurred. These effects were blocked by atropine.
After pilocarpine, given at the dose of 0.15 mg/kg, an approximately
similar effect was obtained as with arecoline, but the EEG activation
was followed by an increase in paradoxical sleep. Again the effects
could be blocked by atropine, but not with the nicotinic antagonist
mecamylamine.

The induction of a regular theta-rhythm in the hippocampus has
been observed by different authors. In studying photically-evoked
after-discharges in rat, Bigler and Fleming (1976) found that 5 mg/kg
of pilocarpine given s.c. induced arousal, regular 'rhythmic slow
activity' (RSA) in the hippocampus during which well developed photically-evoked after-discharges occurred. The latter confirmed earlier
findings by Fleming (1972) using 10 mg/kg s.c. of pilocarpine.

The involvement of cholinergic receptors in the generation of RSA
in the hippocampus has been studied by Malish and Ott (1982) by intra-
hippocampal application of arecoline in rat, demonstrating an increase
in the amount of RSA and a decrease of its dominant frequency.

2.5. Muscarinic Antagonist: Atropine

As was first thoroughly reviewed by Longo (1966), the effects
obtained with atropine were broadly similar in various species such
as rat (Meyers et al., 1964), rabbit (Herz, 1962), cat (Bradley and
Elkes, 1957), dog (Wikler, 1952) and monkey (Domino and Hudson, 1959):
a sleep pattern consisting of 2 to 5 Hz/sec slow waves and 8 to 12
Hz/sec spindles in cortical derivations and slow waves in the subcortex. Similar effects were seen after scopolamine, but with 4 times
(Exley et al., 1958) to 20 times (White and Boyaju, 1960) lower doses.
Further, a dissociation between the EEG effects and behavior has been
observed, in that slow waves occurred in an apparently awake or even
excited animal. Though, Longo (1966) asked for caution in the interpretation of this phenomenon, he nevertheless emphasized that slow
waves in the EEG do not necessarily imply sleep.

The first discussion of the phenomenon of dissociation was by
Wikler (1952). He gave morphine or atropine (2 to 8 mg/kg, s.c.) to
dogs. Though both produced a sleep-like state, characterized by 2 to
6 Hz/sec slow waves and 8 to 12 Hz/sec spindles, atropine caused a
markedly different behavior: the dogs were excited. This showed that
the mechanisms of sleep are different from those producing slow waves.
Such pharmacological dissociation between EEG and behavior has aroused
continuous interest up to the present day.

Domino and Hudson (1959) extensively studied two isomers of atropine: 1-hyoscyamine and the much less potent d-hyoscyamine, in dogs
and monkeys. In dogs an i.v. injection of 2 to 8 mg/kg of d-hyoscyamine, induced EEG synchronization in a similar way as 0.125 to 0.5
mg/kg of 1-hyoscyamine. Arousal could be produced by electrical stimulation of the sciatic nerve, the duration depended on the dose of the

two isomers used, 0.5 mg/kg of l-hyoscyamine being best in shortening
the duration of the arousal.

In monkeys, cumulative doses (1, 2, 4,. 8 mg/kg of both isomers of
atropine were given intravenously. At 1 mg/kg of l-hyoscyamine, excitation was seen: with 2 mg/kg, some high voltage slow waves were
found in frontal and visual cortices, whereas the behavior alternated
between excitement and drowsiness. The threshold for EEG arousal was
elevated. With d-hyoscyamine, excitement was only seen at 8 mg/kg,
with a concomitant general slowing of the EEG. Thus also in this
study a dissociation was seen, though the effects were less marked
than those described by Wikler (1952).

Haranath et al. (1967) did not find a dissociation in dogs upon
injecting 50 µg of atropine into the carotid arteries: EEG and behavioral sleep was observed simultaneously. On the other hand, Frankenheim (1982), carrying out a power spectrum analysis of the effects of
atropine in Beagle dogs, found that 0.1 mg/kg in two dogs and 1 mg/kg
in two other dogs produced urination, vomiting, ataxia and lethargy,
but the total EEG spectral power increased, the percentage of delta
and theta power increased and the percentage of beta power decreased.
Thus no evidence of dissociation was found, but these effects were
probably overshadowed by strong peripheral effects. This might be
related to the route and dose used, though lower doses not producing
the symptoms also did not change the EEG.

Careful studies of the relationship between behavior and EEG in
rabbits (e.g., Sadowski and Longo, 1962; Blozovski and Blozovski,
1973) have suggested that the dissociation to a certain extent is only
apparent after atropine treatment when the animals are capable of
mostly low level elementary behaviors, and not when highly skilled and
conditioned behaviors are involved.

Much discussion thus concerns the definition of the term 'dissociation,' as was also emphasized in a study by Fairchild et al.
(1975). They found that 0.5 mg/kg i.p. of atropine in cats tended to
increase slow waves, with little effect on high frequency waves,
regardless of the behavior of the animal; whereas 2 mg/kg of atropine
produced behavioral excitement persisting for the total observation
period of five hours. This was associated with large amplitude slow
waves in the prepyriform cortex, and increased amplitude of the ventral hippocampus, a suppression of high frequency waves in the lateral geniculate and reticular formation, and little 'specific alterations' of the frequency spectra of the dorsal hippocampus. From the
fact that the frequency spectra induced by atropine differed from
those commonly observed during the sleep-wake cycle, the authors
concluded that there was no true dissociation.

From the presently mentioned sample of studies it appears that
there is indeed a form of dissociation between the EEG and behavior,

but that the definition requires further specification of the EEG as
well as of the different kind of behaviors induced; associated peripheral effects must also be observed.

A further number of studies more specifically deal with the anticholinergic action. Schaul et al. (1978) carefully studied the delta
waves induced by an i.v. injection of 3 mg/kg of atropine in cats.
Intermittent 1 to 3 Hz/sec delta waves intermingled with waves in the
theta and beta range and occasionally spindle bursts of 7 to 11 Hz/sec
waves were induced lasting for the total recording time of 4 to 6
hours. The surface positive delta waves are probably generated by
intracortical EPSP's, whereas surface negative waves may be generated
by IPSP's at the cell soma. The laminar profiles showed a phase
reversal in depth, but the level at which this reversal occurred
varied considerably. The study emphasized that delta waves are generated by pyramidal neurons, without excluding that subcortical mechanisms may be involved. In general, their findings suggest that the
delta waves are induced by a cholinergic de-afferentation of the
cortex.

Santucci et al. (1981) carried out a quantitative analysis of the
effects of atropine (1, 3, 10, 30 and 100 mg/kg, i.p.) in rats. They
differentiated between state 1 and state 2: state 1 corresponds with
low voltage fast activity as found during wakefulness or REM sleep,
and state 2 is characterized by high voltage low frequency waves typical for slow wave sleep. Increasing doses of atropine increased the
duration of state 2 over the five hour period, being significant at
10, 30, and 100 mg/kg. The effects observed with 10 mg/kg were antagonized by physostigmine (0.1 to 0.3 mg/kg) and amphetamine (1 mg/kg)
and potentiated by haloperidol (0.3 mg/kg). A dissociation between
the hypersynchronous EEG and behavioral activation was seen and interpreted in the light of the finding by Schaul et al. (1978) that
atropine caused a blockade of corticopetal pathways. The antagonism
with amphetamine, conversely the potentiating effect by haloperidol,
might be due to the known cholinergic-catecholaminergic interaction.

In this respect, a differentiation between EEG activity resistant
and non-resistant to atropine is of interest. Vanderwolf (1975) carried out a careful analysis of the relationships between neocortical
and hippocampal activation and behavior following atropine application
in rats. Following an i.p. injection of 25-100 mg/kg of atropine, the
low frequency irregular hippocampal waves occurring during immobility
became more frequent, whereas the rhythmic slow activity (RSA) accompanying waking were not abolished. The spontaneous RSA of hippocampus
was found to have two components: one was related to immobility and
was abolished by 25 to 100 mg/kg of atropine; while another was related to waking and was resistant to atropine. Like the waking RSA,
the behavior elicited by electrical stimulation of the reticular formation was unaffected by atropine. Further, 5 mg/kg i.p. of atropine
in rats or rabbits eliminated the urethrane-induced low frequency

theta activity occurring during ether anesthesia in a similar way as
the theta activity present during immobility (Kramis et al., 1975).

In the neocortex (Vanderwolf, 1975), large doses of atropine produced 2 to 6 Hz waves synchronized over the total cortex, but during
movement these were immediately replaced by slow waves of a higher
frequency, up to 10 Hz. Phenothiazine treatment increased the amount
of slow waves by increasing the proportion of time spent motionless,
thus permitting the appearance of slow waves.

Thus, there appear to be two ascending pathways from the brain
stem capable of generating rhythmic hippocampal waves. The RSA
occurring during behavioral immobility is selectively sensitive to
atropine, suggesting that this wave form is dependent on activity in
muscarinic receptors of a cholinergic system (Lewis and Shute, 1967).
An atropine-resistant pathway, activated by amphetamine and inhibited
by phenothiazines, suggests that this pathway may depend on monoaminergic transmission. The neocortical activation is similarly controlled by two systems, one of which is related to movement and the other
to immobility.

2.6. Cholinesterase Inhibitors: Physostigmine and Neostigmine

Physostigmine is a centrally active reversible cholinesterase inhibitor with a short duration of action. Neostigmine, being a quaternary amine, is largely unable to cross the blood-brain barrier and,
therefore, has mainly peripheral cholinergic effects.

The predominant effect observed with physostigmine is EEG
arousal. Often it is associated with signs of strong peripheral cholinergic stimulation, such as profuse secretions in dogs (Haranath et
al., 1967). However, since EEG arousal pattern has been observed in
an otherwise resting animal, it has been stated that physostigmine
caused a 'dissociation' between EEG and behavior. This was not observed in rats following an i.p. injection of 0.3 and 1 mg/kg of
physostigmine (Irmis, 1974).

Rather than describing the effects of physostigmine on its own,
different authors used physostigmine to reverse the effects of other
substances. Santucci et al. (1981) described how the high amplitude
slow wave EEG, and also the associated spindles, were reduced by an
i.p. injection of 0.01, 0.1 and 0.3 mg/kg of physostigmine in rats.
It antagonized this EEG state induced by atropine. An i.v. injection
of 0.05 and 0.3 mg/kg of physostigmine in rats reversed the EEG synchrony induced by ethanol (Erickson and Chai, 1976); and Roy and
Stullken (1981) found that 0.03 mg/kg i.v. of physostigmine converted
the high amplitude EEG induced by halothane in dogs to a low amplitude
EEG.

On sleep, Hill et al. (1979) described how 1 mg/kg of physostigmine given i.p. to rats prolonged the latency of non-REM sleep and

reduced the total sleep time. Further, it shortened the REM sleep latency prolongation found after different doses of imipramine (Hill et al., 1980). This suggested to these authors that an anticholinergic property of imipramine is responsible for the effects on REM sleep induction, not for its maintenance.

However, an induction of REM sleep by physostigmine has been described in the decerebrate and decerebellate cat (Kingsley and Barnes, 1973), though Hill et al. (1979) found no alteration of the REM sleep latency in rats and Karczmar et al. (1970) found an induction of REM sleep in reserpine-pretreated cats only if they were awake.

Haranath and Venkatakrishna-Bhatt (1977) found also that physostigmine given in the inferior horn of the lateral ventricle in dogs produced sleep: 1 μg produced sleep, whereas 10 μg produced REM sleep. Both cholinergics and anticholinergics were found to produce sleep in their study. According to these authors, these findings fitted with the concept of an increased cholinergic activity in wakefulness and REM sleep.

The fact that neostigmine given at a dose of 0.05 mg/kg i.p. in rats treated with chlorpromazine (2.5 mg/kg, i.p.) to a certain degree restored paradoxical sleep, which was suppressed by chlorpromazine, led Khazan et al. (1967) to conclude that central cholinergic mechanisms had a role in precipitating REM sleep.

Thus, it appears that physostigmine produces arousal, is able to reverse EEG synchronization induced by various compounds, and in certain circumstances is able to induce REM sleep, probably by affecting a cholinergic trigger mechanism.

2.7. Conclusions

Because of its poor brain penetration, systemic injections of acetylcholine appeared to induce EEG changes only when cardiovascular changes were induced. Upon direct application to the brain, especially along the medial forebrain bundle, sleep was induced, which suggested the involvement of a cholinergic limbic substrate in sleep. However, ACh is released from the cortex during wakefulness and REM sleep when the brain is activated, rather than during slow-wave sleep. It might be that direct ACh application blocked rather than excited ACh receptors. However, if ACh receptors were excited, it might be that the hypnogenic effects were specifically elicited from the limbic structures. This would then be the opposite of the effects expected from cortical activation. Unless experimental evidence is gathered for such a differential site-specific role of ACh, these ideas remain speculative.

Nicotine produced a biphasic action; an initial EEG desynchronization, related to a predominant central action of nicotine, followed by EEG synchronization and sleep, which is probably related to an action on other transmitter systems.

Neuromuscular blockers such as tubocurarine may produce sleep but this is caused by immobilization, or may induce a short-lasting EEG activation only when the blood brain barrier is disturbed.

Muscarinic agonists such as pilocarpine or arecoline desynchronize the cortical EEG and have a synchronizing action in the hippocampus, but only for a short time. Thus, ACh, nicotine, and muscarinic agonists are all predominantly related to an activated brain, which is expressed in EEG desynchronization.

The effects obtained with the muscarinic antagonist atropine have received considerable attention, mainly because it seems to produce a 'dissociation' between EEG and behavior. In the cortex, slow waves are seen while theta activity is generated in the hippocampus. During this 'sleep-like' pattern, the animals are behaviorally awake or even excited. However, it appears that the term 'dissociation' requires further specification and its meaning attenuated. In some studies it was demonstrated that the EEG effects produced by antimuscarinics had a different frequency spectrum from those seen during sleep. At the same time, the rhythmic slow activity in the hippocampus appears to have two components: one which is sensitive to atropine and related to immobility, and another which is resistant to atropine and related to movement. The slow wave cortical EEG produced by atropine may reflect a de-afferentation of the cortex, and only the theta activity in the hippocampus associated with immobility may depend on activity in muscarinic cholinergic receptors.

The overall conclusion is that cholinergic transmission at the cortical level (together with other transmitters and possibly also peptidergic systems) is involved in the maintenance of high cerebral activity during wakefulness, as well as during paradoxical sleep. Much remains to be done to reveal a more precise role of ACh in the organization of various phases and components of wakefulness and REM sleep. In other words, besides the overall setting of the degree of activity, a distinct site-specific functional role of ACh warrants further study.

3.   CHOLINERGIC MECHANISMS IN LEARNING AND MEMORY

3.1. Developmental Aspects

As in humans, neurological development in the rat is not completed at birth but continues for some time in the postnatal period. The general importance of the cholinergic systems in the control of behavior is illustrated by the correlation observed between postnatal developmental changes in the cholinergic system and the concomitant

changes in behavior. Campbell and Randall (1975) observed that isolated rats become hyperactive from about ten days postpartum and reach
a maximal level at fifteen days. Subsequently the hyperactivity gradually disappears until the animals reach normal adult activity levels
between day twenty and twenty-five. The hyperactivity occurs during
a period in the development where acetylcholine synthesis in the neostriatum and the cortex is poor. The hyperactivity disappears again
when adult levels of acetylcholine are reached. When passive avoidance is used as a learning task, it was demonstrated by Schulenburg
et al. (1971) that the acquisition of the task was dependent upon the
age of the animals. Adults proved to have better retention as compared to young animals. These types of studies suggest that a fully
developed cholinergic system has an inhibitory function with respect
to spontaneous behavior.

    More direct evidence for the involvement of neurotransmitter-
receptor complexes on behavior can be obtained by drug studies that
specifically affect the neurotransmitter system under study. These
drugs can intervene at different levels in the sequence from synthesis
to release and break down of the transmitters involved.

    By using the acetylcholine antagonist scopolamine, Campbell et
al. (1969) were able to prove that the observed hyperactivity in ten
to fifteen day-old rats was mediated by the developmental state of
the cholinergic system. Scopolamine injections had no motor effects
on ten to fifteen day-old animals, but they increased spontaneous
activity from day twenty on. In another experiment, Egger et al.
(1973) found no disruption with scopolamine nor facilitation by
physostigmine prior to the age of twenty-four days on spontaneous
alternation behavior.

    Pilocarpine, a direct acetylcholine agonist, failed to induce
catalepsy in animals younger than fifteen days, that is, during the
period when the cholinergic system was not completely matured (Baez
et al., 1976). These experiments provide further evidence that the
cholinergic system develops in the postnatal period and that a completely functional cholinergic system plays a general role in behavioral inhibition.

3.2. Modulatory Effect of Cholinergic Drugs on Retention

    Very early it was recognized that manipulation of the cholinergic
system with drugs, strongly influenced learning and memory. The evidence comes from both human and animal studies but we shall limit our-
selves to the discussion of mainly animal studies. Already in 1906
Gauss observed that scopolamine was an amnesia-inducing agent in
patients. Amnesic effects were also observed in a number of animal
studies using different learning tasks. When injected before training, the anticholinergic atropine impaired discrimination learning
(Whitehouse, 1964) and passive avoidance learning (Buresova et al.,

1964) in the rat. Bohdanecky and Jarvik (1962), using one-trial passive avoidance in mice, showed that scopolamine or physostigmine injected before training also impaired memory. Similar results were
also obtained by Davis et al. (1971). When cholinergic transmission
was enhanced by application of anticholinesterases, learning was
facilitated when injections were given just prior to (Bures et al.,
1962) or just after (Stratton and Petrinovick, 1963) training for maze
learning in mice. Given these results it is logical that drugs affecting the central cholinergic system were going to be used to investigate the substrates that underlie memory and learning.

3.3. The Role of Cholinergic Mechanisms in Memory Storage

     The observation of retrograde amnesia leads to the suggestion
that the substrates of memory are synaptic changes. Hence pharmacological treatments have been widely used to investigate how the brain
stores information and which transmitter systems are the substrates
for memory holding. Unfortunately, learning and memory have to be
inferred from behavioral performances. Hence, it is often difficult
to evaluate whether changes in performance after drug treatment are
mediated by changes in memory storage and holding itself, or by
changes in neuronal systems that have an indirect influence on memory.
This problem refers to the concepts of intrinsic and extrinsic neural
systems employed in the neurobiological investigation of memory
(Squire and Davis, 1981). Intrinsic neuronal systems refer to those
pathways where the information is actually stored. This is presumably
accomplished by changes in the synaptic properties of neurons belonging to the pathway. Extrinsic neuronal systems do not contain the
memory but they can influence to a large extent the development, read
out, and life time of memory.

     The role that cholinergic synapses have as part of the intrinsic
systems have been investigated by using anticholinesterase and anticholinergic drugs to modulate neurotransmission by acetylcholine in
the brain. In a first series of experiments (Deutsch et al., 1966;
Deutsch and Leibowitz, 1966) discriminated escape learning was used
to investigate the effects of enhanced neurotransmission by intracerebral application of the anticholinesterase diisopropyl fluorophosphate
(DFP). By using different training-injection intervals it was found
that DFP disrupted memory when injections were given shortly (30 minutes) after training, had no effect when training-injection intervals
were between one and three days, and impaired the memory again beyond
a four-day period. Hamburg (1967) could confirm these effects by
using systemic injections (i.p.) of physostigmine, another anticholinesterase drug. In a later experiment, Wiener and Deutsch (1968)
proved that the observed effects were not restricted to negatively
motivated behavior since essentially the same results were obtained
in an appetitive task (sugar water as reward). In addition, it was
found that increase of cholinergic activity by DFP could enhance the
memory twenty-eight days after training when the task was completely
forgotten by control animals. This facilitatory effect was replicated

and further documented by Squire et al. (1971) in an escape task with
mice who were treated with physostigmine on different time intervals
after training. To prove that the effects of anticholinesterase drugs
are directly related to the efficacy of cholinergic transmission,
Wiener and Deutch (1968) blocked the postsynaptic receptor sites with
the anticholinergic scopolamine at different time intervals after a
learned task. The results obtained were almost a complete mirror
image of those seen after anticholinesterase treatment. Scopolamine
enhanced memory at specific time points where DFP disrupted memory.
Based on these experiments, Deutsch (1971) suggested that learning
stimulates a particular group of cholinergic synapses in such a way
that their conductivity was increased. The validity of this hypothesis was further strengthened by experiments indicating that the same
dose of physostigmine impairs memory for well-learned responses but
enhances memory when learning was poor. The original observation of
this phenomenon was made by Deutsch and Lutzky (1967) and has been
replicated and expanded by Stanes et al. (1976) in Y-maze discrimination learning. To test whether or not the observed effects could be
attributed to changes in postsynaptic receptors and not to increased
acetylcholine release, Deutsch (1971) used carbachol, a cholinomimetic
resistant to acetylcholinesterase. He found that a seven day-old
memory was blocked by carbachol but that no effects were observed when
the same dose was used when the memory was three days old. Deutsch
(1971) has integrated the results of different experiments as follows:
"The hypothesis is that, as a result of learning, the postsynaptic
endings at a specific set of synapses become more sensitive to transmitter. This sensitivity increases with time after initial learning
and then declines. The rate at which such sensitivity increases
depends on the amount of initial learning. If the curve of transmission plotted against time is displaced upward with anticholinesterases
then the very low portions will show facilitation, and the high portions will cause block. The middle portions will appear unaffected.
If the curve of transmission is displaced down with anticholinergics,
then the middle portion will appear unaffected and only the very early
or late components will show block." As a conclusion one can say that
central cholinergic synapses or at least some of them have changed
functional states as a result of a learning process. As such they
belong to the intrinsic neuronal substrates responsible for memory
holding.

Very early in the search for the involvement of the central cholinergic system in behavior, Grossman (1962) found that very specific
behaviors can be induced by stimulating cholinergic neural circuits.
Direct cholinergic stimulation in the hypothalamus induced drinking
behavior in satiated rats. Hence the question may be asked whether
all central cholinergic pathways are involved in the holding mechanism
for memory. The experiments by Haycock et al. (1973) clearly demonstrate that different cholinergic pathways can have completely opposite functions in memory processes. In a series of experiments with
avoidance learning, he injected physostigmine into the dorsal hippocampus. This manipulation disrupted avoidance learning. If the same

drug was injected into the caudate putamen, no effects were found.
Injection of scopolamine in the same site, however, attenuated retention, but the injection of the anticholinergic in the dorsal hippocampus resulted in normal retention. These experiments point towards the
fact that morphological localization can be important for the relation
between cholinergic pathways and memory processes.

3.4. Indirect Involvement of Cholinergic Mechanisms in Learning and Memory

In addition to the cholinergic involvement in intrinsic neuronal
systems for learning and memory, cholinergic mechanisms may possibly
affect learning and memory through extrinsic systems that are not directly involved in memory holding. A good example of this is the relation between cholinergic pathways and arousal and information processing (for review see Warburton, 1981). Acetylcholine release in
the cortex is related to electrocortical desynchronization (Jasper and
Tessier, 1971) and it is enhanced by sensory stimulation. However,
the release of neurotransmitter is not restricted to the parts of the
cortex related to the modality of the sensory input. The pathway
responsible for the release originates in the mesencephalic reticular
formation and projects to large areas of the cortex. Microinjections
of the cholinergic agonist carbamylcholine chloride into sites close
to the ventral tegmental area induce electrocortical arousal. The
importance of the ascending cholinergic pathway as a modulator for
sensory activity at the cortex is illustrated by behavioral studies
testing vigilance and discrimination performance (Warburton and Brown,
1972). When rats were tested for responding to infrequent stimuli in
the course of a long session, it was found that doses of physostigmine
which induce electrocortical arousal improve the stimulus detection.
Scopolamine had opposite effects on stimulus discrimination but did
not affect motor performance. The cholinergic agonist carbamylcholine
chloride also improved stimulus detection by mimicking acetylcholine
release. Vigilance and attention seem to be controlled at least in
part by an ascending cholinergic pathway. This means that cholinergic
transmission is involved in the selection of stimuli that are relevant
to the organism. As such, it is involved in mechanisms that are essential for learning and memory to occur, apart from the actual storage of the input information. If stimuli go unnoticed due to reduced
arousal and vigilance they are useless for information processing and
memory retrieval.

The idea that acetylcholine has a general support function in
learning and memory is further strengthened by the suggestion that
memory problems during the aging process are related to some dysfunction in the synthesis of acetylcholine. Jenden (1979) has suggested
that pathological or functional states can result in a deficient choline supply. Since choline is a precursor necessary for acetylcholine
synthesis in the brain it might affect the function of central cholinergic pathways when a shortage in supply occurs. Bartus et al. (1980)
tried to modulate the rate at which memory deficiency related to aging

begins by manipulating the free choline available in diets. Mice were kept on a choline deficient or enriched diet for four and a half months. Subsequently they were trained in a one-trial passive avoidance task and the results were compared with those from animals kept on a normal diet. Animals fed with an enriched diet (13 months-old) performed as well as three month-old animals. Those kept on a choline deficient diet performed poorly and could be compared with senescent animals which received a normal diet. This type of experiment clearly illustrates the general role of cholinergic functioning in memory problems related to age.

3.5. Conclusion

From the experimental evidence presented, we can infer the cholinergic pathways control to some extent the information input to the brain since they are involved in the processes of arousal and attention. The latter functions determine to which stimuli an organism will react by processing the incoming information or by responding to it by means of a motor response. In addition it has been clearly shown that cholinergic mechanisms are involved in the actual storage of information and that the holding capacity is probably closely related to morphological aspects of the cholinergic pathways. That such morphological specificity may be very important has been recently demonstrated by studying how learning itself affects cholinergic mechanisms instead of looking for behavioral effects by manipulating cholinergic transmission through pharmacological interventions. Bürgel and Rommelspacher (1978) showed that animals trained during nine days in an operant response for food reward had enhanced choline transport in hippocampal tissues as compared to animals that received no training. Striatal homogenates however did not show significant differences. This line of research approach should perhaps be extended to investigate which specific cholinergic substrates are related to learning and memory for specified tasks using different types of reinforcers.

4.   OPERANT BEHAVIOR

Carlton (1963) was one of the first to suggest that brain cholinergic systems fulfilled an inhibitory function on behavior. This idea was further developed by, for instance, Stein (1968) who suggested an interaction between noradrenergic and cholinergic systems in forebrain. Margules and Margules (1973), on the basis of intracranial injections into the ventromedial hypothalamus of atropine, physostigmine and carbachol, and studying lever pressing behavior for milk reward, found evidence for a cholinergic receptor involvement determining operant strength. They suggested that a cholinergic system is particularly apt to provide an important inhibitory control over behavior: "This is a system of inhibitory polysynaptic chains of short neurons open to a variety of synaptic inputs, and is capable of discrete action in separate portions of the forebrain." (p. 1479). The major function would consist in suppressing facilitation of unrewarded responses.

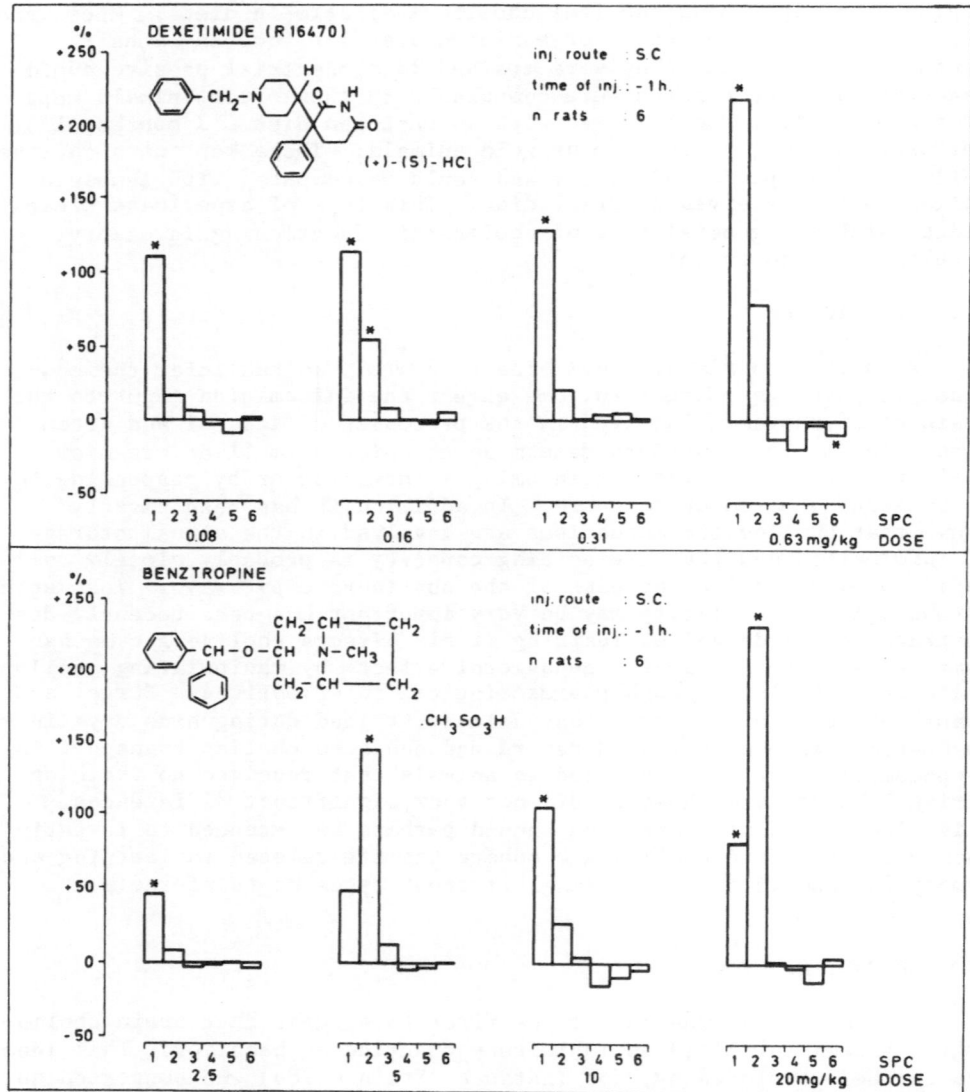

Such an idea is also found in the "balance hypothesis," for example of Pradhan (1976). He suggested that the enhanced responding of intracranial self-stimulation following anticholinergics is due to a blockade of the cholinergic system, thereby unmasking the facilitatory noradrenergic system.

A differentiation, however, needs to be made between the cholinergic involvement in motor organization (pyramidal and extrapyramidal) and in reinforcement. Pradhan (1976) considers that ACh is involved

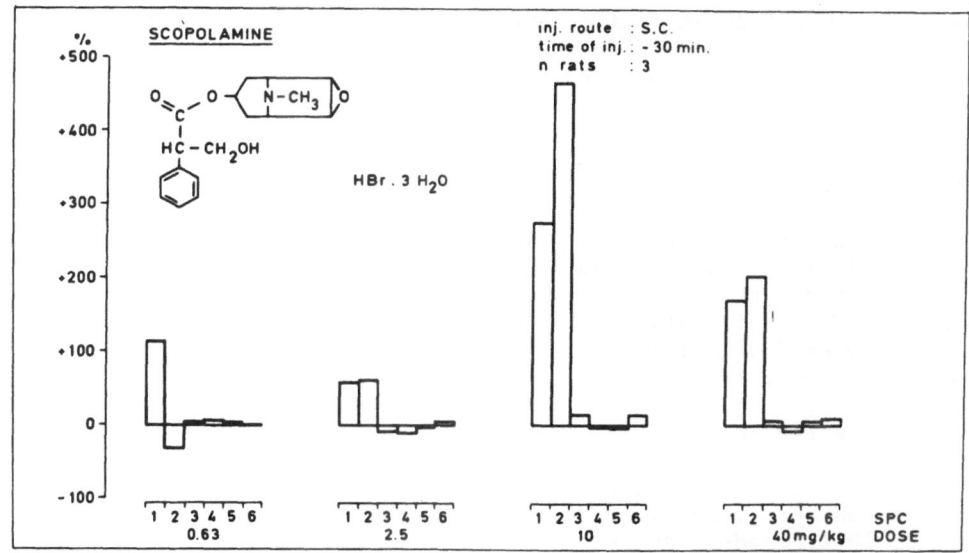

Fig. 1. Response Rates (All Rats Combined) in Percentages of the
Respective Control Response Rates, Obtained with Different
Doses (mg/kg) and for Each Stimulus Parameter Combination
(SPC) with Dexetimide, Benztropine and Scopolamine. Chemical
structure, injection route, time of injection and number of
rats tested are indicated at the top of the figure. $SPC_{1,2}$
elicited low, $SPC_{3,4}$ intermediate and $SPC_{5,6}$ high control
response rates.

in creating an optimal arousal level, allowing an optimal functioning
of motivation and reinforcement, and thus affecting the expression of
behavior. Anticholinergics may, therefore, be expected to facilitate
behavior whether reinforced or non-reinforced through a rather "nonspecific" facilitatory action (4.1). At the level of the caudate
nucleus a direct interaction between dopaminergic and cholinergic
neurons exist. A site-specific interaction can be studied by drugs
acting at these neurons (4.2). Because the previous section dealt
with a number of operant studies and because most of the drug-
interaction studies with cholinergics and anticholinergics have been
carried out on intracranial self-stimulation (ICS), the majority of
the present section will deal with ICS.

4.1. Cholinergics and Anticholinergics

Cholinergic muscarinic agonists exert a response depressant
effect on self-stimulation behavior. With the ACh analogue pilocarpine, the response inhibition was dose-related, peaking 20 to 30 minutes after injection (Newman, 1972). The cholinesterase-inhibitor

physostigmine, induced a time- and dose-related inhibition of lever-pressing (Newman, 1972; Olds and Domino, 1969a,b). Arecoline, a cholinergic agonist, also induced inhibition (Olds and Domino, 1969a,b; Pradhan and Kamat, 1972). The onset of the inhibition was rapid and the recovery was quick. The quaternary amine, neostigmine, which is mainly a peripherally-active cholinesterase inhibitor, was virtually without effect (June and Boyd, 1966; Newman, 1972).

The results obtained with nicotine were contradictory. Olds and Domino (1969a,b) found a transient and variable response inhibition, whereas other authors (e.g., Bowling and Pradhan, 1967), were able to demonstrate a facilitation of ICS. This was most prominent in so-called low self-stimulators and the effects were time- and dose-related (Newman, 1972).

Only a few authors have tested the influence of anticholinergics on ICS, and much of the work has been with scopolamine (Olds and Domino, 1969a,b; Domino and Olds, 1972; Olds, 1972a,b; Newman, 1972; Pradhan and Kamat, 1972, 1973) and atropine (Jung and Boyd, 1966; Newman, 1972; Pradhan and Kamat, 1973). We studied the effects of different doses of dexetimide, benztropine and scopolamine on rats self-stimulating in the lateral hypothalamus for different stimulation parameters which elicited low, intermediate or high response rates (detailed methodology in e.g., Wauquier, 1979).

Fig. 1 shows the number of lever-pressings as percentage of the control after various doses of the anticholinergics tested, for each different stimulus parameter combination (SPC) tested. SPC 1 and 2 elicited low self-stimulation, SPC 3 and 4 moderate self-stimulation and SPC 5 and 6 elicited high self-stimulation.

Dexetimide (top Fig. 1) induced a dose-related facilitation of self-stimulation. The response enhancement was observed on the SPC's inducing a low control self-stimulation (SPC 1 and 2). The lack of a significant effect on other SPC's was mainly due to a high interindividual variability.

Benztropine (middle Fig. 1) induced a rather irregular dose-response effect. The response enhancement was highest at the SPC 1 with 10 mg/kg of benztropine and at SPC 2 with 40 mg/kg. In contrast to dexetimide, which increased responding most when the frequency of the stimulation was low (SPC 1), benztropine increased responding most when the intensity of the stimulation was low (SPC 2). At the other SPC's, a slight inhibition of responding was observed, but the statistical significance was low, which, again, was due to a high interindividual variability.

With scopolamine (bottom Fig. 1), the number of animals tested was small, but the effects seen were comparable to those observed with the other anticholinergics. The dose-response curve appeared irregular, but this might have been due to the small number of rats tested.

There appeared no preferential response enhancement for either the low frequency or the low intensity stimulation parameter.

Muscarinic anticholinergics induce peripheral and central effects (Janssen and Niemegeers, 1967). It appears that relatively high doses of the anticholinergics are required to observe an enhancement of ICS. A central action is required, since peripherally-acting anticholinergics do not affect self-stimulation. The facilitation of self-stimulation is often not clearly dose-related and the interindividual variability is pronounced.

Muscarinic agonists cause depression of self-stimulation. This is due to a central action, because cholinergics which do not cross the blood-brain barrier fail to change self-stimulation performance. Domino and Olds (1968) have shown that the depression of self-stimulation is associated with rise in the ACh level. It could be expected that lowering the ACh level, for instance by means of anticholinergics, would facilitate self-stimulation. It was subsequently confirmed that muscarinic antagonists chiefly produce response enhancement.

The effects of self-stimulation are probably not only due to an anticholinergic activity, since muscarinic anticholinergics also affect catecholamines. Scopolamine and benztropine increase the turn-over of noradrenaline (NA) and decrease the turnover of dopamine (DA) (Corrodi et al., 1972). Benztropine and dexetimide also block the up-take of DA (Coyle and Snyder, 1968; Leysen, personal communication). The effects of anticholinergics on DA and NA are indirect and can be demonstrated most easily in those structures in which cholinergic neurons are supposed to interact with aminergic neurons, such as the striatal structures. Such an interaction between dopaminergic and cholinergic neurons can be demonstrated behaviorally in experiments in which anticholinergics are shown to reverse the inhibition of self-stimulation produced by neuroleptics. The latter effect is assumed to be due to a blockade of DA-receptors (Van Rossum, 1966). (The action of nicotine also might depend on NA, since depletion of NA, for instance by reserpine, prevents nicotine from facilitating self-stimulation.) In order to obtain measurable effects on self-stimulation, high doses of the anticholinergic are required. As measured in the anti-pilocarpine test in rats (Janssen and Niemegeers, 1967), the ED_{50}-dose of central anticholinergic activity (e.g., tremor, chewing) is obtained with 0.016 mg/kg of scopolamine, 0.080 mg/kg of benzetimide and 0.24 mg/kg of benztropine. The doses used in the self-stimulation experiments largely exceed the centrally active doses of the anticholinergics. So, the effects of the anticholinergics might not be due to an effect on ACh but on DA (or NA) via cholinergic neurons. This led to the question of whether a central muscarinic cholinergic system is functional during self-stimulation. The absence of significant changes in neuronal responses measured in various parts of the brain (hypothalamus, preoptic, cingulate and midbrain) after administration of anticholinergics, suggests the cholinergic systems modulate diffusely (Olds and Ito, 1973).

The type of modulation would be inhibitory. The concept of inhibition plays an important role in the description of behavior. Loss
of inhibitory control has been shown in experiments in which various
limbic structures are lesioned (e.g., McCleary, 1966).

Stein (1964, 1967) assigned the inhibitory role in self-stimulation to the periventricular cholinergic system (which he termed "no-go
system"). The ventromedial nucleus of the hypothalamus would be an
important link in a cholinergic system mediating behavioral suppression (Margules and Stein, 1969). This system would interact with a
facilitatory noradrenergic system (termed a "go-system"). Both systems would be mutually inhibitory and determine behavioral output.
Such an interaction was shown in, for instance, experiments by Olds
and Olds (1964) in which they described how stimulation in "aversive"
brain areas, such as the tegmentum, significantly depressed self-
stimulation.

Although the idea of a dual system feeding a final common pathway
is interesting, there is little evidence for the cholinergic mediation
of a suppressive system. It is not known whether "aversive" stimulation depressed self-stimulation merely by stimulation of cholinergic
neurons or by some other means. The behavioral deficits occurring
after lesioning limbic structures can be interpreted in terms of a
loss of inhibitory control. However, lesions do not only affect cholinergic systems and it is hard to accept that a general cholinergic
blockade interferes with all inhibition-related mechanisms (Grossman,
1972). Further, limbic structures do not serve identical behavioral
purposes. Finally, findings on lesioning or locally administered cholinergics and anticholinergics cannot unequivocally be interpreted in
terms of response modulation. Colpaert (1975) proposed that lesions
of the ventromedial hypothalamus and of other limbic structures as
well, caused a failure in the acquisition of fear as a secondary drive.

On a hypothetical basis, one could assume that cholinergic
systems are one source of inhibitory control, whereas other systems
subserved adaptation to the environment by way of fear acquisition.
These systems could modulate behavioral output and function in balance
with aminergic transmitter systems sustaining self-stimulation.

4.2. Studies on Drug Interaction

Self-stimulation behavior depends, at least partly, on catecholaminergic and cholinergic interactions. Olds (1972b) showed that scopolamine (0.5 mg/kg) antagonized about 60 percent of the inhibition of
self-stimulation induced by chlorpromazine (2.5 mg/kg). Our studies
have been aimed at elucidating the functional interaction between
dopaminergic and cholinergic neurons.

Since DA neural transmission appears to be involved in the
neuroleptic-induced inhibition of self-stimulation, one would expect
anticholinergics to antagonize the inhibitory effects of specific

DA-blocking neuroleptics and not those of narcotic analgesics
(Wauquier et al., 1975).

Haloperidol and morphine have a number of similarities: they
increase the turnover of striatal DA (Puri and Lal, 1974); they
release prolactin (Dickerman et al., 1972); they inhibit the release
of luteinizing hormone (Dobrin and Mares, 1974); and they produce a
state of immobility that can be reversed with apomorphine (Puri et al.
1973). They differ, however, in many respects; haloperidol lacks
analgesic effects and tolerance (Lal and Puri, 1973) and neuroleptics
cause catalepsy, whereas morphine-like drugs cause catatonia.

The inhibition of self-stimulation obtained with 0.16 mg/kg of
fentanyl or with 40 mg/kg of morphine could not be reversed by the
centrally acting anticholinergic dexetimide (2.5 mg/kg). The associated catatonia was not reversed either. Naloxone, on the other hand,
reversed the self-stimulation inhibition and catatonia induced by the
former drugs (Wauquier et al., 1974). These experiments showed that
some actions induced by morphine-like agents are reversed by a specific antagonist. Since DA-receptors appear to be involved in causing
morphine- or neuroleptic-induced effects, one would expect different
mechanisms of action (see also Broekkamp and Van Rossum, 1975).

In Wauquier and Niemegeers (1975) and Wauquier et al. (1975) it
was studied whether there was a dose-related antagonism of haloperidol-induced inhibition. A dose of 0.08 mg/kg of haloperidol given
s.c. one hour before the session caused a nearly complete suppression
of self-stimulation. Dexetimide gradually reinstated self-stimulation
in a dose-related manner. Isopropamide, a peripherally acting anticholinergic drug, at a dose (10 mg/kg) 1000 times higher than those
producing peripheral anticholinergic activity (Janssen and Niemegeers,
1967), did not antagonize the haloperidol-induced inhibition.

The reversal of the inhibition by dexetimide suggests that the
haloperidol effect was due to some altered relationship between dopaminergic and cholinergic activity in the striatum (Klawans, 1973;
Sigwald, 1971).

The reversal of the haloperidol-induced inhibition of self-
stimulation was not an exclusive property of dexetimide. Benztropine
(10 mg/kg) likewise antagonized the inhibition brought about by haloperidol (Wauquier et al., 1974). This was later repeated in a study
by Carey (1982), in which it was also shown that diphenylhydramine
(10 mg/kg) reversed haloperidol-induced inhibition of self-stimulation.

In another study (Wauquier, 1979), we compared the antagonism of
penfluridol (5 mg/kg) and clopimozide (1.25 mg/kg)-induced inhibition
by three antiparkinsonian agents; dexetimide (0.63 mg/kg), benztropine
(10 mg/kg) and trihexyphenidyl (10 mg/kg).

At the doses used, penfluridol and clopimozide significantly

inhibited self-stimulation 4, 24, and 48 hours after injection. The
inhibition was most pronounced four hours after neuroleptic treatment,
and self-stimulation gradually recovered during the following four
days. The three antiparkinsonian drugs, which by themselves did not
significantly affect self-stimulation, completely reversed the self-
stimulation inhibition obtained four hours after neuroleptic treatment. Self-stimulation was completely normalized (not significantly
different from controls), except for the combination of penfluridol
with trihexyphenidyl. However, during the following days, self-stimulation rates did not differ from the rates obtained after neuroleptic
treatment alone.

     This study showed that the self-stimulation inhibition induced
by specific neuroleptics could be reversed by different antiparkinsonian drugs at a time when maximum inhibition could be expected.

     The question of whether the antagonism by antiparkinsonian drugs
of neuroleptic-induced inhibition of ICS related mainly to DA mechanisms or to both the DA and NA mechanisms has been investigated
(Wauquier and Niemegeers, 1975).

     Three different neuroleptics were selected: pimozide, haloperi-
dol and pipamperone. Pimozide and haloperidol are both specific DA-
blocking neuroleptics; haloperidol, however, also blocks NA receptors
at high dose levels. Pipamperone, on the other hand, blocks DA and
NA receptors at approximately equal dose levels (Anden et al., 1970).
Four doses of each neuroleptic were given, the second dose being
approximately the ED_{50}-value for inhibition, the fourth dose being 16
times higher. All rats were also given the combination of the neuroleptic and 0.63 mg/kg of dexetimide (Wauquier and Niemegeers, 1975).

     Dexetimide completely reversed the self-stimulation inhibition
induced by pimozide, and self-stimulation was normalized to control
levels. The haloperidol-induced inhibition was also significantly
antagonized at all dose levels, but self-stimulation was not normalized to control levels with the combination of dexetimide with
0.16 mg/kg and 0.63 mg/kg of haloperidol. The pipamperone-induced
inhibition was not antagonized by dexetimide. The inhibition of self-
stimulation induced by pimozide and haloperidol is probably due to the
DA-blocking activity, whereas the pipamperone-induced inhibition is
related to the DA- and NA-blocking activity. It follows that dexetimide reversed the DA-blocking effect, whereas the NA-blocking effect
would not be antagonized. This conclusion was further examined by
using different neuroleptics, which preferentially block NA receptors
(Wauquier, 1979).

     Sedative neuroleptics (ratio NA/DA < 1) could not be antagonized
with the anticholinergic dexetimide, whereas specific (DA-blocking)
neuroleptics were. However, most anticholinergics, apart from their
anticholinergic activity, are also DA-uptake blockers. It is possible
that the reversal of the effects of the specific neuroleptics requires

an action on synaptic DA-mechanisms, i.e., potentiation of the synaptic action of DA might overcome the receptor blockade. The reversal of the sedative neuroleptics (blocking DA and NA) probably requires an action on both NA and DA.

To test this hypothesis, several compounds, i.e., piribedil and apomorphine (DA-agonists), dexetimide (anticholinergic and DA-uptake blocker), cocaine and nomifensine (DA- and NA-uptake blockers), and amphetamine (releaser of NA and DA), were tested for their ability to restore self-stimulation inhibited by pimozide or chlorpromazine (Wauquier, 1979; Wauquier and Niemegeers, 1976).

The results indicate the anticholinergics (non-competitive antagonism) or drugs that enhance endogenous catecholaminergic neurotransmission by increased release or uptake blockade (competitive antagonism) are able to reverse the neuroleptic-induced inhibition of self-stimulation more effectively than receptor agonists.

Pimozide and chlorpromazine induced an almost complete suppression of self-stimulation. The pimozide-induced inhibition of self-stimulation was significantly antagonized by all compounds tested, but marked quantitative differences were observed: cocaine, dexetimide, and nomifensine restores self-stimulation to more than 85 percent of the control levels, amphetamine restored self-stimulation to about 50 percent of normal levels, whereas the two DA-agonists, piribedil and apomorphine, showed very little antagonism.

The chlorpromazine-induced inhibition of self-stimulation was not antagonized by dexetimide, but was completely reversed by amphetamine and nomifensine ($p > 0.05$ as compared to the controls). Cocaine restored self-stimulation to about 50 percent of normal levels. Apomorphine had no effect on chlorpromazine-induced inhibition, whereas piribedil was slightly antagonistic.

The differential antagonism reported here shows that reversal properties are not necessarily dependent upon the inherent facilitatory effects of the antagonists (Wauquier, 1976; Wauquier and Niemegeers, 1974). It appears that the DA-uptake blocking activity, rather than the central anticholinergic action of dexetimide, may be responsible for its antagonism of specific DA-blocking activity, since the two DA-uptake blockers, cocaine (Ross and Renyi, 1967) and nomifensine (Hunt et al., 1974), completely restored self-stimulation inhibited by pimozide.

4.3. Discussion

The results reported are evidence that anticholinergics and DA-uptake blockers are able to overcome the inhibition induced by neuroleptics. Additional experiments are required to show that the antagonism obtained with dexetimide is competitive (at the DA-receptor sites) or a mixture of competitive and non-competitive (at the site of the cholinergic neurons) mechanisms.

Dexetimide did not restore self-stimulation inhibited by chlorpromazine, a neuroleptic that blocks NA at lower doses than DA.   Nomifensine, which blocks DA and NA-uptake (Schacht and Heptner, 1974),
however, completely reversed the chlorpormazine-induced inhibition of
self-stimulation.   The partial antagonism of the pimozide-induced
effects and the complete restoration of the chlorpromazine-induced
effects achieved with amphetamine can be ascribed to its ability to
increase the release of both DA and NA.

Apomorphine is able to restore the inhibition of self-stimulation
obtained after blockade of the synthesis of DA by α-methylparatyrosine
or depletion by reserpine (Stinus et al., 1976).   This points to a
direct receptor activation.

DA-agonists have been used with varying success in the treatment
of parkinsonism: both apomorphine (Cotzias et al., 1970, 1972) and
piribedil (Sweet et al., 1974; Vakil et al., 1973) affected tremor and
rigidity.   These two direct receptor stimulating agents were not able
to antagonize the neuroleptic-induced self-stimulation inhibition.
These results point to the difference between the receptor blocking
activity and parkinsonism, the latter being due to a degeneration of
the nigrostriatal DA-pathway (Hornykiewicz, 1971), resulting in a lack
of DA-input to the striatum and a distorted balance between the transmitters operating in the caudate-putamen (Cools et al., 1975).

The results with nomifensine clearly indicate that the anticholinergic activity, in itself, is not a prerequisite for antagonism of
specific DA antagonism.

The results of the interaction of pimozide with various antagonists favor the supposed connection between DA and ACh neurons.   The
interaction could be explained by an interference with inhibitory DA-
neurons.

Neuroleptic treatment increases homovanillic acid (HVA) content
in the striatum and in the limbic structures, an effect suggesting an
increased DA-turnover.   Neuroleptics also increase the release of ACh
and decrease its content in the striatum (Guyenet et al., 1975; McGeer
et al., 1974; Stadler et al., 1973) but not in the limbic system
(Andén, 1972; Bartholini et al., 1973; Lloyd et al., 1973) or other
brain structures, such as the cortex and the hippocampus (Sethy and
Van Woert, 1974).   Furthermore, in the striatum, but not in other
brain structures, the neuroleptic-induced increase of HVA content is
effectively antagonized by anticholinergics (Consolo et al., 1974;
Stadler et al., 1973), whereas cholinergic drugs have been found to
increase striatal HVA concentrations (Andén, 1974).   A functional
interaction between DA and ACh is indicated both by this study and by
biochemical experiments.   Both these types of study point to an interaction in the basal ganglia; however, the precise site of this

interaction has not been determined.

One approach to this problem is the use of intracerebral microinjection techniques. In one such experiment, Stephens and Herberg (1979) found that scopolamine injected into the nucleus accumbens partially restored spiroperidol-inhibited self-stimulation. Scopolamine had no antagonistic effects, however, when injected into the caudate. Since a direct interaction between DA and ACh neurons in the accumbens is absent, the authors interpreted their findings on indicating that DA and ACh systems function independently, producing opposite effects effects on self-stimulation. This was further supported by the finding that scopolamine restored performance suppressed by non-reward as well.

In an unpublished study we were able to show that dexetimide injected into the substantia nigra partially restored self-stimulation inhibited by pimozide. The ventral midbrain, including the substantia nigra, is thus a putative site of ACh and DA-interaction, as there are projections both to the caudate nucleus and the accumbens from this area. "Autaptic" DA-receptors may be located here and cholinergic neurons may synapse at the nigral cells. The restoration of self-stimulation after systemic injection of antagonists may thus depend on a high local concentration of the antagonists in this area, causing a "concerted action" involving the nigrostriatal as well as mesolimbic systems.

It is conceivable that anticholinergic drugs influence striatal, limbic and cortical structures, because in all these structures cholinesterase and acetylcholinesterase are present (Lewis and Shute, 1967; Shute and Lewis, 1967). This influence is of particular relevance when it can be shown that in these structures monoaminergic-containing systems produced effects contrary to those of the cholinergic system (Shute and Lewis, 1967). Many biochemical experiments substantiate the dopaminergic-cholinergic link in the caudate nucleus. A direct interaction in the limbic structures was, however, not evidenced. An interaction at the origin of the dopaminergic systems is not excluded and remains, therefore, a subject for further experimentation.

5. CONCLUSIONS

An analysis at the level used in the variety of studies described above, would definitively lead to a confusing picture of the role of acetylcholine in input and output control mechanisms of behavior. The involvement in the control of a large number of behaviors, ranging from innate responses to complex learned responses, requires a discussion of the role of acetylcholine in input-output systems in such a way that its general function emerges from a large amount of detailed research on specific behavioral categories and physiological functions.

One of the primary characteristics of the cholinergic system is that its full development is a necessary condition for normal functioning. An example of this general property is the lack of motor inhibition in young animals at a moment when this cholinergic system is not fully developed. An adequate cholinergic functioning is required for the optimalization of normal behavior. For example, a cholinergic hypofunctioning may lead to memory disturbances, as seen with aging.

On the input side, the cholinergic system seems to control to a large extent the information flow that will be subsequently processed. Its role in vigilance and attention and its relation to brain electrical desynchronization suggests that it is the substrate for tuning optimal information input. As such it has a significant role in the selection of the stimuli that an organism will attend to or react to.

In studying sleep-wakefulness, it appears that cholinergic systems are involved in maintaining high cerebral activity during wakefulness and paradoxical sleep. The fact that sleep can be induced by direct brain application of acetylcholine may not be in contradiction to the above, and rather would suggest that the limbic cholinergic system has a different role than the cortical cholinergic system in the regulation of wakefulness and sleep. A study of distinct site-specific roles for acetylcholine in the regulation of the different phases of wakefulness and REM needs still to be done.

The large impact of central cholinergic pathways on behavior seems to be related to their presence at almost all levels of the central nervous system. Here the sometimes very specific function of cholinergic pathways in eliciting specific behaviors, e.g., drinking, are probably more related to a "morphological" specificity of the controlling structure than to the general properties of the cholinergic pathways. The same conclusion probably holds true for the involvement of cholinergic synapses in memory-holding mechanisms. Not all central cholinergic synapses are involved in the holding and different brain areas might be involved, depending on the information that is stored. Much remains to be done to reveal the morphological specificity.

It is also obvious that none of the transmitter systems on its own sustains behavior. A safe conclusion in this respect has been formulated by Russell (1982): "The cholinergic system is essential to normal behavior, but it is not sufficient to support any behavior on its own."

REFERENCES

Abood, L. G., Lowy, K., Tometsko, A., and MacNeil, M., 1979, Evidence for a noncholinergic site for nicotinic action vs brain: psychopharmacological, electrophysiological and receptor binding studies, Arch. Int Pharmacodyn. Ther. 237:213-229.

Andén, N. E., 1972, Dopamine turnover in the corpus striatum and the limbic system after treatment with neuroleptic and antiacetylcholine drugs, J. Pharm. Pharmacol. 24:905-906.

Andén, N. E., 1974, Effects of oxotremorine and physostigmine on the turnover of dopamine in the corpus striatum and the limbic system, J. Pharm. Pharmacol. 26:738-740.

Andén, N., Butcher, S. G., Corrodi, H., Fuxe, L., and Ungerstedt, U., 1970, Receptor activity and turnover of dopamine and noradrenaline after neuroleptics, Eur. J. Pharmacol. 11:303-314.

Ashorobi, R. B., Guha, D., and Pradhan, S. N., 1979, Electrophysiological correlates of the behavioral effects of tubocurarine in conscious rats, Psychopharmacology 64:349-353.

Baez, L. A., Eskridge, N. K., and Schein, R., 1976, Postnatal development of dopaminergic and cholinergic catalepsy in the rat, Eur. J. Pharmacol. 36:155-162.

Bartholini, G., Stadler, H., and Lloyd, K. G., 1973, Cholinergic-dopaminergic relation in different brain structures, in "Frontiers in Catecholamine Research," E. Usdin and S. H. Snyder, eds., pp. 741-745, Pergamon Press, New York.

Bartus, R. T., Dean, G. L., Goas, J. A., and Lippa, A. S., 1980, Age-related changes in passive avoidance retention: modulation with dietary choline, Science 209:301-303.

Bhattacharya, I. C., and Goldstein, L., 1970, Influence of acute and chronic nicotine administration on intra- and inter-structural relationships of the electrical activity in the rabbit brain, Neuropharmacology 9:109-118.

Bigler, E. D., and Fleming, D. E., 1976, Pharmacological suppression of photically evoked after-discharges in rats: incremental dose, hippocampal EEG and behavioral activity correlates, Psychopharmacologia 46:73-82.

Blozovski, D., and Blozovski, M., 1973, Effets de l'atropine sur l'exploration, l'apprentissage et l'activité électrocorticale chez le rat au cours du développement, Psychopharmacologia 33:39-52.

Bohdanecky, Z., and Jarvik, M. E., 1962, Impairment of one-trial passive avoidance learning in mice by scopolamine, scopolamine methylbromide, and physostigmine, Int. J. Neuropharmacol. 6:217-222.

Bowling, C., and Pradhan, S. N., 1967, Interaction of some drugs on nicotine-induced facilitation of self-stimulation in rats, Fed. Proc. 9:201.

Bradley, P. B., and Elkes, J., 1957, The effect of some drugs on the electrical activity of the brain, Brain 80:77-117.

Broekkamp, C. L. E., and Van Rossum, J. M., 1975, The effects of micro-injections of morphine and haloperidol into the neostriatum and the nucleus accumbens on self-stimulation behaviour, Arch. Int. Pharmacodyn. Ther. 217:110-117.

Bureš, J., Bohdanecky, Z., and Weiss, T., 1962, Physostigmine induced hippocampal theta activity and learning in rats, Psychopharmacologia 3:254-263.

Buresova, O., Bureš, J., Bohdanecky, Z., and Weiss, T., 1964, Effect of atropine on learning, extinction, retention and retrieval in rats, Psychopharmacologia 5:255-263.

Bürgel, P., and Rommelspacher, H., 1978, Changes in high affinity choline uptake in behavioral experiments, Life Sci. 23:2423-2428.

Campbell, B. A., Lytle, L. D., and Fibiger, H. C., 1969, Ontogeny of adrenergic arousal and cholinergic inhibitory mechanisms in the rat, Science 166:635-637.

Campbell, B. A., and Randall, P. K., 1975, Paradoxical effects of amphetamine on behavioral arousal in neonatal and adult rats: a possible animal model of the calming effect of amphetamine on hyperkinetic children, in "Aberrant Development in Infancy: Human and Animal Studies," N. R. Ellis, ed., pp. 105-112, Erlhaum Association, Hillsdale, New Jersey.

Carey, R. J., 1982, A comparison of atropine, benztropine and diphenhydramine on the reversal of haloperidol induced suppression of self-stimulation, Pharm. Biochem. Behav. 17:851-854.

Carlton, P. L., 1963, Cholinergic mechanisms in the control of behavior by the rat, Psychol. Rev. 70:19-39.

Celesia, C. G., and Jasper, H. H., 1966, Acetylcholine released from cerebral cortex in relation to state of activation, Neurology 16:1053-1064.

Cohen, S. L., Morley, B. J., and Snead, O. C., 1981, An EEG analysis of convulsive activity produced by cholinergic agents, Progr. Neuro-Psychopharmacol. 5:383-388.

Colpaert, F. C., 1975, The ventromedial hypothalamus and control of avoidance behavior and aggression: fear hypothesis versus response suppression theory of limbic function, Behav. Biol. 15:27-44.

Consolo, S., Ladinsky, H., and Garattinni, S., 1974, Effect of several dopaminergic drugs and trihexyphenidyl on cholinergic parameters in the rat striatum, J. Pharm. Pharmacol. 26:275-277.

Cools, A. R., Hendriks, G., and Korten, J., 1975, The acetylcholine-dopamine balance in the basal ganglia of rhesus monkeys and its role in dynamic dystonic, dyskinetic and epileptoid motor activities, J. Neural Transm. 36:91-105.

Corrodi, H., Fuxe, K., and Lidbrink, P., 1972, Interaction between cholinergic and catecholaminergic neurons in rat brain, Brain Res. 43:397-416.

Cotzias, G. C., Lawrence, W. H., Papavisiliou, P. S., Duby, S. E., Ginos, J. Z., and Menor, I., 1972, Apomorphine and parkinsonism, Trans. Am. Neurol. Assoc. 97:156-158.

Cotzias, G. C., Papavisiliou, P. S., Fehling, C., Kaufman, B., and Menor, I., 1970, Similarities between neurologic effects of L-dopa and apomorphine, N. Engl. J. Med. 282:31-33.

Coyle, J. T., and Snyder, S. H., 1969, Antiparkinsonian drugs: inhibition of dopamine uptake in the corpus striatum as a possible mechanism of action, Science 166:899-901.

Davis, J. W., Thomas, R. K., Jr., and Adams, H. E., 1971, Interactions of scopolamine and physostigmine with ECS and one trial learning, Physiol. Behav. 6:219-222.

Deutsch, J. A., 1971, The cholinergic synapse and the site of memory, Science 174:788-794.

Deutsch, J. A., Hamburg, M. D., and Dahl, M., 1966, Anticholinesterase induced amnesia and its temporal aspects, Science 151:221-223.

Deutsch, J. A., and Leibowitz, S. F., 1966, Amnesia or reversal of forgetting by anticholinesterase, depending simply on time of injection, Science 153:1017.

Deutsch, J. A., and Lutzky, H., 1967, Memory enhancement by anticholinesterase as a function of initial learning, Nature 213:742.

Dickerman, S., Clark, J., Dickerman, E., and Meites, J., 1972, Effect of haloperidol on serum and pituitary prolactin and on hypothalamic PIF in rats, Neuroendocrinology 9:332-340.

Dobrin, E. I., and Mares, S. E., 1974, Effects of morphine on serum gonadotrophin levels in rats and monkeys, in "Drug Addiction 4," J. Singh and H. Lal, eds., International Book Corp., New York.

Domino, E. F., 1967, Electroencephalographic and behavioral arousal effects of small doses of nicotine: a neuropsychopharmacological study, Ann. N.Y. Acad. Sci. 142:216-244.

Domino, E. F., and Hudson, R. D., 1959, Observations on the pharmacological actions of the isomers of atropine, J. Pharmacol. Exp. Ther. 127:305-312.

Domino, E. F., and Olds, M. E., 1968, Cholinergic inhibition of self-stimulation behavior, J. Pharmacol. Exp. Ther. 164:202-211.

Domino, E. F., and Olds, M. E., 1972, Effects of d-amphetamine, scopolamine, chlordiazepoxide and diphenylhydantoin on self-stimulation behavior and brain acetylcholine, Psychopharmacology 23:1-16.

Dunlop, C. W., Stumpf, C., Maxwell, D. S., and Schindler, W., 1960, Modification of cortical, reticular and hippocampal unit activity by nicotine in the rabbit, Am. J. Physiol. 198:515-518.

Egger, G. J., Livesay, P. J., and Dawson, R. G., 1973, Ontogenetic aspects of central cholinergic involvement in spontaneous alternation behavior, Dev. Psychobiol. 6:289-299.

Erickson, C. K., and Chai, K. J., 1976, Cholinergic modification of ethanol induced electroencephalographic synchrony in the rat, Neuropharmacology 15:39-43.

Exley, K. A., Fleming, M. C., and Espelien, A. D., 1958, Effects of drugs which depress the peripheral nervous system on the reticular activating system of the cat, Br. J. Pharmacol. 13:485-492.

Fairchild, M. D., Jenden, D. J., and Mickey, M. R., 1975, An application of long-term frequency analysis in measuring drug-specific alterations in the EEG of the cat, Electroencephalogr. Clin. Neurophysiol. 38:337-348.

Feldberg, W., and Sherwood, S. L., 1954, Injections of drugs into the lateral ventricle of the cat, J. Physiol. (Lond.) 123:148-167.

Fleming, D. E., Rhodes, L. E., Wilson, C. E., and Shearer, D. E., 1972 Time-drug modulations of photically evoked after-discharge patterns, Physiol. Behav. 8:1045-1049.

Floris, V., Morocutti, G., and Ayala, G. F., 1962, Action of nicotine
    on the bioelectric activity of the cortex of the thalamus and
    of the hippocampus in rabbits. Its "arousal" action and primary
    convulsive action on the hippocampo-thalamic structures, Boll.
    Soc. Ital. Biol. Sper. 38:407-410.
Frankenheim, J., 1982, Effects of antidepressants and related drugs on
    the quantitatively analyzed EEGs of Beagles, Drug Develop. Res.
    2:197-213.
Gauss, C. J., 1906, Gerburten in kunstlichem Dammerschlaf, Arch.
    Gynak. 78:579-631.
Glenn, L. L., Foutz, A. S., and Dement, W. C., 1980, Sleep during
    neuromuscular blockade in cats, Electroencephalogr. Clin.
    Neurophysiol. 50:141-150.
Goldstein, L., Beck, R. A., and Mundschenk, D. L., 1967, Effects of
    nicotine upon cortical and subcortical electrical activity of the
    rabbit brain: quantitative analysis, Ann. N.Y. Acad. Sci.
    142:170-180.
Grossman, S. P., 1968, Behavioral and electroencephalographic effects
    of micro-injections of neurohumors into the midbrain reticular
    formation, Physiol. Behav. 3:777-786.
Grossman, S. P., 1972, Cholinergic synapses in the limbic system and
    behavioral inhibition. Neurotransmitters, Res. Publ. Assoc. Res.
    Nerv. Ment. Dis. 50:315-326.
Grossman, S. P., 1962, Direct adrenergic and cholinergic stimulation
    of hypothalamic mechanisms, Am. J. Physiol. 202:872-882.
Guha, D., and Pradhan, S. N., 1976, Effects of nicotine on EEG and
    evoked potentials and their interactions with autonomic drugs,
    Neuropharmacology 15:225-232.
Guyenet, P. G., Agid, Y., Javoy, F., Beaujouan, J. C., Rossier, J.,
    and Glowinski, J., 1975, Effects of dopaminergic receptor
    agonists and antagonists on the activity of the neo-striatal
    cholinergic system, Brain Res. 84:227-244.
Halpern, L. M., and Black, R. G., 1967, Flaxedil (gallamine triethio-
    dide): evidence for a central action, Science 155:1685-1687.
Hamburg, M. D., 1967, Retrograde amnesia produced by intraperitoneal
    injection of physostigmine, Science 155:973-974.
Haranath, P. S. R. K., and Shyamalakumari, S., 1973, Sleep induced by
    small doses of tubocurarine injected into cerebral ventricles of
    the dog, Br. J. Pharmacol. 48:23-28.
Haranath, P. S. R. K., Sunanda-Bai, K., and Venkatakrishna-Bhatt, H.,
    1967, Intracarotid injections and infusions of cholinomimetic
    drugs and their antagonists in conscious dogs, Br. J. Pharmacol.
    Chemother. 29:42-54.
Haranath, P. S. R. K., and Venkatakrishna-Bhatt, H., 1973, Release of
    acetylcholine from perfused cerebral ventricles in unanesthesized
    dogs during waking and sleep, Jpn. J. Physiol. 23:241-250.
Haranath, P. S. R. K., and Venkatakrishna-Bhatt, H., 1977, Sleep
    induced by drugs injected into the inferior horn of the lateral
    cerebral ventricle in dogs, Br. J. Pharmacol. 59:231-236.

Haycock, J. W., Deadwyler, S. A., Sideroff, S. I., and McGaugh, J. L., 1973, Retrograde amnesia and cholinergic systems in the caudate-putamen complex and dorsal hippocampus of the rat, Exp. Neurol. 41:201-213.

Hernández-Peón, R., Chavez-Ibarra, G., Morgane, P. J., and Timo-Iaria, C., 1963, Limbic cholinergic pathways involved in sleep and emotional behavior, Exp. Neurol. 8:93-111.

Hernández-Peón, R., O'Flaherty, J. J., and Mazzuchelli-O'Flaherty, A. Z., 1967, Sleep and other behavioral effects induced by acetylcholine stimulation of basal temporal cortex and striate structures, Brain Res. 4:243-267.

Herz, A., 1962, On the effect of optic isomers of atropine-like substances on the central nervous system, Naunyn Schmiedeberg Arch. Exp. Path. 242:508-521.

Herz, A., 1963, Excitation and inhibition of cholinoceptive brain structures and its relationship to pharmacological induced behavior changes, Int. J. Neuropharmacol. 2:205-216.

Hill, S. Y., Reyes, R. B., and Kupfer, D. J., 1979, Physostigmine induction of REM sleep in imipramine treated rats, Commun. Psychopharm. 3:261-266.

Hill, S. Y., Reyes, R. B., and Kupfer, D. J., 1980, Imipramine and REM sleep: cholinergic mediation in animals, Psychopharmacology 69:5-9.

Hornykiewicz, O., 1971, Neurochemical pathology and pharmacology of brain dopamine and acetylcholine: rational basis for the current treatment of parkinsonism, in "Recent Advances in Parkinson's Disease," F. H. McDowell and C. H. Markham, eds., pp. 33-65, Davis, Philadelphia.

Hudson, R. D., 1979, Central nervous system responses to cigarette smoke inhalation in the cat, Arch. Int. Pharmacodyn. Ther. 237:191-212.

Hunt, P., Karmengieszer, M. H., and Raynaud, J. P., 1974, Nomifensine: a new potent inhibitor of dopamine uptake into synaptosomes from rat brain corpus striatum, J. Pharmacol. 26:370-371.

Irmis, F., 1974, Correlation between spontaneous behavior and cortical or hippocampal EEG in rats: dissociation after atropine and lack of dissociation after physostigmine, Act Nerv. Super (Praha) 16:48-50.

Janssen, P. A. J., and Niemegeers, C. J. E., 1967, The peripheral and central anticholinergic properties of benzetimide (R 4929) and other atropine-like drugs as measured in a new anti-pilocarpine test in rats, Psychopharmacologia 11:231-254.

Jasper, H. H., and Tessier, J., 1971, Acetylcholine liberation from cerebral cortex during paradoxical (REM) sleep, Science 172:601-602.

Jenden, D. J., 1979, The neurochemical basis of acetylcholine precursor loading as a therapeutic strategy, in, "Chemical Influences on Behavior," K. Brown and S. J. Cooper, eds., Academic Press, London/New York.

Jung, O.H., and Boyd, E. S., 1966, Effects of cholinergic drugs on
    self-stimulation response rates in rats, Am. J. Physiol.
    210:432-434.
Karczmar, A. G., Longo, V. G., and Scotti de Carolis, A., 1970, A
    pharmacological model of paradoxical sleep: the role of
    cholinergic and monoamine systems, Physiol. Behav. 5:175-182.
Khazan, N., Bar, R., and Sulman, F. G., 1967, The effect of choliner-
    gic drugs on paradoxical sleep in the rat, Int. J. Neuropharmacol.
    6:279-282.
Kingsley, R. E., and Barnes, C. D., 1973, Olivo-cochlear inhibition
    during physostigmine induced activity in the pontine reticular
    formation in the decerebrate cat, Exp. Neurol. 40:43-51.
Klawans, H. L., Jr., 1973, "The Pharmacology of Extrapyramidal Move-
    ment Disorders," S. Karger, Basel.
Knapp, D. E., and Domino, E. F. 1962, Action of nicotine on the
    ascending reticular activating system, Int. J. Neuropharmacol.
    1:333-351.
Knapp, D. E., and Domino, E. F., 1963, Species differences in the EEG
    response to epinephrine, 5-hydroxytryptamine and nicotine in
    brain stem transected animals, Int. J. Neuropharmacol. 2:51-55.
Kramis, R., Van der Wolf, C. H., and Bland, B. H., 1975, Two types of
    hippocampal rhythmical slow activity in both the rabbit and the
    rat: relations to behavior and effects of atropine, diethyl
    ether, urethane and pentobarbital, Exp. Neurol. 49:58-85.
Lal, H., and Puri, S. K., 1973, Effect of acute morphine or haloperi-
    dol administration on catalepsy and striatal dopamine turnover in
    rats chronically treated with morphine or haloperidol,
    Pharmacologist 15:259.
Lewis, D. R., and Shute, C. C. D., 1967, The cholinergic limbic
    system: projections to hippocampal formation, medial cortex,
    nuclei of the ascending cholinergic reticular system, and sub-
    fornical organ and supra-optic crest, Brain 90:521-539.
Lloyd, K. G., Stadler, H., and Bartholini, G., 1973, Dopamine and
    acetylcholine neurons in the striatal and limbic structures:
    effect of neuroleptic drugs, in "Frontiers in Catecholamine
    Research," E. Usdin and S. H. Snyder, eds., pp. 777-779, Pergamon
    Press, New York.
Longo, V. G., 1966, Behavioral and electroencephalographic effects of
    atropine and related compounds, Pharmacol. Rev. 18:965-996.
Longo, V. G., 1962, "Electroencephalographic Atlas for Pharmacological
    Research. Rabbit Brain Research, Vol. II," Elsevier, Amsterdam.
Longo, V. G., Giunta, F., and Scotti de Carolis, A., 1967, Effects of
    nicotine on the electroencephalogram of the rabbit, Ann. N.Y.
    Acad. Sci. 42:159-169.
Longo, V. G., Von Berger, G. P., and Bovet, D., 1954, Action of nico-
    tine and of the 'ganglioplegiques centraux' on the electrical
    activity of the brain, J. Pharmacol. 111:349-359.
Malish, R., and Ott, T., 1982, Rhythmical slow wave electroencephalo-
    graphic activity elicited by hippocampal injection of muscarinic
    agents in the rat, Neurosci. Lett. 28:113-118.

Margules, D. L., 1969, Noradrenergic rather than serotonergic basis of reward in the dorsal tegmentum, J. Comp. Physiol. Psychol. 67:32-35.

Margules, D. L. and Margules, A., 1973, Cholinergic receptors in the ventromedial hypothalamus govern operant response strength, Am. J. Physiol. 224:1475-1479.

Margules, D. L. and Stein, L., 1969, Cholinergic synapses of periventricular punishment system in the medial hypothalamus, Am. J. Physiol. 217:475-480.

Mazzuchelli-O'Flaherty, A. L., O'Flaherty, J. J., and Hernández-Peón, R., 1967, Sleep and other behavioral responses induced by acetylcholinic stimulation of frontal and mesial cortex, Brain Res. 4:268-283.

McCleary, R. A., 1966, Response-modulating functions of the limbic system: initiation and suppression, in "Progress in Physiological Psychology," E. Stellar and J. M. Sprague, eds., pp. 209-272, Academic Press, New York.

McGeer, P. L., Grewaal, D. S., and McGeer, E. G., 1974, Influence of noncholinergic drugs on rat striatal acetylcholine levels, Brain Res. 80:211-217.

Meyers, B., Roberts, K. N., Riciputi, R. N., and Domino, E. F., 1964, Some effects of muscarinic cholinergic blocking drugs on behavior and the electroencephalogram, Psychopharmacologia 5:289-300.

Miller, F. R., Stavraky, G. W., and Woonton, G. A., 1940, Effects of eserine, acetylcholine, and atropine on the electrocorticogram, J. Neurophysiol. 3:131-138.

Myers, R. D., 1974, "Handbook of Drug and Chemical Stimulation of the Brain," pp. 651-660 and 759, Van Nostrand, New York.

Nakao, H., Ballin, H. M., and Gellhorn, E., 1956, The role of sinoaortic receptors in the activity of adrenaline, noradrenaline and dietylcholine on the cerebral cortex, Electroencephalogr. Clin. Neurophysiol. 8:413-420.

Newman, L. M., 1972, Effects on cholinergic agonists and antagonists on self-stimulation behavior in the rat, J. Comp. Physiol. Psychol. 79:394-413.

Olds, M. E., 1972a, Alterations by centrally acting drugs on the suppression of self-stimulation behavior in the rat by tetrabenazine, physostigmine, chlorpromazine and pentobarbital, Psychopharmacology 25:299-314.

Olds, M. E., 1972b, Comparative effects of amphetamine, scopolamine and chlordiazepoxide on self-stimulation behavior, Rev. Can. Biol. 31 (suppl.):25-57.

Olds, M. E., and Domino, E. F., 1969a, Comparison of muscarinic and nicotinic cholinergic agonists on self-stimulation behavior, J. Pharmacol. Exp. Ther. 166:189-204.

Olds, M. E., and Domino, E. F., 1969b, Differential effects of cholinergic agonists on self-stimulation and escape behavior, J. Pharmacol. Exp. Ther. 170:157-167.

Olds, M. E., and Ito, M., 1973, Noradrenergic and cholinergic action of neuronal activity during self-stimulation behavior in the rat, Neuropharmacology 12:525-539.

Olds, M. E., and Olds, J., 1964, Pharmacological patterns in subcorti-
    cal reinforcement behavior, Int. J. Neuropharmacol. 2:309-325.
Pokorný, J., and Šterc, J., 1980, Effect of D-tubocurarine immobili-
    zation on the resting electroencephalogram in the rat,
    Electroencephalogr. Clin. Neurophysiol. 48:242-245.
Pradhan, S. N., 1976, Balance of various neurotransmitter actions in
    self-stimulation behavior, in "Brain Stimulation Reward," A.
    Wauquier and E. T. Rolls, eds., pp. 171-185, North Holland
    Publishing Company, Amsterdam.
Pradhan, S. N., and Kamat, K. A., 1972, Action and interaction of cho-
    linergic agonists and antagonists on self-stimulation, Arch. Int.
    Pharmacodyn. Ther. 196:321-329.
Pradhan, S. N., and Kamat, K. A., 1973, Effects of anticholinergic
    agents on self-stimulation, Arch. Int. Pharmacol. 201, 16-24.
Puri, S. K., and Lal, H., 1974, Tolerance to the behavior and neuro-
    chemical effects of haloperidol and morphine in rats chronically
    treated with morphine or haloperidol, Naunyn Schmiedeberg. Arch.
    Pharmacol. 282:155-170.
Puri, S. K., Reddy, C. R., and Lal, H., 1973, Blockade of central
    dopaminergic receptors by morphine: effect of haloperidol, apo-
    morphine or benztropine, Res. Commun. Chem. Pathol. Pharmacol.
    5:389-401.
Ross, S. B., and Renyi, A. L., 1967, Inhibition of the uptake of
    tritiated catecholamines by antidepressants and related agents,
    Eur. J. Pharmacol. 2:181-186.
Roy, R. C., and Stullken, E. N., 1981, Electroencephalographic evi-
    dence of arousal in dogs from halothane after doxapram, physostig-
    mine or naloxone, Anesthesiology 55:392-397.
Russell, R. W., 1982, Cholinergic system in behavior: the search for
    mechanisms of action, Ann. Rev. Pharmacol. Toxicol. 22:435-463.
Ryan, L. J., Barr, J. E., Sanders, B., and Sharpless, S. K., 1979,
    Electrophysiological responses to ethanol, pentobarbital and nico-
    tine in mice genetically selected for differential sensitivity to
    ethanol, J. Comp. Physiol. Psychol. 93:1035-1052.
Sadowski, B., and Longo, V. G., 1962, EEG and behavioral correlates of
    an instrumental reward conditioned response in rabbits. A physio-
    logical and pharmacological study, Electroencephalogr. Clin.
    Neurophysiol. 14:465-576.
Santucci, V., Glatt, A., Demieville, H., and Olpe, H. R., 1981,
    Quantification of slow wave EEG induced by atropine: effects of
    physostigmine, amphetamine and haloperidol, Eur. J. Pharmacol.
    73:113-122.
Schacht, W., and Heptner, W., 1974, Effect of nomifensine (HOE 984)
    a new antidepressant on uptake of noradrenaline and serotonin and
    on release of noradrenaline in rat brain synaptosomes, Biochem.
    Pharmacol. 23:3413.
Schaeppi, U., 1967, Effects of nicotine administration to the cat's
    lower brain stem upon electroencephalogram and autonomic system,
    Ann. N.Y. Acad. Sci. 142:40-49.

Schaul, N., Gloor, P., Ball, G., and Gotman, J., 1978, The electro-
    microphysiology of delta waves induced by systemic atropine,
    Brain Res. 143:475-486.
Schulenburg, C. J., Riccio, D. C., and Stikes, E. R., 1971, Acquisi-
    tion and retention of a passive avoidance response as a function
    of age in rats, J. Comp. Physiol. Psychol. 74:75-83.
Sethy, V. H., and Van Woert, M. H., 1974, Modification of striatal
    acetylcholine concentration by dopamine receptor agonists and
    antagonists, Res. Commun. Chem. Pathol. Pharmacol. 8:13-28.
Shute, C. C. D., and Lewis, P. R., 1967, The ascending cholinergic
    reticular system: neocortical, olfactory and subcortical projec-
    tions, Brain 90:497-519.
Sigwald, J., 1971, Thérapeutique des syndromes extrapyramidaux par les
    traitements classiques, in "Monoamines et Noyaux Gris Centraux,"
    J. De Ajuriaguera and G. Gauthier, eds., pp. 369-378, Georg et
    Masson, Geneva and Paris.
Squire, L. R., and Davis, H. P., 1981, The pharmacology of memory: a
    neurobiological perspective, Ann. Rev. Pharmacol. Toxicol.
    21:323-356.
Squire, L. R., Glick, S. D., and Goldfarb, J., 1971, Relearning at
    different times after training as affected by centrally and peri-
    pherally acting cholinergic drugs in the mouse, J. Comp. Physiol.
    Psychol. 74:41-45.
Stadler, A., Lloyd, K. G., Godea-Civia, M., and Bartholini, G., 1973,
    Enhanced striatal acetylcholine release by chlorpromazine and its
    reversal by apomorphine, Brain Res. 55:476-480.
Stadnicki, S. W., and Schaeppi, U., 1970, Nicotine infusion into the
    fourth ventricle of unrestrained cats: changes in EEG and
    behavior, Arch. Int. Pharmacodyn. Ther. 183:277-288.
Stadnicki, S. W., and Schaeppi, U. H., 1972, Nicotine changes in EEG
    and behavior after intravenous infusion in awake unrestrained
    cats, Arch. Int. Pharmacodyn. Ther. 197, 72-85.
Stanes, M. D., Brown, C. P., and Singer, G., 1976, Effects of physo-
    stigmine on Y-maze discrimination retention in the rat,
    Psychopharmacologia 46:269-276.
Stein, L., 1964, Reciprocal actions of reward and punishment mechanism
    in "The Role of Pleasure in Behavior," R. G. Heath, ed., pp. 113-
    139, Harper and Row, New York.
Stein, L., 1967, Psychopharmacological substrates of mental depression
    in "Antidepressant Drugs," S. Garattini, ed., pp. 130-140,
    Excerpta Med. Foundation, Amsterdam.
Stein, L., 1968, Chemistry of reward and punishment, in
    "Psychopharmacology, A Review of Progress 1957-1967," D. H. Efron,
    ed., pp. 105-123, U.S. Government Printing Office, Washington, D.C.
Stephens, D. N., and Herberg, L. J., 1979, Dopamine and acetylcholine
    "balance" in nucleus accumbens and corpus striatum and its effects
    on hypothalamic self-stimulation, Eur. J. Pharmacol. 54:331-339.

Stinus, L., Thierry, A. M., and Cardo, D., 1976, Pharmacological and
    biochemical studies of intracranial self-stimulation: roles of
    dopaminergic and noradrenergic neuronal systems with electrodes in
    area antrallis tegmenti or in lateral hypothalamus, in "Brain
    Stimulation Reward," A. Wauquier and E. T. Rolls, eds., pp. 280-
    283, North-Holland Publishing Company, Amsterdam.
Stratton, L. O., and Petrinovich, L. F., 1963, Post-trial injection of
    an anticholinesterase drug and maze learning in two strains of
    mice, Psychopharmacologia 5:47-54.
Sweet, R. D., Wasterlain, G. G., and McDowell, F. H., 1974, Pribedil,
    a dopamine agonist in Parkinson's disease, Clin. Pharmacol. Ther.
    16:1077-1082.
Vakil, S. D., Caline, D. B., Reid, J. L., and Seymour, C. A., 1973,
    Pyrimidyl-piperonyl-piperazine (ET 495) in parkinsonism, Advan.
    Neurol. 3:121-125.
Vanderwolf, C. H., 1975, Neocortical and hippocampal activation in
    relation to behavior: effects of atropine, eserine, phenothia-
    zines and amphetamine, J. Comp. Physiol. Psychol. 88:300-323.
Van Rossum, J. M., 1966, The significance of dopamine-receptor block-
    ade for the mechanism of action of neuroleptic drugs, Arch. Int.
    Pharmacodyn. Ther. 160:492-494.
Von Wild, K., 1980, Tierexperimentelle Untersuchungen über die
    Beeinflussung des EEG durch Muskelrelaxantien am Beispiel vom
    Pancuronium und Succinylbischolin, in "Anasthesie bei Zerebralen
    Krampfanfällen und Intensivtherapie des Status Epilepticus," A.
    Opitz and R. Degen, eds., pp. 45-55, Verlagsgesellschaft mbH,
    Erlangen.
Warburton, D. M., 1981, Neurochemistry of behavior, Br. Med. Bull.
    37:121-125.
Warburton, D. M., and Brown, K., 1972, The facilitation of discrimina-
    tion performance by physostigmine sulphate, Psychopharmacologia
    27:275-284.
Wauquier, A., 1979, Neuroleptics and brain self-stimulation behavior
    Int. Rev. Neurobiol. 21:335-403.
Wauquier, A., 1976, The influence of psychoactive drugs on brain self-
    stimulation in rats. A review, in "Brain-Stimulation Reward,"
    A. Wauquier and E. T. Rolls, eds., pp. 123-170, North-Holland
    Publishing Company, Amsterdam.
Wauquier, A., and Niemegeers, C. J. E., 1974, Intracranial self-stimu-
    lation in rats as a function of various stimulus parameters. V.
    Influence of cocaine on medial forebrain bundle stimulation with
    monopolar electrodes, Psychopharmacologia 38:201-210.
Wauquier, A., and Niemegeers, C. J. E., 1976, Restoration of self-
    stimulation inhibited by neuroleptics, Eur. J. Pharmacol.
    40:191-194.
Wauquier, A., and Niemegeers, C. J. E., 1975, The effects of dexeti-
    mide on pimozide, haloperidol and pipampero-induced inhibition of
    brain self-stimulation in rats, Arch. Int. Pharmacodyn. Ther.
    217:280-292.

Wauquier, A., Niemegeers, C. J. E., and Lal, H., 1974, Differential
     antagonism by naloxone of inhibitory effects of haloperidol and
     morphine on brain self-stimulation, Psychopharmacologia
     37:303-310.
Wauquier, A., Niemegeers, C. J. E., and Lal, H., 1975, Differential
     antagonism by the anticholinergic dexetimide of inhibitory
     effects of haloperidol and fentanyl on brain self-stimulation,
     Psychopharmacologia 41:229-235.
Westfall, T. C., 1967, Effects of nicotine and related substances upon
     amine levels in the brain, Ann. N.Y. Acad. Sci. 142:83-100.
White, R. P., and Boyaju, L. D., 1960, Neuropharmacological comparison
     of atropine, scopolamine, benactyzine, diphenhydramine and
     hydroxyzine, Arch. Int. Pharmacodyn. Ther. 127:260-273.
Whitehouse, J. M., 1964, The effects of atropine on discrimination
     learning in the rat, J. Comp. Physiol. Psychol. 57:13-15.
Wiener, N. I., and Deutsch, J. A., 1968, The temporal aspects of anti-
     cholinergic and anticholinesterase induced amnesia for an appeti-
     tive habit, J. Comp. Physiol. Psychol. 66:613-617.
Wikler, A., 1952, Pharmacologic dissociation of behavior and EEG
     "sleep patterns" in dogs: morphine, N-allylnormorphine and atro-
     pine, Proc. Soc. Biol. Med. 79:261-265.
Yamamoto, K. I., and Domino, E. F., 1965, Nicotine-induced EEG and
     behavioral arousal, Int. J. Neurophysiol. 4:359-373.
Yamamoto, K. I., and Domino, E. F., 1967, Cholinergic agonist-antago-
     nist interactions on neocortical and limbic EEG activation, Int.
     J. Neuropharmacol. 6:357-373.

Chapter 4

NEW ASPECTS ON THE FUNCTIONAL ROLE OF ACETYLCHOLINE IN THE BASAL GANGLIA SYSTEM
Interactions With Other Neurotransmitters

Jørgen Scheel-Krüger

Psychopharmacological Research Laboratory
St. Hans Mental Hospital
DK-4000 Roskilde, Denmark

---

1.   INTRODUCTION

      Numerous studies suggest a dynamic interaction between dopamine
and acetylcholine according to the principle of an opponent mechanism
of action.   In the clinic this principle seems true for various diseases such as Parkinsonism, schizophrenia, tardive dyskinesia, mania,
depression and Huntington's disease (see Davis et al., 1978).   The
cholinergic effects in all these diseases suggest multiple and complex
interactions with neostriatal and mesolimbic dopamine systems as well
as other neurotransmitter systems.   In this paper evidence will be
presented that the cholinergic systems can have a differential influence on various dopamine systems and/or type of dopamine receptors.
This conclusion is supported by recent biochemical and behavioral
studies which demonstrate a differential influence and reversal by
scopolamine of the cataleptic and antistereotypic effect in mice and
rats of different types of neuroleptic drugs, i.e., the effect of the
butyrophenones compared with the effect of phenothiazines and
thioxanthenes.

      A new animal model will be presented which can be related to
hyperkinesia, akathisia, and probably to tardive dyskinesia, seen in
the clinic after neuroleptic drugs.   It was found that rats receiving
a high dose of reserpine (which depletes the catecholamines and serotonin) developed a syndrome of immobility, catalepsy and phases of
true hyperactive behavior, i.e., sterotyped locomotion, rearing and
sniffing seen as sudden bursts of activity.   This syndrome of hyperactivity was completely abolished by a series of anticholinergic drugs

or very low doses of dopamine stimulants injected systemically, but dopamine or noradrenaline antagonists did not inhibit them. However, low doses of various cholinergic stimulants (arecoline, oxotremorine or physostigmine) significantly increased hyperactivity in these re-serpinized rat and higher doses of cholinergic agonists elicited oral stereotyped activity in addition.

The anatomical section of this paper discusses the role of ace-tylcholine in the nigrostriatal system. The striatum is traditionally considered as the major anatomical site for the opposed interaction between dopamine and acetylcholine. This traditional point of view is challenged. Furthermore, it is shown that striatal cholinergic mechanisms are considerably more complex and less understood than pre-viously thought.

We have found evidence that acetylcholine induces different effects within separate regions of the nigrostriatal system. Thus apomorphine- and dopamine-dependent, stereotyped behavior was blocked by carbachol in the ventromedial part of the striatum but facilitated in the dorsomedial part of the striatum. The immobility and catalepsy induced by haloperidol in the rat seem independent of cholinergic hyperactivity in the striatum, since intrastriatal injections of methylscopolamine were not antagonistic.

Still other recent results indicate that the zona reticulata of substantia nigra, which receives a major efferent, GABAergic projec-tion from the striatal dopamine output system is the relevant site for the dopamine-acetylcholine-GABA interaction. Muscarinic agonists locally injected into the SNR induced a rigid immobile catalepsia in the rats and antagonism of apomorphine stereotypy. These effects seem related to an effect on the non-dopaminergic, efferent neurons of the substantia nigra. The anticholinergic drug methylscopolamine injected locally into the substantia nigra, zona reticulata (SNR) induced, in-dependently of the dopamine system, behavioral stimulation, amphet-amine-like stereotypy and antagonism of the catalepsy induced by the dopamine antagonist haloperidol.

Finally, there is discussion of the cholinergic neurons which innervate the neocortex and are localized in the basal forebrain and substantia innominata. Since the major output of the nucleus accum-bens is directed towards the substantia innominata, it is suggested that the mesolimbic dopamine system innervating the nucleus accumbens may affect the cholinergic input to the cortex and thus also striatal functions by the corticostriatal efferent system.

2.   SIGNIFICANCE OF ACETYLCHOLINE-DOPAMINE INTERACTION FOR
      NEUROLEPTIC DRUGS AND SCHIZOPHRENIA

In schizophrenic patients receiving neuroleptic drugs with dopamine blocking properties, anticholinergic drugs, (i.e., anti-

Parkinsonism drugs) reduce the extrapyramidal side-effects of
Parkinsonian-like character (tremor, rigidity) and also akathisia.
The antischizophrenic effect of the neuroleptic drugs may also be reduced to some extent (Singh and Kay, 1975, 1979; Singh and Lal, 1979).
In support of these findings it has been reported that a facilitation
of cholinergic transmission may induce a short-lasting improvement of
schizophrenia (see Davis et al., 1978, Janowsky et al., 1973; Singh
and Kay, 1979).

The anticholinergic drugs also induce antagonism of neuroleptic
drugs in various specific animal models. These experiments suggest a
functional opponent interaction between dopamine and acetylcholine.
However, several experiments demonstrate that this interaction is
considerably more complex.

Some excellent studies (Morpurgo and Theobald, 1964; Setler
et al., 1976), have found that the various behaviors influenced by a
neuroleptic drug such as haloperidol are differentially attenuated by
additional treatment with scopolamine. The catalepsy (a syndrome considered related to extrapyramidal side effects in the clinic) was most
markedly inhibited, whereas in decreasing order it was found that the
suppression of amphetamine-induced rotation, amphetamine and apomorphine sterotypy and conditioned avoidance responding were also reduced.

The interaction between dopamine and acetylcholine has been extensively studied in one of the most reliable animal models for
schizophrenia, i.e., the stereotypy syndrome induced in animals by
amphetamine, apomorphine, methylphenidate and other dopaminergic
stimulants (Christensen et al., 1979, 1980, 1981; Scheel-Krüger, 1970,
1971; Scheel-Krüger et al., 1981a,b). This behavior is mainly dependent on stimulation of dopamine receptors in the striatum although
recent experiments also suggest some contribution of limbic dopaminergic structures (Cools, 1977; Costall and Naylor, 1976; Costall et al.,
1977; Scheel-Krüger, 1971; Scheel-Krüger et al., 1981a,b). This behavioral syndrome is enhanced by the systemic injection of anticholinergic drugs and antagonized by cholinomimetics to some degree
(Costall et al., 1972b; Fjalland and Møller Nielsen, 1974; Scheel-
Krüger, 1970). These findings are supported by clinical studies which
have shown that the dopamine stimulant methylphenidate (Scheel-Krüger,
1971) exacerbated various symptoms of schizophrenia and this effect
was reversed by physostigmine (Janowsky et al., 1973).

The antagonism of dopamine induced stereotypy still represents
one of the most predictable screening models in animals for antischizophrenic drugs. This effect is reversed and/or abolished in both
acute and chronic treatment by the additional treatment with anticholinergic drugs (Arnt and Christensen, 1981; Christensen et al., 1979,
1981; Fjalland and Møller Nielsen, 1974; Morpurgo and Theobald, 1964;
Scheel-Krüger, 1970). However, it has recently been found that scopolamine had differential effects on the antistereotypic action (and

cataleptic effect) which depended on the type of neuroleptic drug
(Arnt and Christensen, 1981; Christensen et al., 1979, 1980; Scheel-
Krüger and Christensen, 1980). Neuroleptic drugs of the butyrophenone
type (i.e., haloperidol, spiroperidol) were most sensitive to scopolamine reversal, whereas the group of phenothiazines and thioxanthenes
(inclusive fluphenazine, and cis-flupentixol) were considerably less
affected. These findings may be related to a differential influence
on different types of dopamine receptors by the neuroleptic drugs,
i.e., the preferential affinity for the D-2 dopamine receptor by haloperidol and spiroperidol and for both the D-1 and D-2 receptors by the
thioxanthenes and phenothiazines.

The experiments could not be interpreted in terms of differences
in the intrinsic anticholinergic properties of the neuroleptic drugs.
In previous experiments we have found the same classification of neuroleptic drugs with regard to the influence of GABA agonists on stereotyped behavior (Christensen et al., 1979, 1980; Scheel-Krüger and
Christensen, 1980).

Other experiments also indicate a unique interaction between acetylcholine and a certain type of dopamine receptor and/or neuronal
system. For example McDevitt and Setler (1981) found that scopolamine
differentially affected the action of various types of dopamine agonists on stereotyped behavior and Ehlert et al. (1981) reported that
dopamine and apomorphine induced an enhancement of striatal muscarinic
receptors. This effect was specifically antagonized by the cis-flupentixol and fluphenazine, D-1 and D-2 receptor blockers, but not by
haloperidol, spiroperidol or sulpiride, D-2 dopamine receptor blockers. It seems obvious that all these findings must be taken into
account by future studies evaluating the effect of anticholinergic,
anti-Parkinson drugs on the effects of antipsychotic drugs (see Singh
and Kay, 1975, 1979; Singh and Lal, 1979).

3.   ACETYLCHOLINE AND DYSKINESIA INDUCED BY NEUROLEPTIC DRUGS

The neuroleptic drugs produce a wide variety of "extrapyramidal"
and neurological side effects in the clinic. In addition to tremor
and rigidity, a syndrome of initial hyperkinesia and dystonia has been
reported, most often localized to the oral, eye, and neck regions.
In addition, movements of arms and legs, dystonic posture and gait may
be seen as well as akathisia. Similar syndromes are also observed in
the monkey (Gerlach and Randrup, personal communications). All these
syndromes may develop due to initial doses of the neuroleptic drugs
which are "too high." These syndromes may be ameliorated to a certain extent by anticholinergic drugs and accentuated by cholinergic
drugs (Casey and Denney, 1977; Casey et al., 1980; Gerlach, 1979).
The long-term treatment with neuroleptic drugs may provoke more persistent hyperkinesia, i.e., the tardive dyskinesia. This dyskinesia
may further be increased by anticholinergic drugs and decreased by

cholinergic drugs (Gerlach et al., 1974; Gerlach, 1979; Casey and
Denney, 1977; Casey et al., 1980).

The syndrome of akathisia is among the first of the side effects
and is observed as a state of motor restlessness, often as shuffling
and tapping movements of the legs while sitting on a chair, together
with rocking movements and locomotor activity. This syndrome has been
seen in patients with tardive dyskinesia, who received physostigmine
and in a few cases the syndrome of akathisia was accentuated to a
hyperactive stereotyped locomotor activity (Gerlach et al., 1974;
Gerlach, 1979; Casey and Denney, 1977). These latter studies are discussed in some detail, since it seems that we have found a model,
i.e., "paradoxical" stereotyped hyperactivity in reserpinized rats
which may correspond in symptom and pharmacology to akathisia in the
clinic.

4.   "PARADOXICAL" STEREOTYPED HYPERACTIVITY IN RESERPINIZED RATS:
      AN ANIMAL MODEL OF AKATHISIA?

The most characteristic and dominant behavioral effect of antipsychotic neuroleptic drugs and reserpine in the rat is sedation,
akinesia and catalepsy. However, several years ago we observed that
50 to 60 percent of rats treated with a high dose of reserpine (i.e.,
7.5 mg/kg s.c.) show short or long-lasting episodes of stereotyped
behavior seen as bursts of coordinated locomotion, rearing on the
hindlegs and sniffing. Since this behavior and studies on its mechanism of action have only been described in short communications
(Schiørring and Randrup, 1968; Scheel-Krüger and Randrup, 1968) it is
essential to describe this syndrome in more detail. The locomotor
activity appeared suddenly and was often performed according to a
stereotyped pattern along fixed routes. Frequently we observed a
rearing bout and bursts of sniffing activity when the rat reached a
corner of the cage. These reserpinzied rats often climbed on the
walls and/or the roof of the cage. During the active locomotor phase
the rats retained the hunched back, "bison-posture" characteristic of
reserpinized rats. In the sedated phase catalepsy was seen as
"negativism," immobility and resistance to moving when tested on a
vertical wire netting or by placing the forelegs on a horizontal bar,
9 cm high. More surprisingly the catalepsy was also seen if the rats
were taken out of their familiar home cages during the active locomotor phase or immediately after the return of the immobile, sedative
phase. Indeed most of the time the reserpinized rats sat sedated and
immobile and it was never possible to induce hyperactivity by sensory
stimuli. The syndrome of hyperactivity seen in reserpinized rats was
described as a "paradoxical" stereotyped activity, because it was
mainly observed during the period, i.e., 4 to 20 hours after the injection, when the brain catecholamines were most depleted, i.e., below
5 percent of the normal level, (Scheel-Krüger, in preparation). A
very similar syndrome of "paradoxical" hyperactivity has also been

described by Boissier and Simon (1964) in rats treated with high doses of neuroleptic drugs including reserpine.

In all our experiments the rats were observed continuously for several hours with simultaneous recording of activity. We have not seen "paradoxical" hyperactivity immediately after injection of reserpine 7.5 mg/kg and there was a delay until about 4 to 4.5 hours after the injection of reserpine when about 20 percent of the rats showed short-lasting activity lasting 2 to 4 minutes. Most hyperactivity was seen 5 to 7 hours after reserpine when 50 to 60 percent of all the rats tested showed hyperactivity. Locomotion, rearing and sniffing behavior was 15 to 22 percent of the maximum possible score and occurred in 50 percent of the active rats as bursts of activities in successive periods of 1-2 minutes. However, continuous locomotion, rearing and sniffing activity for periods of 10 to 20 minutes was observed in almost 30 percent of the active rats.

About 24 hours after reserpine, the syndrome of "paradoxical" hyperactivities was not observed and the rats showed only the sedative, immobile and cataleptic phase of behavior.

Table 1. Inhibition by Anticholinergic Drugs of the "Paradoxical" Reserpine Hyperactivity.

Anticholinergic drug (mg/kg)	N	Behavioral counts in % of maximum			
		Locomotion	Rearing	Locomotion	Rearing
		(before drug)		(after drug)	
Benzhexol (10)	6	32	18	0*	0*
Caramiphen (20)	6	15	11	0*	0*
Scopolamine (5)	6	12	7	0*	0*
Metatropine (20)	12	27	19	30	17
Saline	12	28	17	52	33

*p< 0.001. A significant decrease in the activity in comparison with the saline group or the metatropine (= methylatropine) group of rats (chi square). All rats were pre-treated with 7.5 mg/kg s.c. of reserpine. Locomotion and rearing were counted before the subcutaneous injection of anticholinergic drugs, i.e., 4.5 to 5.5 hours after reserpine. Then all the rats received an injection of various anticholinergic drugs or saline. The recording of locomotion and rearing was then continued 10 minutes after the anticholinergic drugs for 1 hour, i.e., 5.75 to 6.75 hours after reserpine. N = number of rats.

4.1. The Syndrome of "Paradoxical" Hyperactivity in Reserpinized
      Rats Depends on a Hyperactive Central Cholinergic System

It was found that the anticholinergic drugs, benzhexol HCL, cara-
miphen HCL and scopolamine HCL induced a complete inhibition of the
"paradoxical" locomotion, rearing and sniffing activity in reserpinized rats (Table 1). However, bursts of activities were seen in the
rats receiving methylatropine, nitrate (a quaternary compound which
does not pass the blood brain barrier) or saline as placebo (Table 1).

In these experiments it was also observed that central anticholinergic drugs did not antagonize catalepsy in the rats depleted of
the catecholamines and the reserpinized rats were completely immobile
for several hours after the anticholinergic drugs. However, these
drugs did induce a clear-cut anticataleptic effect in rats receiving
neuroleptic drugs with dopamine receptor blocking effect such as haloperidol or perphenazine (Scheel-Krüger, unpublished).

As further evidence for a cholinergic mechanism in the "paradoxical" hyperactivity syndrome in reserpinized rats, it was found that
centrally active cholinergic drugs such as arecoline (2 mg/kg s.c.),
oxotremorine (0.10 mg/kg s.c.), and physostigmine (0.10 mg/kg s.c.),
given 4 hours after reserpine, induced a significant increase in the
frequency and incidence of locomotion, rearing and sniffing activities. The quaternary compound carbachol (0.20 mg/kg s.c.) which does
not pass the blood brain barrier did not induce stimulation (Fig. 1).
Scopolamine (5 mg/kg s.c.) when injected 30 minutes before the cholinergic drugs, abolished completely all stimulant effects of the cholinergic drugs in reserpinized rats (data not shown). Cholinergic drugs
given in higher doses i.e., arecoline (5 to 10 mg/kg), oxotremorine
(0.5 to 1 mg/kg) and physostigmine (0.5 to 1 mg/kg) induced no further
increase in the "paradoxical" hyper-activity but induced instead dyskinesia, tremor, body-shaking and oral biting/gnawing in the reserpinized rats (Scheel-Krüger, in preparation).

4.2. Evidence for a Counterbalancing Dopaminergic-Cholinergic
      Mechanism in the Reserpine-Induced "Paradoxical" Hyperactivity

The syndrome of "paradoxical" hyperactivity in reserpinized rats
was not related to an increase in the release of the catecholamines,
since even very high doses of the dopamine antagonists, spiroperidol
and perphenazine or the noradrenaline antagonists aceperone and pheno-
xybenzamide did not induce inhibition (Table 2). However, it was
found that very low doses of apomorphine (0.02 mg/kg s.c.) amphetamine
(0.25 mg/kg s.c.) and phenmetrazine (1 mg/kg s.c.) induced complete
inhibition of the hyperactivity syndrome (Table 2).

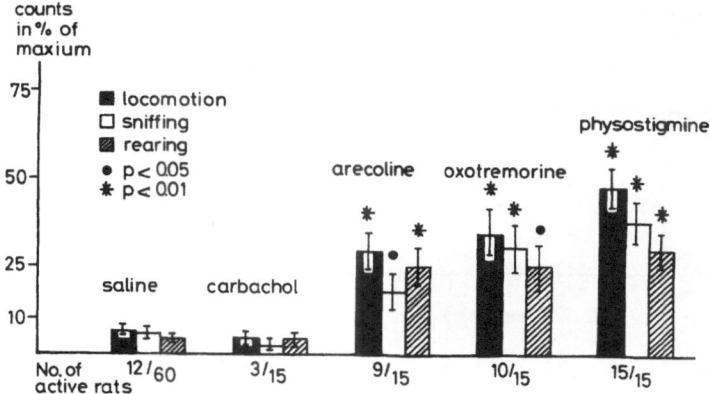

Fig. 1.   Central Stimulant Effects of Cholinergic Drugs in Reserpinized Rats.   All the rats were pretreated with reserpine
(7.5 mg/kg s.c.) injected 3 hours 50 minutes before the cholinergic drugs given subcutaneously: carbachol 0.20 mg/kg,
arecoline 2 mg/kg, oxotremorine 0.10 mg/kg and physostigmine
0.10 mg/kg.   Counting of behavioral activity was then performed 10 minutes later, i.e., 4 to 4.5 hours after reserpine.

        In fact none of the 60 rats which received the dopaminergic
stimulants showed the syndrome, whereas hyperactivity was seen in the
45 control rats receiving saline in addition to reserpine.   It is
known that apomorphine, amphetamine and phenmetrazine activate dopamine receptors and induce dopamine release even after depletion of the
storage pool of the catecholamines by reserpine (Scheel-Krüger, 1971).
The doses of the dopaminergic stimulants in these experiments for the
induction of sedation and immobility in reserpinized rats were critical.   In higher doses, i.e., apomorphine (0.1 to 0.2 mg/kg), amphetamine (1 mg/kg) and phenmetrazine (10 mg/kg), it was found that these
drugs induced a very strong behavioral activation in reserpinized rats
consisting of locomotion, rearing, sniffing and stereotyped licking
and gnawing.   These behavioral effects are correlated with an increase
of dopamine activity in the striatum (Scheel-Krüger, 1971).   The
dopamine-dependent stimulation is qualitatively and quantitatively
different from the reserpine syndrome.   The rats show very strong
continuous and compulsive activities after the dopamine stimulants,
and there are no phases of sedation, immobility or catalepsy.

Table 2. Inhibition by Dopamine Stimulants but not Dopamine or
Noradrenaline Antagonists of the "Paradoxical" Reserpine
Hyperactivity in Rats.

Drug (dose)		N	Behavioral counts in % of maximum		
			Locomotion	Rearing	Sniffing
Apomorphine	(0.02 mg/kg)	15	0.5*	0.2*	0.4*
Amphetamine	(0.25 mg/kg)	30	0.5*	0.1*	0.6*
Phenmetrazine	(1 mg/kg)	15	0*	0*	0*
Perphenazine	(2 mg/kg)	8	21	10	12
Spiroperidol	(2 mg/kg)	8	40	22	37
Aceperone	(5 mg/kg)	8	30	12	18
Phenoxybenzamine	(10 mg/kg)	8	15	10	13
Saline		45	17	11	12

*$p < 0.001$. A significant decrease in activity in comparison with
the saline group (chi square test). All rats were pretreated with
7.5 mg/kg s.c. reserpine. The presence of locomotion, rearing and
sniffing was counted 5.75 to 6.75 hours after the injection of reserpine. N = number of rats. The dopamine stimulants, apomorphine,
amphetamine and phenmetrazine were injected subcutaneously 10 minutes
before measurements of activity. The dopamine antagonists perphenazine and spiroperidol were injected 1.5 and 1 hour before the test,
respectively. The noradrenaline antagonists aceperone and phenoxybenzamine were injected 1.5 and 2 hours before the activity
measurements.

4.3. Conclusions

The results of these experiments provide support for the conclusion that the syndrome of "paradoxical" hyperactivity in reserpinized
rats is correlated with the induction of cholinergic hyperfunction
simultaneous with central dopaminergic (and noradrenergic?) hypofunction. This syndrome is antagonized by anticholinergic drugs and
facilitated by cholinergic agonists. The syndrome is not antagonized
by dopamine or noradrenaline antagonists, but is slightly increased

by spiroperidol and aceperone. However, even a slight increase in the dopaminergic activity induced by very low doses of apomorphine, amphetamine and phenmetrazine abolished the syndrome. Thus the behavior seems critically dependent on a dynamic opposed cholinergic-dopaminergic mechanism. Further support for the existence of a cholinergic-dopaminergic interaction in reserpinized rats was found in a series of experiments shown in Table 3. The syndrome of locomotion, rearing and sniffing was induced and facilitated by the injection of physostigmine (0.10 mg/kg) into reserpine pretreated rats. This effect of physostigmine was almost abolished by additional treatment with dopamine stimulants such as apomorphine (0.04 mg/kg), amphetamine (0.25 mg/kg) or phenmetrazine (2 mg/kg) given in low doses (Table 3). Finally, in previous studies, we have found that a mechanism of cholinergic hyperactivity is also involved in the syndrome of compulsive locomotor and rearing activity seen in the test of tetrabenzine-reversal by thymoleptic drugs of the imipramine group. This study also suggested the involvement of decreased dopamine and noradrenaline function (Scheel-Krüger and Randrup, 1969). It is thus significant and interesting that patients with akathisia have decreased noradrenaline activity (Bartels et al., 1981).

Table 3. A Cholinergic-Dopaminergic Balance in Reserpinized Rats

Drug treatment (mg/kg s.c.)	N	Behavioral counts in % of maximum		
		Locomotion	Rearing	Sniffing
Physostigmine (0.10)	25	35	17	30
Physostigmine (0.10) + Apomorphine (0.04)	15	5*	2*	4*
Physostigmine (0.10) + Amphetamine (0.25)	15	2*	1*	1*
Physostigmine (0.10) + Phenmetrazine (2)	15	5*	3*	5*

*$p < 0.01$. In comparison with the physostigmine treated group (chi square test). N = number of rats. All rats were pretreated with 7.5 mg/kg reserpine. The behavior was measured 5.75 to 6.75 hours after reserpine. Physostigmine was injected simultaneously with the dopamine stimulants and the activity counted 10 minutes later.

5.   ACETYLCHOLINE IN THE STRIATUM AND ITS FUNCTIONAL SIGNIFICANCE

5.1. Localization

It is well established that acetylcholine is localized in striatal interneurons and that the striatum (nucleus caudatus and putamen)
contains a relatively high amount of acetylcholine and the enzymes
involved in its synthesis, choline acetyltransferase (CAT) and metabolism, acetylcholinesterase (AChE), (Brand, 1980; Henderson, 1981;
Kimura et al., 1981; Lehmann and Fibiger, 1978; Lehmann et al., 1980;
Lloyd et al., 1975; Nieoullon and Dusticier, 1980; Takano et al.,
1980). Muscarinic receptors are also present in relatively high concentrations, whereas the number of nicotinic receptors is considerably
lower (Brand, 1980; De Belleroche and Bradford, 1978; Marchand et al.,
1979; McGeer et al., 1979).

Several years ago it was thought that the AChE containing
striato-nigral neurons were cholinergic (Olivier et al., 1970) but
later it was established that the enzyme AChE is not a completely
reliable marker for cholinergic neurons (the nigro-striatal dopamine
neurons also contain AChE (Lehmann and Fibiger, 1978; Lehmann et al.,
1980). It has been possible to visualize the striatal cholinergic
neurons by a new histochemical technique for AChE using DFP (Brand,
1980; Henderson, 1981; Lehmann and Fibiger, 1978; Lehmann et al.,
1980; Parent et al., 1980) and by means of a newly developed immunohistochemical technique for CAT (Kimura et al., 1980, 1981). These
studies have shown that the cholinergic neurons of the striatum are
intrinsic neurons and belong to the so-called large "aspiny" cell type
and not to the medium-sized, spiny cells. These results are in agreement with the biochemical studies on CAT, choline uptake, muscarinic
and nicotinic receptors which have demonstrated that the cholinergic
system is relatively evenly distributed throughout the entire extent
of nucleus caudatus and putamen (Kimura et al., 1980, 1981; Takano
et al., 1980).

The large, or giant, neurons which have only a few long dendrites
with few spines represent only about 1 to 5 percent of the cell population of the striatum (for references, see Divac and Oberg, 1979;
Henderson, 1981; Kimura et al., 1980, 1981). Recently it has been
found that the noncholinergic, medium-sized, spiny neurons which represent about 90 to 95 percent of the neurons of striatum, are efferent neurons (Henderson, 1981; Park et al., 1980; Preston et al., 1980;
Scheel-Krüger et al., 1981a,b). These findings are directly contrary
to previous notions of the neuronal organization of the striatum,
because it was thought that the medium-sized, spiny neurons were interneurons (for discussion, see Graybiel and Ragsdale, 1979; Park et
al., 1980). It also seems that the very extensive dendritic field of
the medium spiny neurons receives neuronal inputs from all the known
afferents to the striatum, i.e., substantia nigra (dopaminergic and
non-dopaminergic inputs), nucleus dorsalis raphe (serotonin), the
intralaminar nuclei of thalamus (transmitters unknown) and the cortex

(glutamic acid). According to Park et al. (1980) and Preston et al. (1980) the major influence on striatal functions is mediated by the extrastriatal afferents innervating the medium spiny neurons together with a mechanism of extensive dendritic and/or collateral inhibition exerted among the medium spiny, GABAergic neurons, whilst the cholinergic interneurons only represent a minor contribution quantitatively. These findings and ideas provide an interesting challenge for future studies of the physiological significance of the cholinergic interneurons of the striatum. It seems likely that the local cholinergic contribution to striatal functions has been overestimated in the past, at least quantitatively.

5.2. Interactions With Other Neurotransmitters

A great deal of attention has been devoted to the intrastriatal mechanisms involved in the regulation of the cholinergic interneurons. In numerous studies it has been found that stimulation of the nigrostriatal dopamine system or the systemic injection of dopamine agonists induces a decrease in the release of acetylcholine in the striatum and blockade of striatal dopamine receptors by antipsychotic drugs facilitates acetylcholine release (Bartholini, 1980; Bartholini et al., 1973; Costa et al., 1978; Stadler et al., 1973; Trabucchi et al., 1975). Tolerance to these effects develops after repeated administration of dopamine agonists or antagonists (Scatton and Worms, 1979; Costa et al., 1978). Serotonin released from the raphe-striatal system inhibits the cholinergic interneurons (Vizi et al., 1981; Samanin et al., 1978), and they are also inhibited by the striatal GABA neurons by a mechanism of action involving the corticostriatal, possibly glutaminergic, neurons (Scatton and Bartholini, 1980a,b). This result is interesting, since in another study it has been found that the turnover of acetylcholine in the striatum is increased by the activity and/or presence of the corticostriatal system (Wood et al., 1979).

5.3. Cholinergic Regulation of Striatal Dopamine Activity

Striatal dopamine release is facilitated by acetylcholine acting on presynaptic nicotinic receptors located on the dopamine nerve terminals (De Belleroche and Bradford, 1978; Giorguieff-Chesselet et al., 1979). The function of muscarinic receptors in the striatum seems to be a more controversial topic since some investigators found reduced dopamine release (De Belleroche and Bradford, 1978), whereas others report facilitation of dopamine release (Bartholini, 1980). Muscarinic receptors located on extrastriatal sites may also increase the striatal dopamine release (Anden and Wachtel, 1977; Taha and Redgrave, 1980).

5.4. Acetylcholine Effect on Striatal Output Neurons

The extensive amount of research on the nigrostriatal regulation of the cholinergic neurons contrasts considerably with the scanty, or

complete lack of, information on the role of acetylcholine in the
striatal efferent neurons. The functional significance of the dopamine agonists decreasing striatal acetylcholine release and antagonists increasing release is not understood at present. The intracerebral injection of methylscopolamine (20 µg) into various regions of
the striatum does not induce amphetamine-like or apomorphine-like
stereotyped behavior but only a modest and shortlasting (15 minutes)
locomotion and rearing activity has been seen (Scheel-Krüger, in preparation). The immobility and catalepsy induced by the neuroleptic,
haloperidol, are not antagonized by the intrastriatal injection of
atropine or methylscopolamine (Costall et al., 1972a, De Montis et
al., 1979; Scheel-Krüger, in preparation).

     There is some indirect evidence that acetylcholine may facilitate
the activity of the striatopallidal/enkephalin neurons (Hong et al.,
1980) but there seems no direct information about the effect of acetylcholine on the major efferent systems of the striatum projecting
to the globus pallidus, the pallido-entopeduncular nucleus (corresponding to the medial segment of globus pallidus in primates) and the
substantia nigra-zona reticulata. It has been found that GABA and
Substance P are transmitters in these striatal efferent systems (for
references, see Jessel et al., 1978; Scheel-Krüger and Magelund, 1981;
Scheel-Krüger et al., 1981a,b; Staines et al., 1980). Recent evidence
strongly suggests that various functions related to stimulation of
striatal dopamine receptors are mediated by a dopamine-induced activation of the striato-pallido-entopenduncular and striatonigral, GABA-
ergic pathways (DiChiara et al., 1981; Scheel-Krüger and Magelund,
1981; Scheel-Krüger et al., 1980, 1981a,b). The significance of the
striatal cholinergic neurons in these striatal output functions still
remains unknown, although recent evidence suggests that muscarinic
receptors may be localized on GABA containing striatal output neurons
(McGeer et al., 1979) and stimulation of muscarinic receptors can
induce a local increase of GABA release in the striatum (Van der
Heyden et al., 1980).

     In many previous reviews the cholinergic interneurons were inter-
spaced in the neuronal circuitry of the striatum between afferent dopaminergic nerve terminals and efferent GABAergic neurons. Today it is
obvious that this model is much too simple to explain many of the
results discussed in this paper. The major significant role of acetylcholine may even be challenged, since the population of interneurons, including cholinergic interneurons, only represents among 1 to 5
percent in total of the striatal neurons (Kimura et al., 1980, 1981).

5.5. Behavioral Functions of Acetylcholine in the Striatum

     In Parkinsonsian patients there is an imbalance between dopamine
and acetylcholine. It is possible that dopaminergic hypofunction and
the relative hyperactive cholinergic system in the striatum contribute
to various syndromes of this disease such as tremor and rigidity (see

Bartholini, 1980; Stadler et al., 1973; Trabucchi et al., 1975). In
support of this hypothesis, intracerebral injection of cholinomimetics
into the caudate nucleus of various animal species induces neurological syndromes such as tremor, limb dystonia, lack of motor coordination, disturbances of posture, head turning and akinesia, (Connor et
al., 1966; Cools, 1977; Hull et al., 1967; Matthews and Chiou, 1978;
McKenzie et al., 1972; Standefer and Dill, 1977; Stevens et al.,
1961).

    The intracerebral injection of cholinomimetics into the substan-
tia nigra also induces symptoms such as tremor (Cox and Potkonjak,
1969; De Montis et al., 1979) and catalepsy-immobility (De Montis et
al., 1979; Scheel-Krüger et al., in preparation) which indicate the
involvement of extrastriatal brain areas for cholinergic symptoms.
However, in contrast to these neurological syndromes induced by the
intracerebral injection of high doses of cholinergic drugs, the intrastriatal injection of lower doses of cholinergic drugs induce quietude
and apparent drowsiness in cats (Stevens et al., 1961) and changes in
conditioned behavior and locomotor activity in rats (Neill and
Grossman, 1970; Neill and Herndon, 1978; Neill et al., 1978; Prado-
Alcala et al., 1980).

5.6.   Striatal Acetylcholine, Parkinsonism, Catalepsy and Immobility
       Induced by Neuroleptic Drugs

    Since the biochemical studies have shown that neuroleptic drugs
with dopamine receptor blocking properties induce an increase of acetylcholine release within the striatum, it has been argued that cholinergic hyperfunction contributes to the Parkinsonian-like, extrapyramidal side effects induced by the systemic injection of neuroleptic drugs (Bartholini, 1980; Bartholini et al., 1973; Costa et al.,
1978; Stadler et al., 1973; Trabucchi et al., 1975). Support for this
hypothesis comes from the results in animals, where the systemic injection of anticholinergic drugs clearly antagonized the extrapyramidal side effects such as tremor, rigidity, immobility and catalepsy
induced by neuroleptic drugs (Arnt and Christensen, 1981; Bartholini,
1980).

    However, there is no experimental support from rat studies that
cholinergic hyperactivity in the striatum is significant for the syndrome of immobility and catalepsy induced by neuroleptic drugs. Later
I will present evidence for a role of the substantia nigra, zona
reticulata in this effect. Several years ago, Costall et al. (1972a)
found that the bilateral injection of atropine into the caudate-
putamen did not modify the catalepsy induced by a systemic injection
of haloperidol and the intrastriatal injection of arecoline did not
produce catalepsy. Systemic injections of muscarinic agonists induced
immobility and catalepsy in rodents but the mechanism of action of
cholinergic catalepsy was distinct from that elicited by neuroleptic
drugs because striatal lesion potentiated cholinergic-induced
catalepsy but abolished the catalepsy induced by neuroleptic drugs.

(Costall and Olley, 1971a,b; Sanberg et al., 1981). However, a lesion
of the substantia nigra abolished the tremor and catalepsy after both
systemically injected arecoline and haloperidol (Costall and Olley,
1971b). The presence of noradrenaline also seems important for cholinergically-induced catalepsy (Mason, 1978).

These studies by Costall et al., have recently been confirmed by
us (De Montis et al., 1979; Scheel-Krüger et al., in preparation).
We injected methylscopolamine (20 µg bilaterally) into the dorsal
or ventral part of the central striatum or the rostral, ventromedial
part of the striatum of rats. The results showed that methylscopolamine given 60 minutes after haloperidol (0.50 mg/kg s.c.) had no significant influence on the haloperidol-induced akinesia, immobility or
catalepsy.

5.7. Differential Functions of Acetylcholine Within Distinct Areas of
     the Striatum

There is a considerable amount of evidence for functional and
regional heterogeneity with respect to the striatal influence on many
behaviors (Cools, 1977; Divac and Oberg, 1979). This heterogeneity
within the striatum is also supported by the heterogeneous anatomical
organization of the various afferent and efferent striatal connections
(Divac and Oberg, 1979; Jessel et al., 1978; Graybiel and Ragsdale,
1979; Staines et al., 1980; Veening, 1980). The available evidence
suggests that the cholinergic system is distributed throughout the
entire extent of the nucleus caudatus and the putamen as seen by the
localization of cholinergic interneurons (Kimura et al., 1980, 1981)
and the biochemical markers for cholinergic functions, i.e., CAT, choline high affinity uptake and muscarinic receptors (Brand, 1980;
Lehmann et al., 1980; Parent et al., 1980: Takano et al., 1980).
These findings indicate that the intrinsic striatal cholinergic systems may influence multiple functions.

However, there are only a few animal studies on the behavioral
role of cholinergic mechanisms within various regions of the striatum.
An excellent review by Cools (1977) discussed two distinct dopaminergic-cholinergic systems localized anatomically in various regions of
the striatum and interconnected by two distinct types of dopamine
systems, i.e., the DAi and the DAe systems. The cholinergic system
responsible for the elicitation of tremor is influenced by the DAi
dopamine system, whereas stimulation of cholinergic receptors within
another striatal region produces effects (contralateral head turning)
identical to those evoked by stimulation of the DAe dopamine system
in the cat. Wolfarth and Kolasiewicz (1977) have also suggested a
cholinergic system in the striatum which acts synergistically with
dopamine for stereotyped behavior in rabbits.

Studies of conditioned behavior or lateral hypothalamus self-
stimulation have found a regional differentiation of cholinergic functions within the caudate nucleus of rats; in fact, it was found that

blockade of cholinergic muscarinic receptors in the dorsal and the
ventral caudate nucleus produced completely opposite effects. Acetylcholine acted antagonistically to dopamine within the ventral anterior
striatum (Neill and Grossman, 1970; Neill and Herndon, 1978; Neill
et al., 1978; Prado-Alacala et al., 1980).

5.8.   Differential Influence of Cholinergic Mechanisms Within the
        Dorsal and Ventral Part of the Striatum on Apomorphine-Induced
        Stereotyped Behavior

In our study it was found that apomorphine-induced stereotyped
behavior was potentiated by a local injection of carbachol into the
dorsal region of the central striatum, whereas carbachol injected into
the ventral region of the central striatum induced a complete blockade
of the apomorphine-induced stimulation. Methylscopolamine injected
into the dorsal and the ventral striatum induced respectively inhibition or facilitation of apomorphine stereotypy. As these experiments
have not yet been published (Scheel-Krüger et al., in preparation)
they are described briefly. Male rats were implanted with cannulae
aimed for the dorsal and the ventral parts of the central striatum
localized immediately rostrally to the globus pallidus. Intracerebral
injections of carbachol chloride or methylscopolamine nitrate were
performed 6 to 10 days after the operation. Apomorphine (0.50 mg/kg)
was injected subcutaneously immediately after the intracerebral injection of drugs or placebo and each rat was then returned to its own
home cage. Each rat was tested only once.

The studies provided no clear-cut or conclusive results when carbachol (2.5 µg) was injected into the most rostral region of the
striatum (data now shown), but significant effects were found when
carbachol was injected more caudally into the central part of the
striatum.

As shown in Table 4, carbachol injected bilaterally into the
dorsal part of the central striatal region (2.5 and 5 µg) induced a
very strong increase in the characteristic stereotyped licking and
gnawing activity produced by apomorphine (0.50 mg/kg s.c.). Such a
strong, continuous licking and gnawing activity is normally only
induced by much higher doses of apomorphine (1.5 to 2.5 mg/kg s.c.)
in our rats (Scheel-Krüger, unpublished results). Carbachol injected
into the dorsal part of the central striatum also decreased the apomorphine-induced locomotion and rearing. These effects also correspond to the behavioral syndrome seen in the rat after apomorphine
given in high doses. In contrast, 2.5 µg carbachol injected into the
ventral part of the central region of the striatum (which is localized
just 2 mm more ventrally than the dorsal injection site) induced a
complete and total blockade of apomorphine-induced activity and all
tested rats remained immobile and sedated for 40 to 50 minutes after
the apomorphine injection. The methylscopolamine data also provided
evidence for a different influence of the dorsal and the ventral parts

of the striatum on apomorphine-induced stereotypy. To some extent
methylscopolamine produced effects which were complementary to the
effects of carbachol. The rats injected with methylscopolamine
(20 µg) into the ventral part of the central region of the striatum
appeared very calm and quiet after apomorphine (0.50 mg/kg s.c.) but
nevertheless all of them showed biting and gnawing activity (Table 4).
In contrast, rats injected into the dorsal part of the striatum showed
more locomotor and rearing activity after apomorphine (0.50 mg/kg
s.c.). Methylscopolamine injected into this region also decreased
the occurrence of stereotyped licking and gnawing activity (Table 4).

The effects of carbachol and methylscopolamine alone on the
gross behavior of the rats have also been tested. Methylscopolamine
(20 µg) produced no obvious behavioral changes after injection into
the dorsal part of the central striatum whereas carbachol (1 to 2.5 µg)
injected at this site induced a small increase of locomotor and rearing activity. Carbachol 1 µg injected into the ventral part of the
central striatum induced a slight sedative effect, whereas methylscopolamine (20 µg) induced a short-lasting (15 minutes) and a small
increase in locomotion, rearing and sniffing.

5.9. Differential Effects on Turning Behavior of Acetylcholine Within
      Various Areas of the Striatum

Recently we found that carbachol (1 µg) injected unilaterally
into the ventral part of the central region of the striatum (localized
immediately rostrally to the globus pallidus) induced a clear ipsiversive postural effect in the rat. Carbachol in a dose of 5 µg was
less active in this region. In contrast, carbachol (especially in the
higher dose range, i.e., 5 µg) injected 2 mm more dorsally into the
striatum produced a contraversive postural effect (Scheel-Krüger), in
preparation.

These findings that different and even opposite effects may be
elicited from different intrastriatal sites may explain much of the
apparent contradictory results published by others. Some studies have
reported ipsiversive head turning and postural effects after unilateral injections of various cholinomimetics into the striatum of the
rat (Costall et al., 1972a; McKenzie et al., 1972), whereas other
investigators found contraversive postural effects in the rat (Dill
et al., 1968; Matthews and Chiou, 1978). Contraversive effects have
also been reported in the cat (Stevens et al., 1961; Hull et al.,
1967; Cools, 1977).

Table 4. Effect of Intrastriatal Injections of Cholinergic Drugs on Apomorphine Stereotypy

			Percentage of rats demonstrating various behavioral effects		Rating groups of stereotypy**			
	(N)	Striatal* Region	Locomotion	Rearing	a	b	c	d
2.5 μg Carbachol	(7)	dorsal	28%	28%	0%	0%	0%	100%
5 μg Carbachol	(7)	dorsal	28%	14%	0%	0%	0%	100%
20 μg Methylscopolamine	(5)	dorsal	80%	40%	60%	20%	0%	20%
Aquadest.	(12)	dorsal	83%	42%	25%	33%	33%	8%
2.5 μg Carbachol	(10)	ventral	10%	10%	0%	0%	0%	0%
20 μg Methylscopolamine	(5)	ventral	20%	20%	0%	0%	60%	40%
Aquadest.	(10)	ventral	90%	40%	30%	40%	30%	0%

N = number of rats. All rats received apomorphine 0.50 mg/kg subcutaneously immediately after the injection of cholinergic drugs into the central part of the striatum (*coordinates Ant. 7-7.4 Lat 2.3-2.6 within the dorsal region DV 1.5-2 or ventral region DV-(0.6-1.2). The rats were observed continuously after the injection of apomorphine and the behavior and stereotypy classified according to the following** rating groups: (a) continuous sniffing, (b) continuous sniffing + episodic licking (c) continuous sniffing + episodic licking and gnawing (d) continuous licking and gnawing.

5.10. Comments and Discussion

The present results provide support for the conclusion that acetylcholine within various regions of the striatum participates in
different behavioral effects and may even have directly antagonistic
functions for certain behaviors (see also Cools, 1977; Neill et al.
1970, 1978; Prado-Alcala, 1980). In the studies by Neill et al.
(1970, 1978), acetylcholine acted antagonistically to dopamine within
the ventral anterior part of the striatum in the rat for lateral hypothalamus self-stimulation or conditioned behavior. In our work the
inhibitory cholinergic system influencing apomorphine and dopamine
dependent stereotyped behavior was localized more caudally in the
ventral part of the central region of the striatum.

The effects of intracerebrally injected carbachol and methylscopolamine on apomorphine stereotypy cannot be interpreted as a cholinergic influence on endogenous dopamine release. The behavioral syndrome of apomorphine is dependent on stimulation of post-synaptic dopamine receptors localized on neurons beyond the dopamine nerve terminals and is thus independent of the presynaptic dopamine system. The
cholinergic effect seems more related to a cholinergic influence on
the striatal output systems mediating dopaminergic functions. Our
results demonstrated that distinct cholinergic mechanism within various regions, i.e., a dorsal and a ventral part of the striatum, mediate opposite functional effects, which are most likely related to a
direct effect on distinct output systems that are involved in the mediation of striatal dopaminergic functions.

6.   PRESENCE AND FUNCTIONS OF ACETYLCHOLINE IN THE SUBSTANTIA NIGRA

For many years, the possible function of acetylcholine in the
substantia nigra has been a very controversial topic. It is known
that acetylcholine, its synthesizing enzyme, choline acetyltransferase
(CAT) and its metabolizing enzyme, acetylcholinesterase (AChE), are
present in the substantia nigra but in lower concentrations than in
the striatum (Collingridge and Davis, 1981; Cross and Waddington,
1980; De Montis et al., 1979; Lehmann and Fibiger, 1978; Lehmann et
al., 1980; Nieoullon and Dusticier, 1980). There is also evidence for
a calcium dependent release mechanism of acetylcholine in the substantia nigra (Massey and James, 1978). Recent studies indicated that
muscarinic receptors are present both on the dopaminergic, zona compacta neurons and the non-dopaminergic, zona reticulata neurons (Cross
and Waddington, 1980; De Montis et al., 1979; Wolfarth, et al., 1979).

It has still not been possible to demonstrate a cholinergic
afferent system to the substantia nigra or intrinsic cholinergic neurons. However, it seems obvious that acetylcholine is not a transmitter in the striatonigral system as originally suggested by Olivier
et al. 1970. For further discussion and references see Lehmann and
Fibiger (1978) and Lehmann et al. (1980).

It has been reported that nigral CAT is strongly decreased in Parkinsonian patients, which suggests a role of nigral actylcholine in extrapyramidal functions (Javoy-Agid and Agid, 1980; Lloyd et al., 1975).

The data we have obtained (see later discussion) provide strong evidence for several distinct behavioral effects of acetylcholine which are related to various regions within the substantia nigra. The results reported by others provide complex and even contradictory results – probably because regional differences within the substantia nigra have not been considered. Biochemical studies indicate an in- hibitory effect of acetylcholine in the substantia nigra on the dop- amine release in the ipsilateral striatum (Javoy et al., 1974; James and Massey, 1978). However other behavioral studies indicate that carbachol injected into the rostral pole of the substantia nigra (zona compacta) elicit behavioral stimulation and stereotyped gnawing as a result of increased dopamine release in the striatum (Taha and Redgrave, 1980; Winn and Redgrave, 1979). Gnawing activity has also been reported after intranigral injection of cholinomimetics (Smelik and Ernst, 1966; Wolfarth et al., 1979).

6.1. The Interaction Between Acetylcholine, Dopamine and GABA in the Substantia Nigra

The substantia nigra has mainly been considered as important due to the presence of the nigrostriatal dopamine neurons. Considerably less attention has been paid to the possible functions of the non- dopaminergic, zona reticulata neurons, which project to the centrome- dial thalamus, the superior colliculus, the tegmental pedunculopontine nucleus, the periaqueductal gray and the reticular formation (for references see DiChiara et al., 1981; Scheel-Krüger, 1981a,b). Very recently, it has been realized that several behavioral effects related to the dopamine function in the striatum are mediated by the striatal GABAergic output neurons projecting to the pars reticulata in the sub- stantia nigra and the pallido-entopenduncular nucleus, corresponding to the medial and inner segment of the globus pallidus in the primates (for references, see DiChiara et al., 1981; Scheel-Krüger and Magelund, 1981; Scheel-Krüger et al., 1981a,b). The efferent neurons located in the pars reticulata and the pallido-entopeduncular nucleus represent the output pathways for various behavioral functions trig- gered by dopamine receptor stimulation in the striatum. Some progress has been made on the specific functions of the efferent projections of the zona reticulata neurons. The nigrothalamic projection seems to be involved in motor hyperfunction, catalepsy and immobility, the superior colliculus and the reticular formation in elements of stereo- typed behavior and turning behavior (for references, see DiChiara et al., 1981; Scheel-Krüger, 1981a,b).

All these studies have shown that the non-dopaminergic zona re- ticulata neurons in the substantia nigra function in opposition to the

dopamine, zona compacta neurons. The inhibition of the zona reticulata neurons by various GABA agonists or their destruction by kainic
acid induces behavioral effects corresponding to stimulation of striatal dopamine receptors (DiChiara et al., 1981; Olianas et al., 1978;
Scheel-Krüger et al., 1981a,b). The dopamine-mediated functions of
the striatum are thought to be mediated by a GABA-induced inhibition
of the non-dopaminergic, zona reticulata neurons in the substantia
nigra and in the pallido-entopeduncular nucleus and triggered by a
dopamine-induced activation of the striatonigral and striato-pallido-
entopeduncular, GABAergic pathways (DiChiara et al., 1981; Olianas et
al, 1978; Scheel-Krüger and Magelund, 1981; Scheel-Krüger et al.,
1981a,b).

    In agreement with this hypothesis we have found that the stimula-
tion of muscarinic receptors in the zona reticulata of the substantia
nigra produces marked behavioral effects such as immobility, catalepsy
and antagonism of apomorphine stereotyped behavior in the rat, like
neuroleptic drugs. Methylscopolamine injected locally into the zona
reticulata gives rise to a syndrome of amphetamine-like and apomorphine-like stimulation and stereotyped behavior independently of dopamine. Methylscopolamine also induced antagonism of haloperidol,
reserpine or α-methyltyrosine induced sedation and catalepsy.

    These findings strongly suggest that the functional and pharmaco-
logical interaction between dopamine and acetylcholine in the basal
ganglia system can be mediated as an interaction between GABA and
acetylcholine at the level of the output site located in the substantia nigra (De Montis et al., 1979; Scheel-Krüger and Arnt, in preparation). Most work previously has studied only the cholinergic influence on the neuronal activity of the dopamine zona compacta, nigrostriatal, neurons (Javoy et al., 1974; James and Massey, 1978). The
significance of our hypothesis is supported by electrophysiological
data which have shown that the nondopaminergic, zona reticulata neurons are excited and are very sensitive to muscarinic agonists, whereas the dopamine zona compacta neurons are relatively insensitive to
acetylcholine (Aghajanian and Bunney, 1975; Collingridge and Davis,
1981).

6.2. Different Behavioral Effects of Cholinergic Drugs Within Regions
     of the Substantia Nigra

    In these experiments in collaboration with Dr. J. Arnt, rats were
implanted with cannulae in the caudal part of the zona reticulata, the
caudal part of the zona compacta and the rostral part of the zona reticulata as in Table 5.

Table 5. Behavioral Effects Induced by Cholinergic Stimulation Within Various Regions of the Substantia Nigra

	N	Catalepsy	Duration	Dyskinetic Biting	Other Effects
Caudal SNR					
Carbachol 2.5 µg	7	100%	34-45 min	29%	Locomotion, rearing, sniffing
Carbachol 5.0 µg	12	100%	45-60 min	25%	(20-30 min) after the cataleptic period.
Oxotremorine 5.0 µg	4	75%	15 min	75%	
Oxotremorine 10.0 µg	8	88%	15-25 min	88%	
Caudal SNC					
Carbachol 2.5 µg	5	80%	10-15 min	0%	Locomotion, rearing, sniffing activity
Carbachol 5.0 µg	8	63%	10-15 min	38%	(25-80 min) after the cataleptic period.
Oxotremorine 10.0 µg	4	0%		0%	Only weak locomotion & sniffing (15-20 min).
Anterior SNR					
Carbachol 5.0 µg	11	27%	10 min	27%	Standing, rearing, episodic locomotion.
Oxotremorine 5.0 µg	5	0%		80%	Standing, rearing, episodic locomotion.
Oxotremorine 10.0 µg	5	0%		100%	

N = Number of rats tested. In the table is shown the percentage of rats showing catalepsy and dyskinetic biting activity after the intranigral injection of carbachol and oxotremorine. The coordinates of the caudal substantia nigra, zona reticulata (SNR) are Ant. 1.2-2, Lat. 2.2-2.6, DV-(2.5-3), caudal substantia nigra, zona compacta (SNC) Ant. 1.2-2 Lat 1.8-2.2 DV-(1.8-2.2) and anterior SNR Ant. 2.6-3 Lat 2-2.4 DV-(2.5-3) according to the König and Klippel (1973) atlas.

6.2.1. The Caudal Part of the Substantia Nigra, Zona Reticulata

Immediately after the injection, carbachol (2.5 and 5 µg) produced a strong and rigid catalepsy which lasted for 45 to 60 minutes
(Table 5). The rats were completely immobile in all of our tests,
i.e., a vertical wire netting, a horizontal bar, and on corks. Later,
i.e., 45 to 60 minutes after the injection of carbachol, these rats
displayed locomotion, rearing and sniffing for 20 to 30 minutes. The
muscarinic agonist oxotremorine (5 and 10 µg) also induced a cataleptic response in the rats immediately after the injection. A few
of the rats injected with carbachol and most of the rats injected with
oxotremorine during the immobile cataleptic period showed oral dyskinetic movements, biting and teeth chattering. However, these rats
showed no repetitive head movements, stereotyped sniffing or licking.

6.2.2. The Caudal Part of the Substantia Nigra, Zona Compacta

Carbachol (2.5 and 5 µg) only produced a short-lasting, immobile cataleptic effect which lasted for 10 to 15 minutes. The rats
then showed locomotion, rearing and sniffing which lasted for 25 to
80 minutes depending on the dose of carbachol (Table 5). Oxotremorine
(10 µg) did not induce catalepsy and only a weak short-lasting locomotion and sniffing was seen.

6.2.3. Anterior Substantia Nigra, Zona Reticulata

Carbachol (5 µg) only induced a short-lasting (i.e., 10 minutes)
cataleptic response in a few rats (3 out of 11 rats) and oxotremorine
(5 and 10 µg) did not induce immobility and catalepsy at all within
this nigral region (Table 5). Most of the rats injected with oxotremorine showed oral dyskinetic activity such as teeth chattering,
whereas this effect was only seen in a few rats injected with carbachol. The most characteristic effect of oxotremorine and carbachol
injected into the rostral SNR was a rearing and standing up towards
the walls with their nose pointing towards the roof of the cages,
leaning and almost falling backwards. Bursts of locomotion were seen.

6.2.4. Anterior Substantia Nigra, Zona Compacta

Recently we became aware of the results by Taha and Redgrave,
(1980); and Winn and Redgrave (1979), who reported that carbachol (1
to 5 µg) injected into the rostral pole of the substantia nigra,
zona compacta, induced behavioral activation and stereotyped licking
and gnawing in rats. These studies emphasize our conclusion (Scheel-
Krüger and Arnt, in preparation) that several distinct behavioral
effects can be ·seen after cholinomimetics are injected into various
regions of the substantia nigra.

Table 6. Methylscopolamine Induces Amphetamine-like Stimulation after Injection into the Caudal Part of Substantia Nigra, Zona Reticulata (SNR)

	N	Stereotyped gnawing/licking	Other effects	Duration
Methylscopolamine 10 μg	8	2/8	Locomotion, stereotyped sniffing	15-20 min
Methylscopolamine 20 μg	8	5/8	Forward/backward locomotion Sterotyped licking/gnawing often on own body	30-35 min

Pretreatments Haloperidol	N	Stereotyped gnawing	Antagonism of catalepsy	Duration	Other effects
+ Methylscopolamine 10 μg	8	3/8	6/8	40-80 min	Forward/backward locomotion (20-30 min) sterotyped sniffing, licking often on own body
+ Methylscopolamine 20 μg	6	5/6	5/6	80-100 min	sterotyped sniffing, licking often on own body
Reserpine + α-MT					
+ Methylscopolamine 5 μg	4	2/4	4/4	20-25 min	Forward/backward locomotion (15-20 min) sterotyped sniffing, licking often on own body
+ Methylscopolamine 10 μg	5	4/5	5/5	20-25 min	sterotyped sniffing, licking often on own body

N = Number of rats. Haloperidol (1 mg/kg) was injected s.c. 1 hour before methylscopolamine and reserpine (5 mg/kg s.c.) and α-methyl-p-tyrosine (α-MT 250 mg/kg) was injected 20 hours and 1.5 hours before methylscopolamine. For further details on the behavioral effects see the text.

6.2.5. Methylscopolamine Injected into the Substantia Nigra

Methylscopolamine injected bilaterally into the caudal part of
the zona reticulata elicited clear cut amphetamine-like behavioral
activation (Table 6). After a 10 µg dose there was locomotion,
rearing and stereotyped sniffing. Licking activity was seen in 2 out
of 8 rats tested. Methylscopolamine (20 µg) induced a short-lasting
locomotor activity and then the rats sat in the crouched posture
typical of high doses of amphetamine (5 to 10 mg/kg) and performed
stereotyped side to side movements of the head. Methylscopolamine
induced also stereotyped sniffing, licking and gnawing of the bottom
of the cage or their own body. Even backward locomotion typical for
amphetamine was seen in some of the rats (4 out of 8 rats) after
methylscopolamine.

The amphetamine-like syndrome induced by methylscopolamine was
completely independent of dopamine activity. We found (Scheel-Krüger
and Arnt, in preparation) that pretreatment with haloperidol in a high
dose (1 mg/kg s.c.) or depletion of the catecholamines by reserpine
(5 mg/kg) +α-MT (250 mg/kg) did not block the behavioral stimulation
induced by intranigrally injected methylscopolamine at all. We found
rather that these pretreatments further enhanced the methylscopolamine
stereotypy (Table 6). The immobility and catalepsy induced by haloperidol or reserpine +α-MT was immediately antagonized by methylscopolamine. The intranigral injection of placebo had no significant
effect on behavior (7 rats tested, data not shown). The muscarinic
receptors in the caudal SNR may thus be a relevant site for the antagonism by anticholinergic drugs of neuroleptic catalepsy seen after
systemic injections (Arnt and Christensen, 1981; Setler et al., 1976;
Morpurgo and Theobald, 1964).

6.3. Cholinergic Influence on Stereotypy

In other studies we have found that intracerebral injections of
carbachol into the caudal SNR induced respectively a partial (2.5 µg)
or complete (5 µg) inhibition of the behavioral activation and stereotypy induced by a systemic dose of apomorphine (0.50 mg/kg). We
have also found (Scheel-Krüger and Arnt, in preparation) that the
apomorphine-like stereotyped stimulation produced by the GABA agonist
muscimol (25 ng) injected into the caudal part of SNR was completely
antagonized by the systemic injection of oxotremorine (0.25 mg/kg
s.c.).

6.4. Concluding Comments

All these findings strongly suggest that the functional antagonism seen after the systemic injection of dopaminergic and choliner-

gic drugs may anatomically be localized at a level beyond the striatal
dopamine nerve terminals (in the ventromedial striatum?) or in the
final output site located in the substantia nigra as an interaction
between GABA and acetylcholine.

Our results cannot be interpreted as a cholinergic influence on
the nigrostriatal dopamine neurons, nor can the carbachol induced catalepsy be interpreted as due to a depression of the nigrostriatal dopamine system, since the injection into the SNC dopamine containing
region induced little or no catalepsy. In fact carbachol injected
into the caudal SNR slightly increased the dopamine metabolite DOPAC
(15 to 50 percent) which depended on the dose (1 to 5 μg) and the
time schedule but had no significant effect on the striatal dopamine
level. It seems that the behavioral effects of carbachol or methylscopolamine are best related to an effect on the efferent zona reticulata neurons (De Montis et al., 1979; Scheel-Krüger et al., 1981a,b;
Wolfarth et al., 1979).

7.   THE INTERACTION BETWEEN DOPAMINE AND ACETYLCHOLINE IN THE LIMBIC
      SYSTEM

The integration of functions related to dopamine and acetylcholine is not restricted to the basal ganglia system. In a recent study
it has been suggested that the mesolimbic dopamine system is involved
in the regulation of the septal-hippocampal cholinergic neurons
(Robinson et al., 1979). Unfortunately, there is no information
available at the moment on the effects of psychotropic drugs on the
extensive cholinergic system localized in the basal forebrain, including "the ventral pallidum," the substantia innominata and the nucleus
basalis magnocellularis. This system constitutes the origin of a
major cholinergic projection to the neocortex (Lehmann et al., 1980;
Mesulam and Geschwind, 1978; Wenk et al., 1980). The importance of
this system to various dopamine-related diseases, including schizophrenia, is obvious when it is considered that the major neuronal output of the mesolimbic and dopamine-rich nucleus accumbens is directed
towards the substantia innominata (Mesulam and Geschwind, 1978;
Scheel-Krüger et al., 1981b). We have found that behavioral effects
related to dopamine receptor stimulation in the nucleus accumbens in
the rat can be induced by a dopamine increase of the nucleus accumbens
- substantia innominata, GABAergic pathway and this effect may influence the cholinergic neurons innervating the neocortex (for further
discussion, see Scheel-Krüger et al., 1981b). Furthermore, since the
cortex provides extensive innervation of the striatum (for references
see Divac and Oberg, 1979; Graybiel and Ragsdale, 1979) it is likely
that the cholinergic neurons localized in the basal forebrain provide
a neuronal link for the integration of functions of the limbic and
striatal systems.

REFERENCES

Aghajanian, G. K., and Bunney, B. S., 1975, Dopaminergic and non-
    dopaminergic neurons of the substantia nigra: Differential
    responses to putative transmitters, in "Neuropsychopharmacology,
    vol. 359, J. R. Boissier, H. Hippius and D. Pichot, eds., pp.
    444-452, Elsevier, Amsterdam.
Anden, N.-E., and Wachtel, H., 1977, Increase in the turnover of brain
    dopamine by stimulation of muscarinic receptors outside the dopa-
    mine nerve terminals, J. Pharm. Pharmacol. 29:435-437.
Arnt, J., and Christensen, A. V., 1981, Differential reversal by
    scopolamine and THIP of the antistereotypic and cataleptic effects
    of neuroleptics, Eur. J. Pharmacol. 69:107-111.
Bartels, M., Gaertner, H.-J., and Golfinopoulos, G., 1981, Acathisia-
    Syndrome: Involvement of noradrenergic mechanism, J. Neural
    Transm. 52:33-39.
Bartholini, G., 1980, Interaction of striatal dopaminergic, cholin-
    ergic and GABAergic neurons: relation to extrapyramidal function,
    TIPS 138-140.
Bartholini, G., Stadler, H., and Lloyd, K. G., 1973, Cholinergic-
    dopaminergic interactions in the extrapyramidal system, Adv.
    Neurol. 3:233-241.
Boissier, J.-R., and Simon, P., 1964, Equivalences experimentales du
    syndrome neurologique des Neuroleptiques, Encephale 53:109-122.
Brand, S., 1980, A comparison of the distribution of acetylcholin-
    esterase and muscarinic cholinergic receptors in the feline
    neostriatum, Neurosci. Lett. 17:113-117.
Casey, D. E., and Denney, D., 1977, Pharmacological characterization
    of tardive dyskinesia, Psychopharmacology 54:1-8.
Casey, D. E., Gerlach, J., and Christensson, E., 1980, Dopamine,
    acetylcholine, and GABA effects in acute dystonia in primates,
    Psychopharmacology 70:83-87.
Christensen, A. V., 1981, Dopamine hyperactivity: Effects of neuro-
    leptics alone or in combination with GABA-agonists, in "Proc. of
    the III World Congress of Biological Psychiatry," B. Jansson, C.
    Perris and G. Strüwe, eds., pp. 828-832, Elsevier/North Holland,
    Amsterdam.
Christensen, A. V., Arnt, J., and Scheel-Krüger, J., 1979, Decreased
    antisterotypic effect of neuroleptics after additional treatment
    with a benzodiazepine, a GABA agonist or an anticholinergic com-
    pound, Life Sci. 24:1395-1402.
Christensen, A. V., Arnt, J., and Scheel-Krüger, J., 1980, GABA-
    dopamine neuroleptic interaction after systemic administration,
    Brain Res. Bull. 5:885-890.
Collingridge, G., and Davies, J., 1981, The influence of striatal
    stimulation and putative neurotransmitters on identified neurons
    in the rat substantia nigra, Brain Res. 212:345-359.
Connor, J. D., Rossi, G. V., and Baker, W. W., 1966, Analysis of the
    tremor induced by injection of cholinergic agents into the caudate
    nucleus, Int. J. Neuropharmacol. 5:207-216.

Cools, A. R., 1977, Basic considerations on the role of concertedly working GABA-ergic, cholinergic and serotonergic mechanisms within the neostriatum and nucleus accumbens in locomotor activity, stereotyped gnawing, turning and dyskinetic activities, in "Cocaine and Other Stimulants, Adv. Behav. Biol., Vol. 21," E. H. Ellinwood and M. M. Kilbey, eds. pp. 97-141, Plenum Press, New York.

Costa, E., Cheney, D. L., Mao, C. C., and Moroni, F., 1978, Action of antischizophrenic drugs on the metabolism of γ-aminobutyric acid and acetylcholine in globus pallidus, striatum and n. accumbens, Fed. Proc. 37:2408-2414.

Costall, B., and Naylor, R. J., 1976, A comparison of the abilities of typical neuroleptic agents and of thioridazine, clozapine, sulpiride and metoclopramide to antagonize the hyperactivity induced by dopamine applied intracerebrally to areas of the extrapyramidal and mesolimbic systems, Eur. J. Pharmacol. 40:9-19.

Costall, B., Naylor, R. J., Cannon, J. G., and Lee, T., 1977, Differential activation by some 2-aminotetralin derivatives of the receptor mechanisms in the nucleus accumbens of rat which mediate hyperactivity and stereotyped biting, Eur. J. Pharmacol. 41:307-319.

Costall, B., Naylor, R. J., and Olley, J. E., 1972a, Catalepsy and circling behavior after intracerebral injections of neuroleptic, cholinergic and anticholinergic agents into the caudate-putamen, globus pallidus and substantia nigra of rat brain, Neuropharmacology 11:645-663.

Costall, B., Naylor, R. J., and Wright, T., 1972b, The use of amphetamine-induced stereotyped behavior as a model for the experimental evaluation of antiparkinson agents, Arzneim.-Forsch. 22:1178-1183.

Costall, B., and Olley, J. E., 1971a, Cholinergic- and neuroleptic-induced catalepsy: Modification by lesions in the caudate-putamen, Neuropharmacology 10:297-306.

Costall, B., and Olley, J. E., 1971b, Cholinergic- and neuroleptic-induced catalepsy: Modification by lesions in the globus pallidus and substantia nigra, Neuropharmacology 10:581-594.

Cox, B., and Potkonjak, D., 1969, An investigation of the tremorgenic effects of oxotremorine and tremorine after stereotaxic injection into rat brain, Int. J. Neuropharmacol. 8:291-297.

Cross, A. J., and Waddington, J. L., 1980, ^{3}H-Quinuclidinyl benzylate and ^{3}H-GABA receptor binding in rat substantia nigra after 6-hydroxy-dopamine lesions, Neurosci. Lett. 17:271-275.

Davis, K. L., Berger, P. A., Hollister, L. E. and Barchas, J. D., 1978, Cholinergic involvement in mental disorders, Life Sci. 22:1865-1872.

De Belleroche, J. S., and Bradford, H., 1978, Compartmentation of synaptosomal dopamine, in "Adv. Biochem. Psychopharmacol., Vol. 19," P. J. Roberts, G. N. Woodruff and L. L. Iversen, eds., pp. 57-73, Raven Press, New York.

De Montis, G. M., Olianas, M. C., Serra, G., Tagliamonte, A. and
    Scheel-Krüger, J., 1979, Evidence that a nigra GABAergic-
    cholinergic balance controls posture, Eur. J. Pharmacol.
    53:181-190.
DiChiara, G., Morelli, M., Imperato, A., and Porceddu, M. L., 1981,
    Substantia nigra as an efferent station for dopaminergic
    behavioral syndromes arising in the striatum, in "Apomorphine and
    Other Dopaminomimetics Vol. 1: Basic Pharmacology," G. L. Gessa
    and G. U. Corsini, eds. pp. 41-64, Raven Press, New York.
Dill, R. E., Nickey Wm. Jr., and Little, M. D., 1968, Dyskinesia in
    rats following chemical stimulation of the neostriatums, Tex.
    Rep. Biol. Med. 26:101-106.
Divac, I., and Öberg, R. B., 1979, "The Neostriatum," Pergamon Press
    Oxford, U.K.
Ehlert, F. J., Roeske, W. R., and Yamamura, I., 1981, Striatal muscar-
    inic receptors: Regulation by dopaminergic agonists, Life Sci.
    28:2441-2448.
Fjalland, B., and Møller Nielsen, I., 1974, Methylphenidate antago-
    nism of haloperidol, interaction with cholinergic and anticholin-
    ergic drugs, Psychopharmacologia 34:111-118.
Gerlach, J., 1979, Tardive Dyskinesia (Thesis), Dan. Med. Bull.
    26:209-245.
Gerlach, J., Reisby, N., and Randrup, A., 1974, Dopaminergic hypersen-
    sitivity and cholinergic hypofunction in the pathophysiology of
    tardive dyskinesia, Psychopharmacologia 34:21-35.
Giorguieff-Chesselet, M. F., Kemel, M. L., Wandscheer, D., and
    Glowinski, J., 1979, Regulation of dopamine release by
    presynaptic nicotinic receptors in rat striatal slices; Effect
    of nicotine in a low concentration, Life Sci. 25:1257-1262.
Graybiel, A. M., and Ragsdale, C. W., 1979, Fiber connections of the
    basal ganglia, Prog. Brain Res. 51:239-283.
Henderson, Z., 1981, Ultrastructure and acetylcholinesterase content
    of neurons forming connections between the striatum and substantia
    nigra of rat, J. Comp. Neurol. 197:185-196.
Hong, J. S., Yang, H. T., Gillin, J. C., and Costa, E., 1980, Effects
    of long-term administration of antipsychotic drugs on enkephalin-
    ergic neurons, in "Long-term Effects of Neuroleptics, Adv.
    Biochem. Psychopharmacol., Vol. 24," F. Cattabeni, ed., pp.
    223-232, Raven Press, New York.
Hull, C. D., Buchwald, N. A., and Ling, G., 1967, Effects of direct
    cholinergic stimulation of forebrain structures, Brain Res.
    6:22-35.
James, T. A., and Massey, S., 1978, Evidence for a possible dopa-
    minergic link in the action of acetylcholine in the rat substantia
    nigra, Neuropharmacology 17:687-690.
Janowsky, D. S., El-Yousef, M. K., Davis, M., and Sekerke, H. J.,
    1973, Antagonistic effects of physostigmine and methylphenidate
    in man, Am. J. Psychiatry 130:1370-1376.

Javoy-Agid, F., Agid, Y., 1980, Is the mesocortical dopaminergic system involved in Parkinson's disease?, Neurology 30:1326-1330.

Javoy, F., Agid, Y., Bouvet, D., and Glowinski, J., 1974, Changes in neostriatial DA metabolism after carbachol or atropine microinjections into the substantia nigra, Brain Res. 68:253-260.

Jessel, T. M., Emson, P. C., Paxinos, G., and Cuello, A. C., 1978, Topographic projections of substance P and GABA pathways in the striato- and pallido-nigral system: A biochemical and immunohistochemical study, Brain Res. 152:487-498.

Kimura, H., McGeer, P. L., Peng, F., and McGeer, E. G., 1980, Choline acetyltransferase-containing neurons in rodent brain demonstrated by immunohistochemistry, Science 208:1057-1059.

Kimura, H., McGeer, P. L., Peng, J. H., and McGeer, E. G., 1981, The central cholinergic system studied by choline acetyltransferase immunohistochemistry in the cat, J. Comp. Neurol. 200:151-201.

König, J. F. R. and Klippel, R. A., 1963, "The Rat Brain: A Stereotaxic Atlas of the Forebrain and Lower Parts of the Brain Stem," Williams and Wilkins, Baltimore.

Lehmann, J., and Fibiger, H. C., 1978, Acetylcholinesterase in the substantia nigra and caudate-putamen of the rat: properties and localization in dopaminergic neurons, J. Neurochem. 30:615-624.

Lehmann, J., and Fibiger, H. C., 1979, The localization of acetylcholinesterase in the corpus striatum and substantia nigra of the rat following kainic acid lesion of the corpus striatum: A biochemical and histochemical study, Neuroscience 4:217-225.

Lehmann, J., Nagy, J. I., Atmadja, S., and Fibiger, H. C., 1980, The nucleus basalis magnocellularis: The origin of a cholinergic projection to the neocortex of the rat, Neuroscience 5:1161-1174.

Lloyd, K. G., Mohler, H., Heitz, Ph., and Bartholini, G., 1975, Distribution of choline acetyltransferase and glutamate decarboxylase within the substantia nigra and in other brain regions from control and parkinsonian patients, J. Neurochem. 25:789-795.

Mao, C. C., Cheney, L., Marco, E., Revuelta, A., and Costa, E., 1977, Turnover times of gamma-aminobutyric acid and acetylcholine in nucleus caudatus, nucleus accumbens, globus pallidus and substantia nigra: effects of repeated administration of haloperidol, Brain Res. 132:375-379.

Marchand, C. M.-F., Hunt, S. P., and Schmidt, J., 1979, Putative acetylcholine receptors in hippocampus and corpus striatum of rat and mouse, Brain Res. 160:363-367.

Mason, S. T., 1978, Pilocarpine: noradrenerigc mechanism of a cholinergic drug, Neuropharmacology 17:1015-1021.

Massey, S. C., and James, T. A., 1978, The uptake of ^{3}H-choline and release of ^{3}H-acetylcholine in the rat substantia nigra, Life Sci. 23:345-350.

Matthews, R. T., and Chiou, C. Y., 1978, Cholinergic stimulation of the caudate nucleus in rats: a model of parkinson's disease. Neuropharmacology 17:879-882.

McDevitt, J. T., and Setler, P. E., 1981, Differential effects of
    dopamine agonists in mature and immature rats, Eur. J. Pharmacol.
    72:69-75.
McGeer, P. L., McGeer, E. G., and Innanen, V. T., 1979, Dendro axonic
    transmission. I. Evidence from receptor binding of dopaminergic
    and cholinergic agents, Brain Res. 169:433-441.
McKenzie, G. M., Gordon, R. J., and Viik, K., 1972, Some biochemical
    and behavioral correlates of a possible animal model of human
    hyperkinetic syndromes, Brain Res. 47:439-456.
Mesulam, M.-M., and Geschwind, N., 1978, On the possible role of
    neocortex and its limbic connections in the process of attention
    and schizophrenia: clinical cases of inattention in man and
    experimental anatomy in monkey, J. Psychiatr. Res. 14:249-259.
Morpurgo, C., and Theobald, W., 1964, Influence of antiparkinson
    drugs and amphetamine on some pharmacological effects of pheno-
    thiazine derivatives used as neuroleptics, Psychopharmacologia
    6:178-191.
Neill, D. B., and Grossman, S. P., 1970, Behavioral effects of
    lesions or cholinergic blockade of the dorsal and ventral caudate
    of rats, J. Comp. Physiol. Psychol. 71:311-317.
Neill, D. B., and Herndon, J. G., 1978, Anatomical specificity within
    rat striatum for the dopaminergic modulation of DRL responding
    and activity, Brain Res. 153:529-538.
Neill, D. B., Peay, L. A., and Gold, M. S., 1978, Identification of a
    subregion within rat neostriatum for the dopaminergic modulation
    of lateral hypothalamic self-stimulation, Brain Res. 153:515-528.
Nieoullon, A., and Dusticier, N., 1980, Choline acetyltransferase
    activity in discrete regions of the cat brain, Brain Res.
    196:139-149.
Olianas, M. C., DeMontis, G. M., Concu, A., Tagliamonte, A., and
    DiChiara, G., 1978, Intranigral kainic acid: Evidence for nigral
    non-dopaminergic neurons controlling posture and behavior in a
    manner opposite to the dopaminergic ones, Eur. J. Pharmacol.
    49:223-232.
Olivier, A., Parent, A., Simard, H., and Poirier, L. J., 1970, Cholin-
    esterasic striatopallidal and striatonigral efferents in the cat
    and the monkey, Brain Res. 18:273-282.
Parent, A., O'Reilly-Fromentin, J., and Boucher, R., 1980, Acetylcho-
    linesterase-containing neurons in cat neostriatum: A morphologi-
    cal and quantitative analysis, Neurosci. Lett. 20:271-276.
Park, M. R., Lighthall, J. W., and Kitai, S. T., 1980, Recurrent
    inhibition in the rat neostriatum, Brain Res. 194:359-369.
Prado-Alcala, R. A., Cruz-Morales, S. E., and Lopez-Miro, F. A., 1980,
    Differential effects of cholinergic blockade of anterior and
    posterior caudate nucleus on avoidance behaviors, Neurosci. Lett.
    18:339-345.
Preston, R. J., Bishop, G. A., and Kitai, S. T., 1980, Medium spiny-
    neuron projection from the rat striatum: An intracellular
    horseradish peroxidase study, Brain Res. 183:253-263.

Robinson, S. E., Malthe-Sorensen, D., Wood, P. L., and Commissiong, J., 1979, Dopaminergic control of the septal-hippocampal cholinergic pathway, J. Pharmacol. Exp. Ther. 208:476–479.

Samanin, R., Quattrone, A., Peri, G., Ladinsky, H., and Consolo, S., 1978, Evidence of an interaction between serotonergic and cholinergic neurons in the corpus striatum and hippocampus of the rat brain, Brain Res. 151:73–82.

Sanberg, P. R., Pisa, M., and Fibiger, H. C., 1981, Kainic acid injections in the striatum alter the cataleptic and locomotor effects of drugs influencing dopaminergic and cholinergic systems, Eur. J. Pharmacol. 74:347–357.

Scatton, B., and Bartholini, 1980a, Increase in striatal acetylcholine levels by GABAergic agents: dependence on corticostriatal neurons, Brain Res. 200:174–178.

Scatton, B., and Bartholini, G., 1980b, Modulation of cholinergic transmission in the rat brain by GABA, Brain Res. Bull. 5:223–229.

Scatton, B., and Worms, P., 1979, Tolerance to increases in striatal acetylcholine concentrations after repeated administration of apomorphine dipivaloyl ester, J. Pharm. Pharmacol. 31:861–863.

Scheel-Krüger, J., 1970, Central effects of anticholinergic drugs measured by the apomorphine gnawing test in mice, Acta Pharmacol. Toxicol. 28:1–16.

Scheel-Krüger, J., 1971, Comparative studies of various amphetamine analogues demonstrating different interactions with the metabolism of the catecholamines in the brain, Eur. J. Pharmacol. 14:47–59.

Scheel-Krüger, J., Arnt, J., Magelund, G., Olianas, M., Przewlocka, B., and Christensen, A. V., 1980, Behavioral functions in GABA in the basal ganglia and limbic system, Brain Res. Bull. 5:261–267.

Scheel-Krüger, J., and Christensen, A. V., 1980, The role of gamma-aminobutyric acid in acute and chronic neuroleptic action, Adv. Biochem. Psychopharmacol. 24:233–243.

Scheel-Krüger, J., and Magelund, G., 1981, GABA in the entopeduncular nucleus and the subthalamic nucleus participates in mediating dopaminergic striatal output functions, Life Sci. 29:1555–1562.

Scheel-Krüger, J., Magelund, G., and Olianas, M. C., 1981a, Role of GABA in the striatal output system: globus pallidus, nucleus entopenduncularis, substantia nigra and nucleus subthalamicus, Adv. Biochem. Psychopharmacol. 30:165–186.

Scheel-Krüger, J., Magelund, G., and Olianas, M. C., 1981b, The role of GABA in the basal ganglia and limbic system for behavior, Adv. Biochem. Psychopharmacol. 29:23–36.

Scheel-Krüger, J., and Randrup, A., 1968, Pharmacological evidence for a cholinergic mechanism in brain involved in a special stereotyped behavior of reserpinized rats, Br. J. Pharmacol. 34:217P.

Scheel-Krüger, J., and Randrup, A., 1969, Evidence for a cholinergic mechanism in brain involved in the tetrabenazine reversal by thymoleptic drugs, J. Pharm. Pharmacol. 21:403–406.

Schiørring, E., and Randrup, A., 1968, "Paradoxical" stereotyped activity of reserpinized rats, Int. J. Neuropharmacol. 7:71–73.

Setler, P., Sarau, H., and McKenzie, G., 1976, Differential attentua-
    tion of some effects of haloperidol in rats given scopolamine,
    Eur. J. Pharmacol. 39:117-126.
Singh, M. M., and Kay, S. R., 1975, A comparative study of haloperidol
    and chlorpromazine in terms of clinical effects and therapeutic
    reversal with benztropine in schizophrenia. Theoretical implica-
    tions for potency differences among neuroleptics, Psychopharma-
    cologia 43:103-113.
Singh, M. M., and Kay, S. R., 1979, Therapeutic antagonism between
    anticholinergic antiparkinsonism agents and neuroleptics in
    schizophrenia, Neuropsychobiology 5:74-86.
Singh, M. M., and Lal, H., 1979, Dysfunctions of cholinergic processes
    in schizophrenia in "Biological Psychiatry Today," J. Obiols, C.
    Ballus, E. Gonzalez Monclus and J. Pujol, eds., pp. 434-438,
    Elsevier/North-Holland Biómedical Press, Amsterdam.
Smelik, P. G., and Ernst, A. M., 1966, Role of nigro-neostriatial
    dopaminergic fibers in compulsive gnawing behavior in rats, Life
    Sci. 5:1485-1588.
Stadler, H., Lloyd, K. G., Gadea-Ciria, M., and Bartholini,. G., 1973
    Enhanced striatal acetylcholine release by chlorpromazine and its
    reversal by apomorphine, Brain Res. 55:476-480.
Staines, Wm. A., Nagy, J. I., Vincent, S. R., and Fibiger, H. C.,
    1980, Neurotransmitters contained in the efferents of the stria-
    tum, Brain Res. 194:391-402.
Standefer, M. J., Dill, R. E., 1977, The role of GABA in dyskinesias
    induced by chemical stimulation of the striatum, Life Sci.
    21:1515-1520.
Stevens, J. R., Kim, C., and MacLean, P. D., 1981, Stimulation of
    caudate nucleus, Arch. Neurol. 4:47-54.
Taha, E. B., and Redgrave, P., 1980, Neuroleptic suppression of
    feeding and oral sterotypy following microinjections of carbachol
    into substantia nigra, Neurosci. Lett. 20:357-361.
Takano, Y., Kohjimoto, Y., Uchimura, K., and Kamiya, H-O, 1980,
    Mapping of the distribution of high affinity choline uptake and
    choline acetyltransferase in the striatum, Brain Res. 194:583-487.
Trabucchi, M., Cheney, D. L., Racagni, G., and Costa, E., 1975, In
    vivo inhibition of striatal acetylcholine turnover by L-DOPA,
    apomorphine and (+)-amphetamine, Brain Res. 85:130-134.
Van der Heyden, J. A. M., Venema, K., and Korf, J., 1980, In vivo
    release of endogenous γ-aminobutyric acid from rat striatum:
    Effects of muscimol, oxotremorine, and morphine, J. Neurochem.
    34:1648-1653.
Veening, J. G., Cornelissen, F. M., and Lieven, P. A. J., 1980, The
    topical organization of the afferents to the caudatoputamen of the
    rat. A horseradish peroxidase study, Neuroscience 5:1253-1268.
Vizzi, E. S., Harsing, L. G., and Zsilla, G., 1981, Evidence of the
    modulatory role of serotonin in acetylcholine release from
    striatal interneurons, Brain Res. 212:89-99.

Wenk, H., Bigl, V., and Meyer, U., 1980, Cholinergic projections from
    magnocellular nuclei of the basal forebrain to cortical areas in
    rats, Brain Res. Rev. 2:295-316.
Winn, P., and Redgrave, P., 1979, Feeding following microinjection
    of cholinergic substances into substantia nigra, Life Sci.
    25:333-338.
Wolfarth, S., and Kalasiewicz, W., 1977, The effects of intrastriatal
    injections of atropine and methacholine on the apomorphine
    induced gnawing in the rabbit, Pharmac. Biochem. Behav. 6:5-10.
Wolfarth, S., Wand, P., and Sontag, K. H., 1979, The effects of intra-
    nigral injections of picrotoxin and carbachol in cats with a
    lesioned nigrostriatal pathway, Neurosci. Lett. 11:197-200.
Wood, P. L., Moroni, F., Cheney, D. L., and Costa, E., 1979,
    Cortical lesions modulate turnover rates of acetylcholine and
    γ-aminobutyric acid, Neurosci. Lett. 12:349-354.

Chapter 5

CENTRAL CHOLINERGIC INVOLVEMENT IN LEARNING AND MEMORY

David G. Spencer, Jr. and Harbans Lal

Department of Pharmacology
Texas College of Osteopathic Medicine
Camp Bowie at Montgomery
Forth worth, Texas 76107, U.S.A.

1. INTRODUCTION

Drugs affecting cholinergic transmission in the brain have long been known to disrupt learned behaviors in rather specific ways. Several different theoretical formulations of cholinergic function have been developed focusing primarily on concepts such as behavioral inhibition (Carlton, 1963), discrimination (Milar et al., 1978), learning (Deutsch, 1973), and memory (Bartus and Johnson, 1976). Their differences seem to be due to differential emphasis on various

groups of experimental findings. In this review, we will examine
several experiments using cholinergic drugs to produce changes in
learning and/or memory performance, with the goal of generating a
hypothesis of central cholinergic function in cognitive processing.
In so doing, our discussion will be largely focused on the effects of
muscarinic receptor antagonists for two reasons. First, the vast
majority of acetylcholine (ACh) receptors in the mammalian brain are
of the muscarinic type. The predominance of muscarinic receptors is
also apparent in brain structures that seem specifically involved with
attentional, acquisitional, or memorial function, such as the hippocampus. Second, the effects of systemic muscarinic blockade on performance in memory tasks are much more striking than those of nicotinic stimulation or blockade. The discussion will also be limited
to cholinergic drug effects on behaviors requiring learning and/or
memory since it is clear that cholinergic transmission also participates in sensory processing (the auditory pathway), motor function
(the extrapyramidal motor system), and the alerting response, for
example. The implicit assumption is therefore that in focusing on
learning and memory performance, drug effects on the subset of cholinergic circuits dealing with such cognitive processes will predominate.

Much of the controversy over cholinergic function has to do with
whether ACh is directly involved with the acquisition (learning)
and/or maintenance (memory) of associative links between stimuli, or
between stimuli and responses, or whether it mediates processes that
are only indirectly involved in learning and memory. Such attendant
processes that have been implicated include perceptual discrimination,
selective attention, or regulation of overall excitatory-inhibitory
response "tone" (the general tendency to emit or withhold a response:
behavioral inhibition). Significant effects on any one of these hypothetical constructs will produce performance deficits in most situations. Accordingly, we will review and summarize the effects of cholinergic manipulations on animals performing different types of associative tasks. Drug effects on the development (learning) and maintenance (memory) of associative strength will be estimated through
their effects on stimulus control: i.e., the degree of relationship
between experimental variations in conditioned or discriminative stimuli and variations in the subsequent response accuracy. Drug effects
on behavioral inhibition will be estimated by the occurrence of specific drug-induced changes in (1) previously extinguished or non-reward-
ed discriminative responses, (2) previously punished responses, and
(3) responses to stimuli to which habituation has previously occurred.
It is recognized, however, that these three types of behavioral inhibition may be functionally and physiologically distinct.

In discussing the evidence on cholinergic manipulations, data
will be presented in procedurally-defined units, starting with the
classical conditioning paradigm. Spontaneous alternation (proposed
by Douglas and Isaacson [1966] to be based on habituation), passive
avoidance, and conditioned suppression will be considered next,
followed by active avoidance, discrimination, and memory procedures.

Memory procedures will be split into two main categories: delayed
response and delayed conditional discrimination. In the former, the
correct response to be made at the end of the retention interval is
specified by a stimulus presented before the interval. In the latter,
the type of correct response is unspecified until a comparison stimulus is presented at the end of the retention interval. The response
is, however, often specified in terms of the stimulus (e.g., go to the
red).

2.   CLASSICAL CONDITIONING

        In classical (Pavlovian) conditioning, a previously neutral stim-
ulus such as a tone is presented immediately before a stimulus that
unconditionally provokes a response from the organism (e.g., presentation of food, resulting in a salivation response). After a number of
such pairings, the preceding neutral stimulus begins by itself to
evoke a response usually quite similar to that produced by the unconditioned stimulus. The first systematic examination of the central
cholinergic role in the acquisition, maintenance, and extinction of
classical conditioning, was performed by Downs and coworkers (1972).
Using the rabbit nictitating eye membrane (NM) preparation, shock to
the outer eyelids was the unconditioned stimulus (US) for NM extension
(the unconditioned response, UR) while tones of varied frequency
served as either the conditioned stimulus correlated with shock (CS+)
or that uncorrelated with shock (CS-). Injection of atropine sulfate
(a centrally active muscarinic receptor blocker), but not of atropine
methylnitrate (a quaternary ammonium form of atropine that does not
readily pass the blood-brain barrier) or saline, retarded the rate of
acquisition of conditioned responses to the CS+ in dosages from 10 to
26 mg/kg. However, the frequency of URs throughout acquisition was
uninfluenced by the drug. Atropine was also found to reduce or abol-
ish the occurrence of conditioned heart rate changes in response to
the CS+ and CS-. When a separate group of rabbits first received extensive conditioning with no drug and were then exposed to it after
asymptotic conditioning had occurred, atropine sulfate, but not atropine methylnitrate or saline, markedly decreased conditioned NM responses (CRs) to the CS+ and did not affect CRs to the CS-, which were
almost nonexistent under control conditions. Finally, these experi-
menters conditioned previously untreated rabbits and extinguished the
conditioning (presented CS+s and CS-s without the USs) either under
atropine sulfate, atropine methylnitrate, or saline. Although atropine sulfate reduced the percent of CRs to both CSs in the first two
extinction sessions as compared to either control treatment, when saline was administered on the third extinction session, the percent of
CRs was no different from that during asymptotic conditioning sessions.
These data indicate that while central muscarinic blockade did not
affect expression of the NM response itself (since percent URs were
unaffected), atropine did retard acquisition of stimulus control by
CS+ and CS-, as well as extinction of stimulus control. Moreover,

atropine disrupted the expression of a previously conditioned response
to the CS+.

Moore et al. (1976) also used classical conditioning of NM response to investigate the effects of another muscarinic antagonist,
scopolamine hydrobromide. In their first experiment, these investigators found that scopolamine (1.5 mg/kg) failed to affect expression
of the UR to a low-intensity US (0.25 mA), thus agreeing with Downs
et al. (1972). In addition, scopolamine did not affect habituation
to the US (shock). Also in agreement with Downs et al. were their
findings that scopolamine hydrobromide (but not scopolamine methylbromide, a form that does not readily penetrate the blood-brain barrier)
markedly retarded acquisition of the CR. In an effort to discover
whether central muscarinic blockade affected registration of the CS
("input" processes), Moore and coworkers determined the threshold intensities of the tonal CS in producing a CR. While scopolamine hydrobromide did increase the CS threshold intensity from 48 to 58 dB SPL,
thresholds were still lower than the CS intensity used in conditioning
(75 dB SPL). In order to determine whether these effects were specific to auditory CSs, acquisition of CRs to visual CSs and corresponding
CS threshold intensities were studied. Although scopolamine hydrobromide again retarded acquisition, no significant increase in visual
CS threshold intensity was noted. Moore et al. attributed this audi-
tory-visual threshold discrepancy to the fact that several cholinergic
pathways are known to exist in regions of the central nervous system
known to be involved in auditory processing.

Most recently, Harvey et al. (1983) have reported a thorough analysis of the effects of scopolamine hydrobromide and methylbromide
on classical conditioning of the rabbit NM response, using both auditory and visual CSs. These authors examined a wide range of scopolamine doses (0.005 to 1.6 mg/kg, i.v.) and tried to define more pre-
cisely the behavioral mode of action. They first supported previous
findings by showing that scopolamine retarded acquisition at doses not
affecting UR or threshold intensity of the US. In addition, scopolamine was again found to increase the auditory CS intensity necessary
to produce a CR. Finally, Harvey et al. demonstrated that the retardation of acquisition produced by several pre-exposures to the CS alone
was not affected by scopolamine. Therefore, scopolamine did not appear to produce its effects through interfering with other non-associative processes, such as "the development of habituatory decrements
during unpaired stimulus presentations" (i.e., latent inhibition).
This demonstration of a lack of effect by scopolamine on the development of latent inhibition also indicates that scopolamine could not
have blocked the registration (or "unconditioned" excitatory effects)
of the CS.

Taken together, the data presented above lead to the following
conclusions on central muscarinic blockade. First, the motoric expression of the UR ("output") is unaffected. This is unlikely to be

due to the possibility that UR expression was at ceiling or that the
US was far from suprathreshold since Moore et al. (1976) found the
same result using low-intensity USs. Second, although the registration ("input") of auditory CSs may be reduced, this effect is certainly not strong enough to account for the reduction in the acquisition
and maintenance of stimulus control by the CS produced by antimuscarinics since (a) the latent inhibition experiment by Harvey et al. indicates unimpeded stimulus registration, and (b) although visual CS
thresholds are unaffected, scopolamine produced the same reduction in
associative stimulus control by visual CSs as by auditory CSs. Third,
Leaton (1968) and others have implicated the cholinergic system in the
mediation of habituation, yet non-associative changes in the unconditioned excitation produced by CSs (latent inhibition) and USs (habituation) were unaffected in these classical conditioning studies.
Fourth, Meyers (1965), among others, has proposed that antimuscarinics
chiefly interfere with the process mediating suppression of punished
responses. If this type of behavioral inhibition were involved in
suppressing CRs to the CS- in either the Downs et al. (1972) or the
Moore et al. (1976) study, one would therefore expect either atropine
or scopolamine to increase the occurrence of CRs to the CS-. Such was
not observed to be the case. Fifth, Milar et al. (1978) hypothesized
that antimuscarinics disrupt the discriminatory process - the ability
to tell stimuli apart and differentiate responses to them. Thus, if
the discriminatory process were impaired in the absence of any changes
in overall behavioral excitation/inhibition, CRs to the CS+ would be
expected to decrease AND CRs to the CS- would be expected to increase.
Again, this pattern of results was not observed. Thus, antimuscarinics would seem to produce their behavioral disruption by specifically
interfering with the maintenance and perhaps even formation of the
association between CS and US. It must be noted that the fact that
antimuscarinics retard acquisition does not logically require that
formation of associative links be interfered with; an ongoing interference with maintenance or expression of the forming association
would suffice. Therefore, the most parsimonious working hypothesis
of the role of the central cholinergic system in aversive classical
conditioning of the NM response in rabbits is that it may be involved
in the maintenance or expression of associative links. The cognitive
equivalent of this hypothesis is that either retention or retrieval
of previously formed associations is mediated by the central cholinergic system.

3.   SPONTANEOUS ALTERNATION

     In the spontaneous alternation (SA) paradigm, subjects are typi-
cally given two to three unrewarded trials per day in a T- or Y-maze.
Untreated naive rats display a significant tendency to alternate arm
choices over trials. The occurrence of spontaneous alternation has
been shown to increase as a direct function of the time subjects are
detained in the previously chosen arm (Kirkby et al., 1967) and to
depend on olfactory and vestibular cues (Douglas, 1966; Rosen and

Stein, 1969). It has been hypothesized by Glanzer (1953) that SA is a
function of satiation or habituation to previously encountered stimuli. However, it should be clear that habituation alone cannot account
for SA; the habituated stimulus must also be associated with either
the response of turning toward that stimulus or the olfactory stimulus
paired with approaching that stimulus.

Several investigators have demonstrated that both atropine and
scopolamine can potently decrease and physostigmine increase the rate
of SA (Douglas and Isaacson, 1966; Leaton, 1968; Squire, 1969;
Swonger and Rech, 1972; Drew et al., 1973). The fundamental nature
of the scopolamine disruption of SA is emphasized by the finding that
even when genetic differences in mouse strains lead to opposite responses to scopolamine in activity and exploration (e.g., object sniffing and rearing), scopolamine uniformly disrupts SA (Van Abeelan and
Strijbosch, 1969; Anisman, 1975; Anisman and Kokkinidis, 1975).

However, there is good evidence that scopolamine does not disrupt
SA performance when additional stimulus information is presented during the trials. Leaton and Buck (1968) showed that when, on trial one
in a T-maze, one arm was black and one white and then both arms became
either black or white on trial two, rats entered the arm that was
changed in color whether treated with saline or scopolamine. Similarly, Leaton and Utell (1970) showed that SA was unimpaired by scopolamine when on trial one, subjects were "forced" into one arm (a door
covered the entry into the other arm). Since SA occurred even following scopolamine treatment in these cases, it could be argued that the
effects of antimuscarinics on SA reported in the preceding discussion
are due to a partial disruption of either habituation or retention/
retrieval of the associative link between the previously chosen arm
and the corresponding odor or response. Defects in formation or
acquisition of the association cannot be the sole effect produced by
the drug since Squire (1969) demonstrated that physostigmine and
scopolamine had significant and opposite effects when given either
before or after trial one. However, both drugs had less effect on SA
when given 60 or 120 minutes after trial one. Squire interpreted
this finding as indicative of an effect on "consolidation" of memory.
The next section will present more evidence on putative consolidation
effects.

4.   PASSIVE AVOIDANCE

The passive avoidance (PA) procedure has two main variations.
In the first, called "step-through" avoidance, subjects are placed
into one compartment of a chamber and access to another compartment
is allowed. Once the subject enters the second compartment, a door
is closed and the floor bars are mildly electrified. The second is
called "step-down" avoidance. Subjects are placed on a platform above
floor bars in a chamber. When the subject steps down from the platform to the floor bars, it receives a mild foot shock.

PA is referred to as a one-trial learning procedure because one brief exposure (trial) to the paradigm is usually enough to produce significant increases in the latency to step-through or step-down on a second trial as much as seven days later. As such, the procedure is well suited for evaluating potential drug effects on the consolidation of memory for the training trial.

When either scopolamine or physostigmine is administered before the first trial, trial two response latency is reduced (Burešova et al., 1964; Meyers, 1965; Bohdanecky and Jarvik, 1967; Glick and Zimmerberg, 1972; Hamburg and Fulton, 1972). While Meyers (1965) found that scopolamine given just prior to a tenth training session produced a retention deficit, Burešova et al. (1964) found no such retention deficit when they administered atropine before trial two.

Another area of controversy lies in the effects of cholinergic drugs on consolidation when given immediately after the first (training) trial. Glick and Zimmerberg (1972) demonstrated that, when given at this time, scopolamine hydrobromide (and not methylscopolamine hydrobromide) disrupted retention test latencies one, two, and seven days after training. However, Bohdanecky and Jarvik (1967) found no such effect. Both studies employed a one-trial step-through procedure in which mice were placed in a small, brightly-lit compartment and were allowed access to a large, dark compartment. The only apparent difference was that the former study used a scopolamine dose of 10 mg/kg and the latter, only 1 mg/kg. Ten mg/kg of scopolamine is an extremely high dose for mice, and it is likely that some nonspecific effects were produced, perhaps accounting for the disagreement. At any rate, the lower dose was sufficient to produce large decreases in trial two latency when given before trial one. Similarly, using an atropine dose (6 mg/kg) high enough to produce a large trial two effect when given immediately before either trial one or trial two, Burešova et al. (1964) found no evidence for a consolidation effect.

Thus, the evidence supporting an effect of antimuscarinics on the so-called consolidation phase of memory in the PA procedure is inconclusive. Moreover, the elusiveness of the consolidation effect as compared to the inarguable effects of pre-trial administration indicates that "consolidation disruption" is not the primary effect of cholinolytics. Furthermore, the demonstration by Hamburg and Fulton (1972) that physostigmine-induced "amnesia" in the PA procedure could be reversed by a brief re-exposure ("reminder") to any facet of the task (the chamber, step-down platform, or shock alone), indicates that the deficit is a matter of retrieval, rather than retention. Indeed, the findings in the SA paradigm, that an increase in the number of or exposure to stimuli reduces the effects of cholinergic drugs, also indicates that disruption of retention is not the principal drug effect.

Taking the strong cholinergic effects on acquisition into account it is apparent that a slightly more complex conceptualization is

necessary. Antimuscarinics and anticholinesterases seem to exert the
most disruption during acquisition and upon retest. Therefore, cho-
olinergic transmission may mediate the dynamic processes of encoding
(storing in retrievable form) and retrieving associations: input/
output transfers to and from memory storage. This notion is consistent with the evidence presented to this point, but excludes cholinergic involvement in behavioral inhibition, memory storage, discrimina-
ation, and selective attention.

5.   CONDITIONED SUPPRESSION

Berger and Stein (1969) examined the effects of scopolamine on
mice in a one-trial conditioned suppression procedure, quite similar
to PA. Subjects were trained to drink a fixed amount of water from a
tube in a chamber with an electrifiable floor. Conditioning involved
delivering a foot-shock after drinking on trial one. Retention on
trial two was measured by the latency required to consume that fixed
amount of water. When scopolamine (1 mg/kg) was given before trial
one, latency to drink on trial two was markedly reduced. When given
solely before trial two, scopolamine had no effect when trial one
shock was relatively intense (1 mA). When trial one shock was reduced
to 0.5 and 0.4 mA, pre-trial two injection of scopolamine decreased
the latency to drink. The same pattern of results over shock intensity occurred when scopolamine was given prior to both trials one and
two.

Thus, Berger and Stein's data support the acquisition half of the
encoding/retrieval hypothesis formulated in the last section. An interesting sidelight is the partial tendency towards state dependence
in Berger and Stein's results. That is, under high shock conditions,
scopolamine had no effect when administered before both trial one and
trial two. This was not observed in the PA studies discussed previously, but is still not inconsistent with the current hypothesis.
If scopolamine perturbed encoding on trial one in a certain way, it
is conceivable that a similar perturbation in retrieval on trial two
would aid performance. The current hypothesis does not demand this,
however.

6.   ACTIVE AVOIDANCE

6.1. One-way and Shuttlebox Avoidance

One-way avoidance typically involves placing subjects in one part
of a two compartment chamber and providing a number of pairings between either an auditory or visual CS and a shock US. Subjects even-
tually learn to avoid the shock by crossing over into the opposite
compartment when the CS predictive of shock is presented. Shuttlebox,
or bidirectional avoidance, is similar, except that animals are

to shuttle back and forth over trials - the previous start box becoming goal box and vice-versa. Anisman (1973) examined the effects of scopolamine (1.0 mg/kg) and physostigmine (0.5 mg/kg) when injected before the second 50-trial session of either type of avoidance. In agreement with other reports, scopolamine was found to increase the number of avoidance responses in the bidirectional procedure but did not affect performance in the one-way task. Physostigmine reduced the number of avoidance responses in both tasks.

Baseline performance of one-way avoidance has often been found to be better than that in shuttlebox avoidance (as it was in Anisman's study) and the one-way task is acquired more rapidly. These findings have been ascribed to the theoretical consideration that in shuttlebox avoidance, the subject must repeatedly extinguish the association between shock and the compartment just departed from (developed often in acquisition, when an avoidance response is not emitted in time) in order to emit an avoidance response back to that same compartment. It is therefore understandable that scopolamine could improve avoidance performance by interfering with the encoding or retrieval of compartment-shock associations. Data from previous sections have shown that when associations are "overlearned" they are less vulnerable to disruption by antimuscarinics. Since nearly all acquisition trials contribute to the strength of the CS (auditory or visual signal)--US (shock) association in this paradigm, it would be expected that dynamic interaction with the CS-US association subserving the avoidance response would be less disrupted by scopolamine than that with the more transitory and rapidly shifting association between compartment and shock.

The understanding of cholinergic drug effects on performance in this paradigm becomes more complete when the motor effects of these drugs are taken into account. Cholinergic drugs have well-recognized effects on the balance of the extra-pyramidal motor system (see for example Janowsky et al., 1972; Wolfarth and Kolasiewicz, 1977). Scopolamine has been reported to produce hyperactivity in the open field (Anisman et al., 1975; Wolthuis et al., 1975), thus providing another mechanism whereby active avoidance performance could be improved by scopolamine (hyperactivity leading to more rapid crossing over in a shuttlebox) and decreased by physostigmine.

6.2. Aversively-Motivated Discrimination

This categorization refers to procedures in which animals are trained to discriminate stimuli in order to avoid shock. Typically, subjects are placed in a Y- or T-maze with a floor that is electrified everywhere except for the arm that is illuminated. Subjects learn over several trials to approach the lit arm. Both shuttlebox avoidance and aversively-motivated discriminations have been used to examine the Kamin effect, a phenomenon in which retention performance following a training session is found to first decline and then improve

over the course of 10 to 20 days. While it is not the purpose of this
review to summarize the extensive work done in order to support or
question Deutsch's (1973) theory relating cholinergic function to the
Kamin effect, some generalizations on the effects of cholinergic drugs
on performance of aversively-motivated discriminationscan be made.

Deutsch and coworkers have shown that antimuscarinics impair
performance when given before a retention test which falls a few days
after initial learning, while physostigmine or DFP (an irreversible
anticholinesterase) impair performance most when given before a retention test that comes 5 to 10 days after the initial learning.
Signorelli (1976) demonstrated that the effects of physostigmine
lasted only as long as the drug was in the body, again indicating an
effect on some dynamic component of performance rather than on memory
storage. Flood et al. (1981) found that when anticholinergic drugs
were centrally injected immediately after training, and retention was
tested a week later, performance declined. When cholinergic agonists
(e.g., arecoline, oxotremorine, muscarine) or anticholinesterases were
tested the same way, and baseline was adjusted to be low, some doses
improved retention test performance. Deutsch and coworkers, as well
as Stanes et al. (1976) have also extended Deutsch's cholinergic model
to apply to the effects of physostigmine on appetite Y-maze discrimination.

Thus, drugs that increase cholinergic function can increase or
decrease performance depending on dose and retention interval; antimuscarinics either do not affect or degrade performance. Interestingly, however, when anticholinesterases disrupt performance, concurrent
administration of muscarinic receptor blockers can antagonize this
disruption. These data may indicate that while decreasing cholinergic
function usually impairs acquisition or retest performance, increasing
it does not necessarily improve performance.

7.   APPETITIVELY-MOTIVATED DISCRIMINATION

Hearst (1959) provided the first report of the effects of scopolamine on go/go discriminated responding in the rat. Subjects were
trained to press one of two levers for water reinforcement in the presence of one stimulus (either a clicker or a tone) and the other lever
during presentations of the other stimulus. Subjects were trained to
an asymptotic level of correct performance and then occasionally given
scopolamine (0.2 to 1.0 mg/kg). Pre-session drug treatment resulted
in a decreased percent of correct responding (from 94.5 to 63.6) and
increased the number of responses on either lever emitted when neither
stimulus was present. In addition, subjects developed a marked lever
preference on drug sessions. Although this led to an increased occurrence of repeated responses on a given lever as opposed to alterna-
tions between levers, it did not result in true perseveration, i.e.,
the tendency to repeat a previous response regardless of which

response it was. When these subjects were given extinction sessions, scopolamine increased responses on both levers, even when no stimuli were presented or subjects were sated with water.

These data would seem to indicate that in addition to disrupting discrimination performance (perhaps through interference with retrieval of stimulus response associations), scopolamine increases non-reinforced and extinguished responding, and the overall tendency to respond is increased. However, subsequent discrimination studies have not borne this out. Milar et al. (1978) conducted a series of auditory (1000 and 3000 Hz tones) and visual (panel light) discrimination experiments in order to evaluate the effects of prior scopolamine (0.0625 to 0.5 mg/kg) treatment. Rats were trained to perform a go/no go discrimination: lever presses were reinforced with sucrose solution in the presence of one stimulus and not reinforced in the presence of another. Another stimulus (white noise) was established as a conditioned inhibitor through presentation during extinction sessions. In all experiments, excitatory as well as inhibitory stimulus control were decreased by scopolamine. Rats given scopolamine responded more on no go trials and less on go trials.

Milar (1981) studied the effects of scopolamine (0.125 to 0.50 mg/kg) on a go/no go brightness discrimination in rats. Reinforcement probabilities were manipulated for both correct responses and correct omission of responses in order to vary the degree of baseline excitatatory and inhibitory stimulus control. A signal detection analysis of the data was used in order to obtain independent estimates of drug (and behavioral manipulation) effects on sensitivity (the subject's absolute ability to discriminate the stimuli) and bias (relative preference for responding, or not responding, in the case of a go/no go task). Scopolamine was found to decrease sensitivity in a more difficult discrimination (less intensity difference between the discriminative stimuli) and to not affect sensitivity in a simpler intensity discrimination, in which the degree of baseline stimulus control was at ceiling. Bias was unaffected by the drug and manipulations of reinforcement probabilities did not alter drug effects.

The latter two experiments thus do not support perseverative or disinhibitory actions of antimuscarinics. Rather, they are consistent with the current encoding/retrieval hypothesis in that stimulus control of all types, which is dependent upon retrieval of previously established stimulus-response associations, is disrupted. Thus, the central discrimination processess allowing for comparison of the sample stimulus with a previously established internal representation of the rewarded (positive) discriminative stimulus may not be affected by anticholinergic drugs. Rather, cholinolytics may disrupt retrieval of the internal stimulus representation, along with its correct response associations. In this way, alterations in cholinergic function may disrupt performance in discrimination tasks while leaving the discriminatory processes intact.

8.   DELAYED RESPONSE

Two sorts of procedures exist which can provide measures of
memory for recent events in animals. The first is delayed response,
in which correct responding at the end of a retention interval is
dependent upon retaining memory for the response-type specified before
the interval. The second is delayed conditional discrimination, in
which a stimulus presented at the beginning of the retention interval
must be remembered and compared to the post-interval stimulus in order
to determine the correct response.

8.1. Free-Operant Procedures

Schedules of reinforcement such as fixed-interval (FI) and differential reinforcement of low rate (DRL) can be thought of as delayed
response procedures. The degree of stimulus control by the schedule
can be related to the degree to which responses are most efficiently
partitioned over time and reinforcements received are maximized.
There have been many reports of disruption of the pattern of responding on these schedules and others by atropine and scopolamine (e.g.,
Boren and Navarro, 1959; Herrnstein, 1958). Brown and Warburton
(1971) applied signal detection analysis to the effects of scopolamine
on DRL-15 seconds responding by rats. Signal detection analysis revealed drug-induced changes in sensitivity but not in bias, indicating
an overall reduction in control by the schedule contingencies, but not
disinhibition of responding.

Several other investigators have noted that free-operant responding under simple or multiple time-based schedules is not only more
accurate under "external" (presence of an exteroceptive discriminative
stimulus correlated with opportunity for reinforcement) than under
"internal" (no environmental cue given to signal reinforcement opportunity) control, it is also less affected by antimuscarinic agents
(Laties and Weiss, 1966; Wagman and Maxey, 1969). Ksir and Slifer
(1982) have demonstrated a similar effect of scopolamine on performance of an appetitive operant discrimination. These data cannot be
unambiguously interpreted, however. Degree of "internality" covaries
with baseline level of response accuracy and, as has been previously
discussed, cholinergic drug effects may vary depending on degree of
training and resultant level of accuracy.

8.2. Eight-Arm Radial Maze Peformance

In this procedure, food-deprived subjects are placed on a central
platform from which eight arms (walkways) radiate. Usually, a bit of
food is placed at the end of each arm and subjects are trained to
travel to the arms in order to obtain all of the available food. The
optimal behavior in such a situation is to enter only those arms that
have not been entered before. Entering previously selected arms
before all eight have been visited is considered an error. The development and maintenance of extremely accurate win-shift behavior in

rats placed in an eight-arm radial maze has been used by several researchers to study the effects of hippocampal lesions and antimuscarinics on "working memory." Eckerman et al. (1980) produced the first
systematic study of drug effects on this behavior. When administered
before a test session, scopolamine reduced both the accuracy and
number of arm entries. The drug did not increase response perseveration (tendency to repeat entries consecutively into the same arm).
Finally, scopolamine reduced the accuracy of arm choice performance
by about the same amount from the fourth choice to the eighth choice.
Eckerman et al. interpreted these findings as indicative of a drug
effect on discriminative control by the memorial stimuli of previous
arms entered, as opposed to an effect on memory storage, which would
lead to an acceleration of performance decrement over increasing retention intervals.

    Stevens (1981) and Watts et al. (1981) have supported and extend-
ed these findings to show (1) scopolamine markedly reduces both acquisition and retest performance, and (2) subjects using a non-spatial
strategy (i.e., a response strategy, such as always picking the arm
adjacent in the clockwise direction next) were less impaired by scopolamine.

    Godding et al. (1982) confirmed the hypothesis that scopolamine
did not alter memory storage in this task by slightly altering the
procedure. Rats were allowed to make their first four choices and
were then subjected to a five-hour retention interval. Scopolamine
injections during the interval had no effect on subsequent choice
performance that was not attributable to carry-over performance effects of the drug. This was true regardless of whether subjects exhibited a spatial or non-spatial strategy.

8.3. Discrete Trial Procedures

    Both acquisition (Warburton, 1969) and retest performance of go/
no go and go/go alternation of lever-pressing is disrupted by atropine
and scopolamine (Warburton and Heise, 1972; Ksir, 1974; Heise, 1975;
Heise et al., 1975; Heise et al., 1976; Glick et al., 1979). When
variable retention intervals are used, antimuscarinics reduce accuracy
following all intervals to about the same extent. Since no interaction occurred between drug effects and accuracy after increasing retention intervals, Heise (1975) and others have argued that the drug
does not disrupt memory storage.

    Bartus and Johnson (1976), however, provided evidence that when
measured against delayed response performance in rhesus monkeys, scopolamine disrupted performance more at longer retention intervals.
Furthermore, physostigmine was found to antagonize scopolamine's dele-
terious effects (Bartus, 1978). Since no other studies using a variable retention interval procedure have confirmed these results, it is
possible that the effect might be specific to rhesus monkeys. Another

possibility is that the apparent storage effect was due to a less
scopolamine-induced disruption when performance (memorial stimulus
control) was at ceiling, at the lowest retention intervals. Indeed,
the control- and drug-induced memory functions (accuracy-by-interval
plots) for delayed response performance were less obviously divergent
in the later Bartus (1978) study. Therefore, the cholinergic role in
performance of delayed response tasks would once again seem to be more
closely associated with an input/output function in accessing memory
than with memory retention itself.

9.   DELAYED CONDITIONAL DISCRIMINATION

Delayed matching-to-sample is an example of a delayed conditional
discrimination. In the paired-trial form of task, subjects are usually trained to make an observing response to a stimulus on trial one,
subjected to a variable retention interval, and are then presented
with two stimuli on trial two, one of which is identical to that on
trial one. Subjects are reinforced for a response to that "matching"
stimulus.

Using this procedure with rhesus monkeys as subjects, both
Bohdanecky et al. (1967) and Glick and Jarvick (1969) demonstrated
that scopolamine not only decreased matching accuracy, but that it did
so to the same extent at all inter-trial delays, including no delay
at all. On no-delay trials, subjects were simultaneously presented
with sample and comparison stimuli. Under these conditions, a simple
discrimination was required with no dependence upon working memory
(as the term was defined in the introduction to this chapter), and
yet scopolamine disrupted performance to the same degree.

Spencer (1981) trained one group of rats on a Continous Non-
Matching to sample (CNM) task, in which trials with a bright light
irregularly alternated with dim light trials. Subjects were rewarded
for responding when the stimulus on the current trial was different
than that presented on the previous trial. Retention intervals varied
from 2.5 to 10 seconds. Another group of rats was trained to discriminate bright and dim lights during trials. The light intensity difference was decreased until base-line performance on trials (following
the same inter-trial intervals as in the CNM task) was similar to that
of the rats performing the CNM task. Scopolamine injected pre-session
reduced response accuracy on both discrimination and memory measures
to the same extent. In addition, accuracy on no go trials was reduced
by the drug to the same extent as on go trials. Accuracy in the non-
matching task under drug also declined a constant amount over retention intervals as compared to controls. These data indicate that the
cholinergic system does not mediate memory storage in these tasks;
rather, it is equally involved in the processing of tasks depending
on memory for both recent stimulus occurrences (CNM procedure) and
stimulus-response-reinforcement occurrences (both CNM and discrimination procedures).

10.   CONCLUSION

     Based on the data presented above, the following generalizations
on the effects of cholinergic drugs in animals seem appropriate.
First, behavioral effects of the type discussed in this chapter are
the result of drug action within the central nervous system.   Second,
the various types of behavioral inhibition are not selectively affected by these agents.   Third, cholinergic drugs do not selectively
affect the tendency to repeat a previously-emitted incorrect response
(perseveration).   Thus, theories requiring a specific role for the
cholinergic system in detecting "mismatches" between consequences and
expectations are at odds with the drug effects on discrimination performance summarized above.   Fourth, the types of associational link
(operant or classical), task motivation, and memory requirements do
not seem to modify the pattern of behavioral effects produced by
cholinergic alterations.   Fifth, memory storage itself is rarely
affected.

     It has been proposed that all of the experimental data reviewed
above are best accounted for by the hypothesis that central cholinergic transmission mediates the input (encoding)/output (retrieval) processes involved in dynamic interactions with memory storage.   This is
not to say that other hypotheses might not account more parsimoniously
for certain portions of the reviewed data.   Rather, the current hypothesis is presented as the simplest theoretical construct that is
at least consonant with the results from all of the various behavioral
procedures.

     A further proposition is that the strength or situational gener-
ality of the associative link affects the probability of its successful retrieval during or following exposure to cholinergic drugs.   This
notion was prompted by consideration of the spontaneous alternation
data, which strongly indicate that increasing the differential stimulus salience in T-maze arms or increasing the degree of exposure to
stimuli accompanying an arm choice decreases the effect of antimuscarinic drugs.   If the probability of successful retrieval of a response
depends on the strength and diversity of association to the prompting
stimuli (situational or discriminative cues), and if a certain degree
of cholinergic dysfunction results in an overall depression of the
retrieval process, then it is reasonable to assume that responses with
stronger or more diverse associational links will still be relatively
more easily retrieved while under cholinergic drug influence.   Future
research on central cholinergic function might therefore profit by
devoting additional study 'to the interaction between the number of
exposures to conditional associations, the diversity of situations or
stimuli accompanying such exposures, graded variations in degree of
stimulus control in a particular task, and resulting cholinergic drug
effects.

11. SUMMARY

Experiments investigating the effects of systemically-administer-
ed, centrally-acting cholinergic drugs on animal learning and memory
performance were reviewed. Data were separately analyzed for drug
effects on each one of several types of behavioral procedures. Based
on the resulting pattern of cholinergic drug effects, it was proposed
that the central cholinergic system is involved in dynamic interactions with memory: the input (encoding) and output (retrieval) of
information to and from memory.

ACKNOWLEDGEMENT

We thank George Heise for his excellent critical and editorial
efforts and Jeanne Hudson for her secretarial assistance. Partially
supported by NIA grant number 1 R03 AG03623-01.

REFERENCES

Anisman, H., 1973, Cholinergic mechanisms and alterations in behav-
    ioral suppression as factors producing time-dependent changes in
    avoidance performance, J. Comp. Psysiol. Psych. 83:465-477.
Anisman, H., 1975, Dissociation of disinhibitory effects of scopo-
    lamine: Strain and task factors, Pharmacol. Biochem. Behav.
    3:613-618.
Anisman, H., and Kokkinidis, L., 1975, Effects of scopolamine,
    d-amphetamine and other drugs affecting catecholamines on spon-
    taneous alternation and locomotor activity in mice, Psychopharma-
    cology 45:55-63.
Anisman, H., Wahlsten, D., and Kokkinidis, L., 1975, Effects of
    d-amphetamine and scopolamine on activity before and after shock
    in three mouse strains, Pharmacol. Biochem. Behav. 3:819-824.
Bartus, R. T., 1978, Evidence for a direct cholinergic involvement in
    the scopolamine-induced amnesia in monkeys: Effects of concurrent
    administration of physostigmine and methylphenidate with scopola-
    mine, Pharmacol. Biochem. Behav. 2:833-836.
Bartus, R. T., and Johnson, H. R., 1976, Short-term memory in the
    rhesus monkey: Disruption from the anti-cholinergic scopolamine,
    Pharmacol. Biochem. Behav. 5:39-46.
Berger, B. D., and Stein, L., 1969, Analysis of the learning deficits
    produced by scopolamine, Psychopharmacology 14:271-283.
Bohdanecky, Z., and Jarvik, M. E., 1967, Impairment of one-trial
    passive avoidance learning in mice by scopolamine, scopolamine
    methylbromide, and physostigmine, Int. J. Neuropharmacol.
    6:217-222.
Bohdanecky, Z., Jarvik, M. E., and Carley, J. L. 1967, Differential
    impairment of delayed matching in monkeys by scopolamine and
    scopolamine methylbromide, Psychopharmacology 11:293-299.

Boren, J. J., and Navarro, A. P., 1959, The action of atropine, ben-
     actyzine, and scopolamine upon fixed interval and fixed ratio
     behavior, J. Exp. Anal. Behav. 2:107–116.
Brown, K., and Warburton, D. M., 1971, Attention of stimulus sensitiv-
     ity by scopolamine, Psychon. Sci. 22:297–298.
Buresova, O., Bures, J., Bohdanecky, Z., Weiss, T, 1964, Effect of
     atropine on learning, extinction, retention and retrieval in rats,
     Psychopharmacology 5:255–263.
Carlton, P. L., 1963, Cholinergic mechanisms in the control of behav-
     ior by the brain, Psychol. Rev. 70:19–39.
Deutsch, J. A., 1973, The cholinergic synapse and the site of memory,
     in "The Physiological Basis of Memory," J. A. Deutsch, ed,
     pp. 59–76, Academic Press, New York.
Douglas, R. J., 1966, Cues for spontaneous alternation, J. Comp.
     Physiol. Psych. 62:171–183.
Douglas, R. J., and Isaacson, R. L., 1966, Spontaneous alternation and
     scopolamine, Psychon. Sci. 4:283–284.
Downs, D., Cardozo, C., Schneiderman, N., Yehle, A. L., Van Dercar,
     D. H., and Zwilling, G., 1972, Central effects of atropine upon
     aversive classical conditioning in rabbits, Psychopharmacology
     23:319–333.
Drew, W. G., Miller, L. L., and Baugh, E. L., 1973, Effects of
     delta-9-THC, LSD-25 and scopolamine on continous, spontaneous
     alternation in the Y-maze, Psychopharmacology 32:171–182.
Eckerman, D. A., Gordon, W. A., Edwards, J. D., MacPhail, R. C., and
     Gage, M. I., 1980, Effects of scopolamine, pentobarbital, and
     amphetamine on radial arm maze performance in the rat, Pharmacol.
     Biochem. Behav. 12:595–602.
Flood, J. F., Landry, D. W., and Jarvik, M. E., 1981, Cholinergic
     receptor interactions and their effects on long-term memory pro-
     cessing, Brain Res. 215:177–185.
Glanzer, M., 1953, Stimulus satiation: An explanation of spontaneous
     alternation and related phenomena, Psychol. Rev. 60:257–268.
Glick, S. D., Cox, R. D., Maayani, S., and Meibach, R. C., 1979, Anti-
     cholinergic behavioral effect of phencyclidine, Eur. J.
     Pharmacol. 59:103–106.
Glick, S. D., and Jarvik, M. E., 1969, Amphetamine, scopolamine, and
     chlorpromazine interactions on delayed matching performance in
     monkeys, Psychopharmacology 16:147–155.
Glick, S. D., and Zimmerberg, B., 1972, Amnesic effects of scopolamine
     Behav. Biol. 7:245–254.
Godding, P. R., Rush, J. R., and Beatty, W. W., 1982, Scopolamine does
     not disrupt spatial working memory in rats, Pharmacol. Biochem.
     Behav. 16:919–923.
Hamburg, M. D., and Fulton, D. R., 1972, Influence of recall on an
     anticholinesterase induced retrograde amnesia, Physiol. Behav.
     9:409–418.
Harvey, J. A., Gormezano, I., and Cool-Hauser, V. A., 1983, Effects of
     scopolamine and methylscopolamine on classical conditioning of the
     rabbit nictitating membrane response, J. Pharmacol. Exp. Ther.
     225:42–49.

Hearst, E., 1959, Effects of scopolamine on discriminated responding in the rat, J. Pharmacol. Exp. Ther. 126:349-358.

Heise, G. A., 1975, Discrete trial analysis of drug action, Fed. Proc. 34:1898-1903.

Heise, G. A., Conner, R., and Martin, R. A., 1976, Effects of scopolamine on variable intertrial interval spatial alternation and memory in the rat, Psychopharmacology 49:131-137.

Heise, G. A., Hrabrich, B., Lilie, N. L., and Martin, R. A., 1975, Scopolamine effects on delayed spatial alternation in the rat, Pharmacol. Biochem. Behav. 3:993-1002.

Hernstein, R. J., 1958, Effects of scopolamine on a multiple schedule, J. Exp. Anal. Behav. 1:351-358.

Janowsky, D. S., El-Yousef, M. K., Davis, J. M., and Sekerke, H. J., 1972, Cholinergic antagonism of methylphenidate-induced sterotyped behavior, Psychopharmacology 27:295-303.

Kirby, R. J., Stein, D. G., Kimble, R. J., and Kimble, D. P., 1967, J. Comp. Physiol. Psychol. 64:342-345.

Ksir, C. J., Jr., 1974, Scopolamine effects in two-trial delayed response performance in the rat, Psychopharmacology 34:127-134.

Ksir, C., and Slifer, B, 1982, Drug effects on discrimination performance at two levels of stimulus control, Psychopharmacology 76:268-290.

Laties, V. G., and Weiss, B., 1966, Influence of drugs on behavior controlled by internal and external stimuli, J. Pharmacol. Exp. Ther. 152:388-396.

Leaton, R. N., 1968, Effects of scopolamine on exploratory motivated behavior, J. Comp. Physiol. Psychol. 66:524-527.

Leaton, R. N., and Buck, R. L., 1968, Effect of scopolamine on response by the rat to environmental change, Psychon. Sci. 12:101.

Leaton, R. N., and Utell, M. J., 1970, Effects of scopolamine on spontaneous alternation following free forced trials, Physiol. Behav. 5:331-334.

Meyers, B., 1965, Some effects of scopolamine on a passive avoidance response in rats, Psychopharmacology 8:111-119.

Milar, K. S., 1981, Cholinergic drug effects on visual discriminations: A signal detection analysis, Psychopharmacology 74:383-388.

Milar, K. S., Halgren, C. R., and Heise, G. A., 1978, A reappraisal of scopolamine effects on inhibition, Pharmacol. Biochem. Behav. 9:307-313.

Moore, J. W., Goodell, N. A., and Solomon, P. R., 1976, Central cholinergic blockade by scopolamine and habituation, classical conditioning, and latent inhibition of the rabbit's nictitating membrane response, Physiol. Psychol. 4:395-399.

Rosen, J.J. and Stein, D. G., 1969, Spontaneous alternation behavior in the rat, J. Comp. Physiol. Psychol. 68:420-426.

Signorelli, A., 1976, Influence of physostigmine upon consolidation of memory in mice, J. Comp. Physiol. Psychol. 90:658-664.

Spencer, D. G., 1981, Central cholinergic function and short-term memory in the rat, Soc. Neurosci. Abs. 7:524.

Squire, L. R., 1969, Effects of pretrial and post-trial administration of cholinergic and anticholinergic drugs on spontaneous alternation, *J. Comp. Physiol. Psychol.* 69:69–75.

Stanes, M. D., Brown, C. P., and Singer, G. E., 1976, Effect of physostigmine on Y-maze discrimination retention in the rat, *Psychopharmacology* 46:269–276.

Stevens, R., 1981, Scopolamine impairs spatial maze performance in rats, *Physiol. Behav.* 27:385–386.

Swonger, A. K., and Rech, R. H., 1972, Serotonergic and cholinergic involvement in habituation of activity and spontaneous alternation of rats in a Y-maze, *J. Comp. Physiol. Psychol.* 81:509–522.

Van Abeelen, J. H. F., and Strijbosch, H., 1969, Genotype-dependent effects of scopolamine and eserine on exploratory behavior in mice, *Psychopharmacology* 16:81–88.

Wagman, W. D., and Maxey, G. C, 1969, The effects of scopolamine hydrobromide and methyl scopolamine hydrobromide upon the discrimination of interoceptive and exteroceptive stimuli, *Psychopharmacology* 15:280–288.

Warburton, D. M., 1969, Behavioral effects of central and peripheral changes in acetylcholine systems, *J. Comp. Physiol. Psychol.* 68:56–44.

Warburton, D. M., and Heise, G. A., 1972, Effects of scopolamine on spatial double alternation in rats, *J. Comp. Physiol. Psychol.* 81:523–532.

Watts, J., Stevens, R., and Robinson, C., 1981, Effects of scopolamine on radial maze performance in rats, *Physiol. Behav.* 26:845–851.

Wolfarth, S., and Kolasiewicz, W., 1977, Effects of intrastriatal injections of atropine and methacholine on the apomorphine-induced gnawing in the rabbit, *Pharmacol. Biochem. Behav.* 6:5–10.

Wolthuis, O., DeVroome, H., and Van Wersch, R., 1975, Automatically determined effects of lithium, scopolamine, and methamphetamine on motor activity of rats, *Pharmacol. Biochem. Behav.* 3:515–518.

Chapter 6

CHOLINERGIC MECHANISMS IN
AGGRESSIVE BEHAVIOR
Role of Muscarinic and Nicotinic Systems

Robert Bell and Kenneth Brown

Department of Psychology
The Queen's University of Belfast
Belfast, N. Ireland, U.K.

---

1. THEORETICAL BACKGROUND

It has been suggested (Scott, 1958; Valzelli, 1967) that aggression is not a unitary concept. This premise is based on the fact that stimulus situations eliciting aggression are so diverse and hence

there must be several types of behavior. It followed from this that
there would be a variety of physiological substrates involved in the
mediation of these different aggression types. Only recently, however, has any systematic attempt been made to list the types of
aggression and indicate a basis for classification. Moyer (1968),
suggested that if there were several forms of aggression, then progress in understanding the general phenomenon of this behavior could
be made only when the various types were carefully and operationally
defined. The definitional phase must then be followed by research in
which experimental manipulations are applied to the subjects who are
then tested in a variety of situations which define the various classes of aggression. A given manipulation may very well facilitate one
kind of aggression, suppress another, and have no effect on a third
(Moyer, 1968).

        Moyer (1968), outlined eight kinds of aggression, but emphasized
that they could not be considered mutually exclusive. Outside the
laboratory, behavior may involve several of the different kinds of
aggression, reflecting a possible overlap in the underlying neural and
endocrine controlling mechanisms. Nonetheless, Moyer contended that
the types of aggression are essentially different and that it would be
possible to distinguish the physiological substrates experimentally.
Moyer's classifications are briefly reviewed, accompanied by the various physiological factors believed to be important in the manifestation of each kind of aggressive behavior.

Predatory Aggression is elicited by the presence of a natural object
of prey. The probability of attack is increased by movement on the
part of the prey. The pattern of responses is different from that of
other aggression types in that it involves interaction between members
of different species. It is distinguished from inter-male and irritable aggression on the basis of the object of attack and can be differentiated from fear-induced aggression if the subject is given the
opportunity to escape from the stimulus object. Brain structures
implicated in the mediation of this behavior include the lateral hypothalamus, amygdala and frontal cortex. Sex hormones do not appear to
play any significant role in predatory aggression.

Inter-male Aggression is elicited by the presence of a strange male
conspecific to which the attacker does not become habituated. The
general environment in which the stimulus is presented is not particularly important and the attack is made without provocation on the part
of the victim. Testosterone, a male sex hormone, plays a crucial role
in the development and maintenance of this particular behavior. The
effects of social isolation are known to increase this type of aggression. Little is known of the possible brain structures involved.

Fear-induced Aggression is always preceded by attempts to escape.
Hence one of the components of this form of aggression is a degree of
confinement in which the defensive animal is cornered and unable to

escape (the "cornered rat"). In this situation, the animal turns
and attacks the attacker. The amygdala, septum and hypothalamus are
thought to exert a modulatory influence over fear-induced aggression.

Territorial Aggression is seen in an area in which the animal has established itself by a process of exploration and marking of territory.
Attack is provoked by a conspecific intruding into this area, with the
probability of attack by the "home" animal decreasing as the intruder
retreats from the marked area. It is dependent upon the presence of
testosterone but little is known of the brain mechanism involved.

More recently, Moyer has criticized the usefulness and explana-
tory power of the concept of territoriality. Territorial aggression
may involve inter-male, maternal, sex-related and instrumental aggression. The construct of territoriality has, therefore, been employed
to encompass divergent behavior, so limiting its use in understanding
aggressive behavior (Moyer, 1976).

Maternal Aggression is peculiar to the female of most mammalian species, the stimulus situation involving the proximity of some threatening agent to the young of that female. As the mother moves further
away from the young, the tendency towards aggression decreases.
Reproductive hormones influence the development of maternal aggression, although again very little is known about the underlying neural
mechanisms.

Instrumental Aggression does not appear to have a particular physiological basis. It consists of an increase in the tendency of an organism to engage in destructive behavior in a situation where aggression has been reinforced in the past. If the particular situation
involves another animal, the cue complex of that animal tends to
elicit an aggressive response. As a result, dominance hierarchies
will develop over a period of time, with animals in some species
tending to respond to each other in an aggressive or submissive
manner.

Sex-related Aggression, an example of which is rape, is thought to be
elicited by the same stimuli that produce the sexual response. There
is some experimental evidence to show that the sexual and aggressive
motivations are related (Barclay and Haber, 1965).

Irritable Aggression occurs in the presence of any attackable organism
or object. The epitome of this type of aggression is usually described as anger or rage. It can be elicited by a wide range of stimuli,
e.g., fatigue or pain, and is aggravated by frustration or deprivation.
Irritable aggression is distinguished from fear-induced aggression in
that it is not preceded by attempts to escape. The amygdala, hypothalamus, caudate nucleus and septal area are the main brain structures implicated in the control of the behavior. Testosterone,
again, enhances the occurrence of this type of aggression. A type of

irritable aggressive behavior not defined by Moyer (1968) is shock-
induced defensive fighting (S.I.D.F.).

The S.I.D.F. paradigm was first employed by O'Kelly and Steckle
(1939) when they discovered that when paired rats are subjected to
electrical footshock, a stereotyped fighting reaction is elicited.
The elements of this fighting, which include upright threat posture
and forward attack, are very similar to those displayed in naturally
occurring aggression by rats (Reynierse, 1971) and by mice (Legrand
and Fielder, 1973). The actual measure of aggression taken in this
and other studies is the number of forward attacks made by one animal
on its opponent. This follows the results of a detailed investigation
carried out by Ulrich and Azrin, (1962) who suggested three easily
recordable responses elicited by footshock; no response, upright
threat posture and attack (a well directed forward lunge with fore-
paws/body, which may be accompanied by biting).

The parameters of the stimulus situation are very important to
the occurrence of S.I.D.F. Shock variables such as frequency, intensity and duration of shock, the length of the shock session and the
unpredictability of the shock are all crucial factors (Ulrich and
Azrin, 1962; Azrin et al., 1964; Dreyer and Church, 1968; Creer and
Powell, 1971). Avoidance and escape behavior occur in S.I.D.F. situations only when shock frequency and duration are too great (Azrin et
al., 1967). The size of the test chamber, the number of animals present and sensory input also influence the frequency of S.I.D.F.

Some investigators, (Scott, 1966; Uyeno and White, 1967) have
sought to identify the behaviors observed during S.I.D.F. as more
"defensive" than "offensive." This classification of this type of
aggression was arrived at on the grounds that shock-induced attack
showed no similarity to that displayed by dominant members of wild rat
colonies. Other studies have concluded that the boxing posture displayed during S.I.D.F. is not associated with an attack response or
other factors involved in offensive aggression in the rat or mouse
(Kimbrell, 1969; Knutson and Hynan, 1972).

Blanchard et al., (1975) carried out an analysis of different
behavior patterns of dominant colony animals and of strangers introduced into the colonies. The resuls strongly indicated that the agonistic behavior of domesticated rats may be divided into offensive and
defensive reactions. Further, the analysis suggested that the behaviors observed during S.I.D.F., such as boxing and lying on the back,
are characteristic of colony intruders, rather than of dominant colony
males.

Further studies by Blanchard et al. (1977) provided additional
information indicating that the characterization of behaviors seen in
S.I.D.F., as "aggression," is inaccurate. Results from these experiments indicated that the striking component of behavior in this type

of fighting is reflexive, and need not be considered an aggressive response since it occurs at a high level when there is no other rat (or other animate stimulus) present to fight with.

Whilst the results of these experiments stress the defensive, as opposed to offensive, nature of the behaviors in S.I.D.F., this clarification does not call into question the value of the task itself (Blanchard et al., 1977). Instead, the data from such studies serve to put the behaviors observed in "reflexive fighting" tasks into a more appropriate perspective. Boxing behavior, as it occurs in such tasks, is primarily an unconditioned reaction to shock and should be classified as a defensive response.

Four classes of aggressive behavior commonly employed for study are: S.I.D.F., predatory, isolation-induced fighting (inter-male), and irritable aggression. (For discussion of behavioral topography and cholinergic pathways in the brain see Rodgers, 1979a,b). Investigations into the role of acetylcholine (ACh) for each type are now reviewed.

2.   EVIDENCE FOR MUSCARINIC CHOLINERGIC MEDIATION OF AGGRESSIVE
      BEHAVIOR

2.1. Shock-Induced Defensive Fighting

The role of central cholinergic mechanisms in S.I.D.F. has been investigated in mice and rats, but only to a very limited degree. Grossman (1972a) carried out one of the first reported studies on the effects, on S.I.D.F., of directly injecting cholinergic agents into the brain. He injected either carbachol or scopolamine into the ventromedial hypothalamus and found no consistent effect on this form of aggression. Injections of drugs that altered the levels of norepinephrine (NE) or 5-hydroxytryptamine (5-HT) similary produced no effect on S.I.D.F. From these results, Grossman concluded that, since lesions of the ventromedial hypothalamus increased S.I.D.F. levels in the rat (Grossman, 1972a), yet transmitter agonists and antagonists had no effect, then this region must consist of fibers (passing through) and not cell bodies or synapses. However, as Grossman points out, these data do not prove the null hypothesis. It is possible that different doses of the same drugs or other putative transmitters might have modified aggressive behaviors (Grossman, 1972b).

The data from neurochemical studies on cholinergic mediation of S.I.D.F. have produced conflicting and confusing conclusions. It is suggested that two reasons may be advanced to account for the differing results.

The first reason concerns the lack of control for drugs altering pain sensitivity. Obviously the extent of shock experienced by the

animal will alter levels of S.I.D.F. in relation to the pain levels
generated by altered synaptic levels of neurotransmitters (Leroux and
Myers, 1975). Whilst investigators have controlled for possible nonspecific effects of manipulating central nervous system (CNS) transmitter levels such as locomotor impairment, it seems that alterations
in pain sensitivity are not considered as a possible effect, at least,
not one worth controlling in their experimental designs.

The second reason involves a lack of standardization of experimental paradigms for S.I.D.F. Instead of adhering to one specific
experimental method (e.g., the optimum conditions for S.I.D.F. as suggested by Ulrich and Azrin 1962), many investigators have modified the
original technique to such an extent that they have forfeited the com-
parability of their results. This type of mistake is evident in the
use of widely varying shock intensities, durations and frequencies.
As was pointed out by Ulrich et al. (1969), the level of S.I.D.F. is
heavily dependent upon the shock variable and, presumably, treatment
effects are also influenced by particular situational variables.

Recently, however, some investigations have been made on the cholinergic mediation of S.I.D.F. in the amygdala. These studies employed the optimum shock paramenters for S.I.D.F. and carefully controlled
for changes in pain sensitivity and locomotor activity.

Rodgers and Brown (1976) found that bilateral microinjections of
the cholinolytic, scopolamine hydrobromide, into the basolateral amygdala resulted in a specific reduction in S.I.D.F. Similar cholinergic
blockade in either the dorsal or ventral hippocampus produced a concomitant reduction in S.I.D.F. and pain sensitivity. These results
suggest that it is unlikely that the hippocampus is specifically involved in the cholinergic mediation of S.I.D.F. Microinjections of
physostigmine (an inhibitor of the enzyme acetylcholinesterase) resulted in a significant increase in fighting without altering pain
sensitivity or locomotor coordination. This finding supported the
earlier results of Rodgers and Brown (1973a) who reported increased
S.I.D.F. with peripheral injections of physostigmine.

Rodgers and Brown were further able to demonstrate neuroanatomical specificity, within the amygdala, for the cholinergic mediation of
S.I.D.F. Both scopolamine and physostigmine failed to alter S.I.D.F.
when injected into the corticomedial amygdala. The importance of the
cholinergic amygdaloid influence on S.I.D.F. was demonstrated by the
fact that bilateral electrolytic lesions of the basolateral amygdala
resulted in a specific blockade of S.I.D.F. This indicated that an
intact cholinergic basolateral amygdala is essential for the manifestation of this type of aggression.

. Finally, bilateral injections of scopolamine into the basolateral
amygdala had no consistent effect upon the social attraction between
paired rats in the Latane Test, suggesting that the decrement in

S.I.D.F. following this treatment was not due to nonspecific reduction in social responsiveness (Rodgers and Brown, 1976).

Bell and Brown (1980) reported evidence for cholinergic mediation
of S.I.D.F. in the lateral hypothalamus. Bilateral microinjections of
cholinergic agonists (carbachol and physostigmine) increased aggression, whilst administration of cholinergic antagonist (scopolamine)
reduced S.I.D.F. Behavioral specificity of lateral hypothalamic mediation of S.I.D.F. was demonstrated by the lack of effect of altered
ACh levels on pain sensitivity, motor activity, motor coordination,
social attraction and control injection site. Similar results were
found for the anterior hypothalamus (Bell and Brown, unpublished
results).

There is no information on endogenous acetylcholine levels and
shock-induced defensive fighting. Perhaps we should not expect to
detect changes in biochemical levels, because pain-induced defensive
behavior is a response to an acute stimulus and not a chronic state.

2.2. Predatory Aggression

There seems to be no positive evidence linking endogenous brain
acetylcholine levels with predatory aggression and the only evidence
available is negative (Consolo and Valzelli, 1970). However, Mandel
et al. (1979) demonstrated higher choline acetyltransferase activity
in the amygdala of killer rats and in the amygdala of bulbectomized
rats after they had become killers; a significant different of 33.05
+/- 3.44 non-killers compared with to 41.85 +/1 4.85 in intact killers
and a rise from 36.74 +/- 4.85 to 42.98 +/- 4.85 in bulbectomized
killer rats. This evidence would suggest higher rates of synthesis
and this fact together with the negative evidence on acetylcholine
levels can be interpreted as increased release in killer rats.

The psychological evidence for a cholinergic involvement in the
mediation of interspecific aggression in the rat is abundant, but far
from consistent. Initial attempts to demonstrate cholinergic mediation of muricide were not encouraging. Horovitz et al. (1966) found
that peripherally administered atropine (an ACh blocker) was ineffective as an antimuricidal agent. Subsequently, however, it has been
shown that pilocarpine (a cholinomimetic) can induce muricide in non-
killer rats (McCarthy, 1966; Vogel and Leaf, 1972). Atropine and scopolamine can produce a marked inhibition of this pilocarpine-induced
muricide, whilst methyl atropine (with mainly a peripheral cholinolytic action) potentiates pilocarpine-induced muricide through its inhibitory action on the peripheral side-effects of this cholinomimetic
(Vogel and Leaf, 1972).

Carbachol, injected into lateral hypothalamic attack sites, can
facilitate predatory aggression (Yoburn et al., 1981) whilst methylatropine inhibits this behavior (Bandler, 1969, 1970; Smith et al.,

1970; Albert, 1980). .Carbachol application to the dorsal, medial or ventral hypothalamus was ineffective in eliciting the killing response thus indicating the specific role of the lateral hypothalamus in muricide. Bandler (1970) reported that hypothalamic application of ACh (mixed with physostigmine) could also facilitate the killing response, whilst Smith et al. (1970) demonstrated that neostigmine (an anticholinesterase which indirectly increases ACh) elicited and methyl atropine blocked muricide when applied to hypothalamic attack sites. Although Bandler found that norepinephrine could suppress mouse-killing at some carbachol-effective sites in the hypothalamus, Smith et al. (1970) reported that neither norepinephrine, amphetamine nor serotonin altered muricide.

Carbachol injections into the medial nucleus of the thalamus also facilitates killing whilst atropine suppresses it; neither norepinephrine nor serotonin had any effect in this area (Bandler, 1971a). Bandler also found that atropine, injected into the thalamus, could block muricide induced by carbachol injections into the lateral hypothalamus, but that the reverse treatment did not work. These resuls suggested that some phases of hypothalamic-induced facilitation of muricide are dependent upon the activity of the thalamus, while thalamic induced killing is dependent on neither activity in the hypothalamus nor activity in pathways descending through the hypothalamus. Again, administration of serotonin or norepinephrine to the thalamic sites had no effect on muricide.

The ventral midbrain tegmentum has been implicated in the cholinergic control of mouse-killing, since carbachol application to this area lowers attack and kill latencies (Bandler, 1971b). Atropine, when injected into these effective midbrain sites, blocked carbachol facilitation in the lateral hypothalamus, thus suggesting a link between hypothalamic and midbrain areas possibly via cholinergic neurons in the medial forebrain bundle. Interestingly, norepinephrine injections into these ventral midbrain sites also resulted in increased muricide (Bandler, 1971b).

Leaf et al. (1969) found that scopolamine methylbromide, when injected directly into the amygdala, blocked the killing response, whilst physostigmine induced killing. More specifically, Igic et al. (1970) indicated that the basolateral nucleus of the amygdala was involved in muricide, as local application of amitone (an anticholinesterase) induced killing whilst atropine application resulted in an inhibition of this response. These authors also reported that amitone injections into the septal area could also elicit the muricide response.

Wnek and Leaf (1973) elicited muricide by rats with systemic injections of another muscarinic agonist, pilocarpine. However, other cholinergic agonists including arecoline (a muscarinic agonist), oxotremorine, physostigmine, neostigmine and methacholine were ineffective over a broad range of doses. They were also unable to induce killing in guinea pigs and hamsters with pilocarpine. However, these results must be interpreted cautiously because guinea pigs and hamsters will rarely kill mice. It is quite possible that muscarinic cholinergic stimulation is only effective for some species which have a neurological substrate for predatory aggression.

2.3. Isolation-induced Aggression

In isolation-induced aggression there has been a consistent neurochemical picture obtained. There is some evidence for enhanced synthesis in isolated rats with a 13 percent increase in choline acetylase (ChA) activity in the mesencephalic regions (Garattini and Sigg, 1969). This increase is paralleled by a 10 percent lowering of the levels of ACh in the same regions (Karczmar and Scudder, 1969). These findings suggest strongly that there is a markedly increased release of ACh in the isolated animals, although no studies have been conducted measuring brain acetylcholine turnover.

Peripheral injections of cholinolytics (e.g., scopolamine) have been found to decrease isolation-induced fighting in mice, without producing any significant side-effects (DaVanzo, 1969; Karczmar and Scudder, 1969). Further, DaVanzo reported that scopolamine can potentiate the anti-aggressive properties of chlordiazepoxide at lower doses than those required to produce locomotor impairment. More recently, Krsiak and Tomasikova (1980) have reported that scopolamine, in low doses, reduced aggression whilst increasing social behavior and locomotion. Further investigations revealed that relatively high doses of scopolamine were required to reduce defense and escape behaviors (Krsiak et al, 1981). The authors suggest different mechanisms may be involved in aggression and defense-escape components.

Further detailed analysis of the effects of scopolamine on aggression was carried out by Yoshimura and Ogawa (1982). These authors reported a significant, dose dependent, suppression of offensive sideways posture, tail rattling and biting attack. However, scopolamine also increased locomotor and rearing activity, indicating that nonspecific effects of the drug cannot be ruled out.

Physostigmine appears to have a biphasic effect on aggression; the drug facilitates isolation-induced aggression at low doses (due to increased functional ACh levels) but inhibits fighting at high doses. This last effect is probably due to a depolarization blocking effect produced by an overabundance of synaptic ACh competing for a limited number of post-synaptic receptor sites (Karczmar and Scudder, 1969). Physostigmine may also produce a specific increase in defensive reactions (Mollenauer et al., 1979).

In a study by Charpentier (1969) male mice were isolated in individual cages, situated in quiet surroundings. Aggressiveness was tested by exposing isolated mice to the same adversary. The contact duration was limited to six minutes. For the purpose of the study,

aggressiveness was defined as the delay before first attack; number
of attacks and length of attack period; and passiveness was defined
as the number of squeals after attack; number of spontaneous squeals,
without attack; number of defense movements and number of flights.
The score for the attack is calculated from their intensity as follows: 1, for a movement towards the adversary, with contact; 2, for
an attack without biting; 3, for biting and 4, for continued attack,
with repeated biting.

He used the following drugs to modify the cholinergic systems:
physostigmine salicylate, 0.5. mg/kg i.p. and tested 90 minutes after
injection, because this dose disrupted most behaviors for 30 minutes
and atropine sulphate, 20 mg/kg i.p. and tested 30 minutes after
injection. These doses of drug were given to animals isolated for
four months, well-trained and in well-established aggressive/passive
pairs. The two types of mice, aggressive and passive, had different
sensitivity to the drugs. The drugs were always given in both animals
in a pair. He observed that physostigmine increased and atropine
almost completely inhibited the attack behavior in terms of all the
measures.

2.4.   Irritable Aggression

In cats, Hernández-Peón et al. (1963) found that rage could be
induced by cholinergic stimulation (micorinjections of ACh, ACh +
physostigmine or carbachol) of areas extending from the septum,
through the hypothalamus to the periaqueductal gray matter. Carbachol
injections into the ventromedial hypothalamus also elicit the rage
reaction in both cats and rats (Myers, 1964; Baxter, 1967; Grossman,
1970; Allikmets, 1974; Stokman and Glusman, 1981). These hypothalamic
attack sites correspond to sites at which electrical stimulation has
also produced rage reactions. Other structures where carbachol injections have elicited rage include the caudate nucleus of cats and rats,
(Hull et al., 1967; Grossman, 1970), midbrain (Stockman and Glusman,
1981), amygdala (Baxter, 1967; Grossman, 1970) and the dorsal hippocampus (Baxter, 1967; Grossman, 1970). Grossman also reported that
scopolamine, injected into the rat amygdala, reversed the effect of
carbachol. Intraventricular injections of carbachol (Beleslin and
Samardzic, 1977, 1979a) and arecoline, a muscarinic agonist, (Katz,
1981) increased irritable aggression.

The anti-aggressive effects of cholinolytics have been demonstrated over a wide phylogenetic range; for example, scopolamine has
been reported to inhibit the attack behavior of the ant, Formica rufa,
(Kostowski, 1968), cichlids (Avis and Peeke, 1973) and squirrel monkeys (Plotnik et al., 1975).

However, not all studies have provided clear cut evidence of ACh
mediation of aggression. Stern et al., (1975) found that peripheral
administration of an anticholinesterase called 4-NVP(trans-4-[naphtyl-
vinyl] pyridine) reversibly blocked the mouse-killing response in rats

and depressed fighting behavior in isolated mice. 4-NVP failed to
attentuate the reactivity of rats with septal lesions. The doses of
this compound used did not produce ataxia. These authors also reported that the administration of the purified venom of the female black
widow spider, <u>Latrodectus mactans tredecimguttatus</u>, in non-toxic
doses, induced a mouse-killing response in non-killer rats. Applied
in higher doses, however, the venom depressed isolation-induced
aggression in mice, muricide and septal-lesion induced aggression in
rats due to poisoning. It seems, therefore, that muscarinic cholinergic overactivation depresses and moderate activation facilitates
certain types of aggression.

It is suggested that it is possible to interpret these findings
in terms of a model of the central brain structures involved in aggression as proposed by Karli et al. (1972) for predatory aggression
and extended by Rodgers (1975) for S.I.D.F. In order to understand
the derivation of this model, it is necessary to examine the evidence
for brain structures involved in predatory aggression.

2.5.   Identification of Brain Structures Involved in Control of
        Predatory Aggression

Mouse-killing behavior in the rat may be elicited by stimulation
of the lateral hypothalamus, ventral to the fornix (King and Hoebel,
1968), the anterolateral hypothalamus (Panksepp and Trowill, 1969),
hypothalamic areas above the optic tract, around the fornix and the
lateral border of the ventromedial hypothalamus (Panksepp, 1971) and
the ventral hypothalamus (Woodworth, 1971). Vergnes and Karli (1969,
1970) demonstrated that stimulation of the posterolateral hypothalamus
facilitates muricide in killer rats but not in non-killers. These
authors also reported that ventromedial/dorsolateral stimulation can
elicit killing in non-killer rats. Stimulation of the amygdala (Karli
et al., 1969) and the mesencephalic central gray (Chaurand et al.,
1972) inhibits the killing response whilst stimulation of the dorsomedial thalamus has no effect (Vergnes and Karli, 1972.

Lesions of the olfactory bulbs induce muricide in non-killer rats
(Vergnes and Karli, 1963a; Malick, 1970) but inhibit killing in killer
rats (Bandler and Chi, 1972). Didiergeorges et al. (1966) demonstrated that if the olfactory afferents are severed at various ages then
the inhibitory influence, exerted by the bulbs in killer rats, does
not appear before 3 to 4 weeks. This finding suggests a lack of
olfactory maturation before that age. The result of olfactory bulbectomy appears to be influenced by rearing conditions, since this operation inhibits killing only if the animals are housed in groups
(Didiergoeorges and Karli, 1966); if isolated, the animals show a
greater tendency to kill (Bernstein and Moyer, 1970). Castration has
been found to decrease the percentage of killing, especially in bulbectomized animals (Didiergeorges and Karli, 1967). Sex differences
have also been shown in muricide, since males kill more than female,
whether normal or bulbectomized (Thorne et al., 1973).

Whether olfactory bulbectomy effects are due to bulb damage or
further CNS degeneration has not been fully resolved.   Although
bulbectomy increases killing in non-killers, anosmia produced by zinc
sulphate or olfactory deafferentation has no effect on this response
(Alberts and Friedman, 1972; Spector and Hull, 1972; Cain and Paxinos,
1974).   However, further work by Cain (1974) and Thorne et al. (1974)
on discrete lesions in the olfactory area, yielded results suggesting
that only damage to bulbs rostral to the frontal pole had a selective
effect on killing.   Damage to the caudal areas produced muricide
accompanied by increased emotionality/irritability.

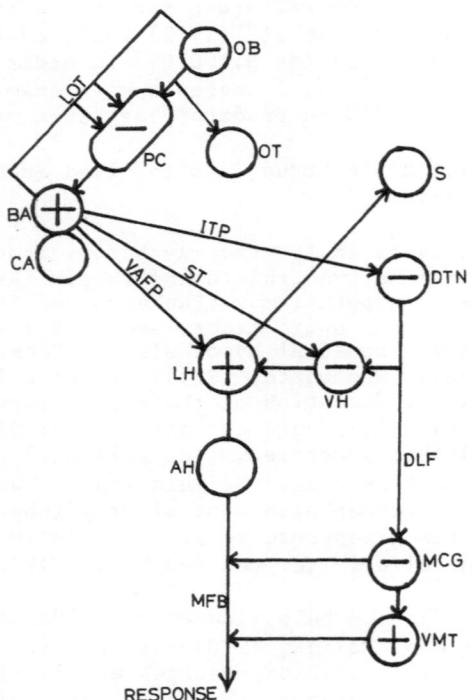

Fig. 1.   Structures Involved in the Facilitation (+) and Suppression
          (-) of Muricide in Rats (after Karli et al., 1972).   AH-anter-
          rior hypothalamus; BA-basolateral amygdala; CA-corticomedial
          amygdala; DLF-dorsal longitudinal fasciculus; DTN-dorsomedial
          thalamic nuclei; ITP-inferior thalamic peduncle; LH-lateral
          hypothalamus; LOT-lateral olfactory tract; MFB-medial fore-
          brain bundle; MCG-mesencephalic central gray; OB-olfactory
          bulb; OT-olfactory tubercle; PC-prepiriform cortex; S-septum;
          ST-stria terminalis; VAFP-ventral amygdalo-fugal pathway;
          VH-ventral hypothalamus; VMT-ventromedial midbrain tegmentum.

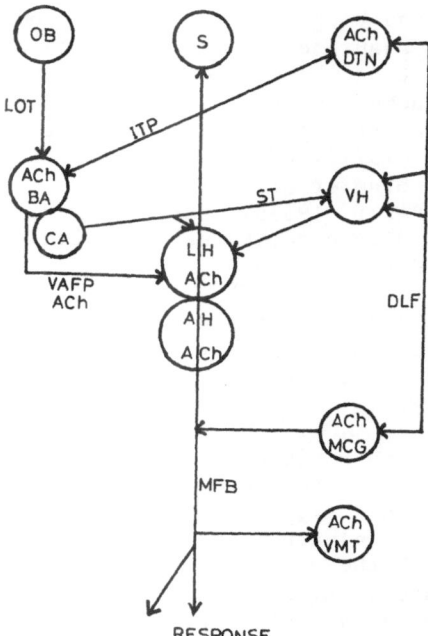

Fig. 2.   The Proposed Cholinergic Facilitatory System for Aggressive
          Behavior.   AH-anterior hypothalamus; BA-basolateral amyg-
          dala; CA-corticomedial amygdala; DLF-dorsal longitudinal
          fasciculus; DTN-dorsomedial thalamic nuclei; ITP-inferior
          thalamic peduncle; LH-lateral hypothalamus; LOT-lateral
          olfactory tract; MFB-medial forebrain bundle; MCG-mesencepha-
          lic central gray; OB-olfactory bulb; OT-olfactory tubercle;
          PC-prepiriform cortex; S-septum; ST-stria terminalis; VAFP-
          ventral amygdalo-fugal pathway; VH-ventral hypothalamus;
          VMT-ventromedial midbrain tegmentum.

        Bilateral amygdalectomy has been shown to abolish mouse-killing
(Karli, 1956).   Subsequently, Karli and Vergnes (1965) demonstrated
that bilateral destruction of the central amygdaloid nucleus was
essential to the abolition of muricide in killer rats.   Also, the
inhibitory effects on muricide, exerted by the olfactory bulbs, are
thought to act directly on the central amygdaloid nucleus (Karli
et al., 1969).

        Other subcortical regions have also been investigated in connec-
tion with mouse-killing.   Bilateral lesions of the posterior lateral

hypothalamus (Karli and Vergnes, 1964) or ventromedial tegmentum (Karli et al., 1972; Chaurand et al., 1973) inhibit muricide. Mouse-killing can be facilitated by bilateral destruction of the dorso-medialthalamus (Eclancher and Karli, 1968, 1969), the mesencephalic central gray (Chaurand and Karli, 1970) or ventromedial hypothalamus (Eclancher and Karli, 1971). Finally, bilateral lesions of the septal area (Karli, 1960; Thorne et al., 1974), caudate nucleus or frontal cortex (Vergnes and Karli, 1963b), periaqueductal gray (Vergnes and Chaurand, 1973) or midbrain reticular formation (Kesner and Keiser, 1973) have been found to have no effect on muricide.

Karli et al. (1972) have provided a schematic summary of central structures involved in the facilitation (+) or suppression (−) of mur-icide. This summary, based on the previously cited experimental data, is illustrated in Fig. 1.

From the literature reviewed on the pharmacology of predatory aggression, it is apparent that a cholinergic "trigger" is responsible for the mediation of this type of agonistic behavior, as proposed by Allikmets, (1974). The electrolytic lesion studies carried out on S.I.D.F. indicate that the same structures involved in S.I.D.F. also play a role in predatory aggression. Further, the pharmacology of S.I.D.F. studies indicates cholinergic facilitation of this type of aggression, consistent with the cholinergic mediation of predatory aggression. Thus Rodgers (1975) "mapped" the cholinergic circuits involved in shock-induced and predatory aggression using the earlier diagram proposed by Karli et al. (1972). The cholinergic "trigger" for these two types of aggression, as proposed by Rodgers (1975) is summarized in Fig. 2.

2.6. A Model for Shock-Induced Defensive Fighting in the Rat

This model proposed that an intact functional cholinergic system, in the basolateral amygdala, is essential for the manifestation of S.I.D.F. The role of this area of the amygdala is a modulatory one, exerting its effect via more basic hypothalamic motivational mechan-isms. The central cholinergic facilitatory mechanism included a neo-cortical − basolateral amygdala − hypothalamic connection, with the amygdala serving as an integrative interface between cortex and hypo-thalamus. Since the amygdala receives input from all sensory modali-ties, the model envisages this structure as a link between past exper-iences, stored in the cortex, and basic hypothalamic effector mecha-nisms. (Rodgers, [1977] subsequently demonstrated a dopamine/seroto-nin balance in the corticomedial amygdala, serving to exert a thresh-hold for the release of aggression by the cholinergic basolateral amygdala.)

The studies reviewed support the prediction that the cholinergic facilitation of S.I.D.F. from the basolateral amygdala is mediated, via the ventral amygdalo-fugal pathway to the lateral and anterior hypothalamus. From the hypothalamus, effector mechanisms, mediated by ACh, may operate through mesencephalic structures such as the midbrain central gray and the ventral midbrain tegmentum. In fact, the midbrain central gray may act as a modal command system on these mechanisms (Edwards and Adams, 1974; Stokman and Glusman, 1981).

It is of interest to compare the roles of the amygdala and the hypothalamus in S.I.D.F. The amygdala is portrayed as an integrating link between the cortex and the hypothalamus, such that it can bias hypothalamic output in accordance with sensory input and past experiences (Rodgers, 1975; Siegel and Edinger, 1981). In addition to its relationship with the hypothalamus, the amygdala is also linked, via the inferior thalamic peduncle, to the dorsomedial thalamus which may also be involved in this system. This structure projects to posterior systems lower by way of the dorsal longitudinal fasciculus. However, it is more likely that the role of the thalamus in aggression is related to its function in sensory evaluation, suggesting that such information may be relayed from there to the amygdala and higher cortical centers for interpretation and integration. This would explain the apparent double-interface function for the amygdala in behavior. The cortical-amygdaloid-thalamic interface is involved in interpreting sensory inputs in the light of past experiences, whilst the cortical-amygdaloid-hypothalamic interface activates basic effector mechanisms (Rodgers, 1975).

The hypothalamus, whilst containing its own inhibitory systems in the lateral and anterior nuclei, appears to be biased by amygdaloid influences. Since hypothalamic output can further be modulated, for example by the midbrain central gray, it is possible to conceive of the limbic system as a series of structures which serve to modulate hypothalamic attack mechanisms (Siegel and Edinger, 1981). However, it may also be the case that the hypothalamus may bias other limbic structures, such as the septal areas and the thalamus. Direct evidence to support this hypothesis is lacking in the literature (Siegel and Edinger, 1981).

Finally, we can say something about the earlier comments by Moyer (1968) that different forms of aggression have different physiological bases. Although Jacobs and Cohen (1976) state that it is an open question whether different types of aggression share a common neurochemical substrate, the results of S.I.D.F. investigations suggest that the occurrence of aggression in a particular situation is dependent upon the activity of a cholinergic trigger mechanism which, in turn, is subject to influences from the counter-balancing inhibitory mechanisms. These central control systems are further influenced by past experience, heredity, olfaction and endocrinology. Therefore, the differentiation between aggression types may only reflect the different stimulus situations which produce them and the final stereotyped, situation-specific responses which result. Indeed, since both cholinergic stimulation and serotonergic depletion facilitate different types of aggression, it can be argued that these two transmitters

and their related pathways are shared by aggression outputs through
common central brain structures.

If this concept of the neural circuits involved in aggression is
applied to a given situation, the relationships between transmitters,
central systems and the resulting type of aggression can be explained.
For example, in the case of territorial aggression, the home animal
detects an intruder and the sensory input is integrated in the amygdala along with past experiences from the cortex. The amygdala biases
the hypothalamic output, which is further modulated in the midbrain
to produce social aggression. The mediation of this aggressive response is brought about by firing of the cholinergic trigger mechanism
and inhibited, where necessary, by monoaminergic systems. In predatory aggression, the sensory inputs, which are mainly olfaction, this
time activate the cholinergic trigger mechanism which, through limbic
integration and interpretation, results in a typical predatory attack.
S.I.D.F. results through the same transmitter-structures system,
except that the important sensory input comes from the vibrissae.
Thus, it is suggested that a common aggression system exists in the
brain which, depending on different sensory inputs, produces different
types of aggressive responses through common neurotransmitters.

3.   EVIDENCE FOR NICOTINIC CHOLINERGIC MEDIATION OF AGGRESSIVE
     BEHAVIOR

In comparison with the literature on muscarinic mechanisms, very
few studies have directly investigated nicotinic influences on attack
or defensive behaviors. No doubt this is partly due to the relative
lack of direct evidence on the nature and distribution of nicotinic
receptors in brain tissue and their functional significance. Recent
advances, e.g., the use of radio-receptor binding techniques, may lead
to greater understanding of CNS nicotinic receptors (Nordberg and
Larsson, 1981). An additional difficulty is the suggestion that,
although the action of nicotine is mediated via cholinergic receptors,
some non-cholinergic sites for nicotine may exist within the brain
(e.g., Abood et al., 1981).

3.1.   Shock-Induced Defensive Fighting

Emley et al. (1971) and Hutchinson and Emley (1973) reported
that nicotine suppressed the biting attack (on a rubber hose) induced
in squirrel monkeys by tail-shock. No further reports appeared until
1979, when Rodgers obtained a dose-dependent inhibition of fighting
following i.p. nicotine (0.25, 0.50 and 1.00 mg/kg) in paired male
rats exposed to foot-shock. None of the nicotine doses had any effect
on jump flinch shock thresholds and locomotor activity in a photocell
activity test was unaffected (with the exception of a reduction in
rearing in the highest nicotine dose). Mecamylamine, a centrally
active nicotinic antagonist, produced a facilitation in fighting at a

dose of 2.5 mg/kg and an inhibitory effect at 10 mg/kg (perhaps not surprising, given such a massive dose). The latter dose reduced both horizontal and vertical activity, but none of the doses had any effect on jump-flinch thresholds. When hexamethonium, a quarternary anti-nicotinic agent which does not penetrate to CNS, was used, the 2.25 and 4.50 mg/kg doses had little effect on fighting while the 9.0 and 18.0 mg/kg doses reduced fighting levels. The last dose significantly increased locomotor activity. Once again there were no alterations in jump-flinch thresholds with the drug.

Further support was provided by Waldbillig (1980) and Driscoll and Baettig (1981). Waldbillig found that both intraperitoneal and intraventricular injections of nicotine (a large dose of 800 µg) suppressed fighting in male rats induced by tail-shock and foot-shock respectively without influencing flinch, vocalization or escape thresholds. Driscoll and Baettig used female as well as male rats and in addition recorded the incidence of posturing behavior, in which the two rats face each other in an upright position, without actually fighting. This type of behavior can play an important part in the shock-induced fighting tests (Blanchard et al., 1977; Knutson and Hynan, 1972). Subcutaneous doses (0.1 and 0.2 mg/kg) of nicotine inhibited fighting in males with high frequency attack baselines by means of a dose-dependent replacement of fighting by posturing. At a dose of 0.4. mg/kg (approximately the maximum effective dose) there was an increase in the 'no reaction' category, particularly freezing. Thus reduced activity may have been partly responsible for the reduction in fighting recorded at that dose. None of the doses had any significant effect on sensitivity to foot-shock. An interesting finding was that nicotine had no effect on fighting in the low frequency fighting males and females were unaffected except at the 0.4 mg/kg level, where a reduction in fighting occurred due to an increase in the 'no reaction' category.

The possibility of important species differences is highlighted by a report by Rolinski and Herbut (1981), in which nicotine (i.p. 0.25 to 2.00 mg/kg and i.v. 5 to 30 µg) increased foot-shock elicited fighting in mice. The central injections affected previously tested animals only while the peripheral administration produced increases in both naive and previously tested mice. At a higher dose (i.p. 4.0 mg/kg) fighting was suppressed. Hexamethonium (2.0 and 4.0 mg/kg) potentiated the aggressive responding as did mecamylamine at low doses (2.0 and 4.0 mg/kg). At a higher dose, 8 mg/kg, the mecamylamine inhibited fighting.

3.2. Predatory Aggression

Although Wnek and Leaf (1973) had elicited muricide by rats with systemic injections of pilocarpine, nicotine was ineffective over a broad range of doses. Bernston et al. (1976) reported that nicotine suppressed, in a dose dependent manner, predatory attack in cats.

Further, pretreatment with nicotine reduced arecoline-induced predatory aggression. The nicotine reduction in attack behavior was
observed in the absence of general behavioral inhibition. On the
basis of these findings, Bernston et al. concluded that muscarinic and
nicotinic compounds can exert antagonistic control over predatory
aggression.

More evidence for the role of nicotinic systems in predatory
aggression was provided by Waldbillig (1980). Intraperitoneal injection of nicotine reduced mouse-killing by rats in a dose dependent
fashion. This suppression of muricide was not blocked by hexamethonium. However, mecamylamine did reduce the inhibition of attack produced by nicotine.

Although there is evidence of the role of nicotine in cat and rat
predatory aggression, there may be major species differences in the
effects of nicotine on aggression. Meierl and Schmidt (1982) found no
evidence for nicotinic cholinergic mechanism in the control of spontaneous predatory behavior in the ferret.

3.3. Isolation-Induced Aggression

Nicotine has been reported to increase the ratio of bound to free
ACh in mouse cerebral cortex. This ratio was decreased in group
housed mice when administered nicotine (Essman, 1971). Hutchinson and
Emley (1981) found that nicotine reduced elevated blood pressures in
rats and squirrel monkeys. These authors suggest that nicotine may be
selectively influential in altering states of aggression.

Silverman (1971) isolated rats for a few days, and then introduced one (the "partner") into the home cage of another which released
their social behavior. Each of the six partners was introduced once
on each of three successive mornings, meeting one saline- and two
(different) drug-injected rats in a counter-balanced order. In some
tests the whole procedure was repeated after a week's interval. Nicotine's effects were studied by comparing the behavior of the drug-
injected with saline-injected rats to the same partners. He found
that 25 μm per kg of nicotine selectively and reversibly reduced
aggression. This dose is comparable to that which a person obtains
from a cigarette.

Higher doses of nicotine clearly disrupted aggression rather than
reduce it. In pilot tests, rats given 50 μg/kg i.p. instead of
25 μg/kg s.c. showed signs which might be interpreted as those of
abdominal pain and of nausea. Pain and other unpleasant sensations
would certainly interfere with an animal's ability to perform any
elaborate and coherent behavior sequence like agonistic behavior.
This fact should clearly be borne in mind when interpreting data with
high doses of nicotine.

3.4. Irritable Aggression

Beleslin and Samardzic (1979a) examined the effects of intraventricular administration of nicotinic ganglionic stimulants on aggression in cats. Nicotine, dimethylphenylpiperazinium iodine (DMPP) and tetramethylammonium bromide (TMA) failed to evoke aggressive behavior. The authors concluded that central nicotinic receptors are not involved in the appearance of aggression in cats.

In a further study, Beleslin and Samardzic (1979b) reported that intraventricularly administered nicotine, DMPP, TMA, hexamethonium, tetraethylammonium and mecamylamine were ineffective in antagonizing muscarine-elicited aggression in cats.

An interesting study on the possible relationship between central nicotinic and muscarinic cholinergic systems in aggression was carried out by Romaniuk and Golebiewski (1977). Pretreatment microinjections of hexamethonium into the anterior medial hypothalamus and midbrain central gray caused a delay in the onset of carbachol-induced aggression in cats. This result was compared to the finding that pretreatment central injections of atropine completely blocked any subsequent carbachol injections effects. These authors concluded that nicotinic, as well as muscarinic, cholinergic systems are involved in carbachol-induced aggression, but muscarinic receptors were more important.

4.   EVIDENCE FOR CHOLINERGIC INTERACTIONS WITH OTHER NEUROTRANSMITTERS IN AGGRESSIVE BEHAVIOR

The evidence considered so far may reflect the effects, on aggression, of direct action on muscarinic and nicotinic cholinergic systems. However, it may well be the case that some of the observations are due to indirect actions on other neurotransmitters.

Several studies have implicated a muscarinic cholinergic interaction with dopamine activity (e.g., Colpaert, 1975; De Souza and Palermo-Neto, 1982). A muscarinic cholinergic interaction has also been suggested with norepinephrine (Egbe, 1982) and serotonin (Ladinsky et al., 1981). Nicotinic cholinergic systems have been shown to interact with catecholamines (Westfall, 1974) and serotonin (Balfour, 1973). Given these findings, what is the evidence for cholinergic interactions with other transmitters in the control of aggressive behavior?

Malick and Barnett (1976) reported that administration of serotonergic antagonists, eyproheptadine, pizotyline and cinanserin, reduced isolation-induced aggression in mice. The doses employed did not alter locomotor activity. Malick and Barnett argued that serotonergic and cholinergic systems are independently involved in the regulation of isolation-induced aggression in mice.

Gianutsos and Lal (1976) demonstrated antagonism of apomorphine-induced aggression in rats using pilocarpine. Cholinergic blockade, produced by dexetimide, intensified this aggression. These authors suggested the existence of a cholinergic system, presumably mucarinic, which is antagonistic to dopamine in drug-induced aggression. In a further study using the model of apomorphine-induced aggression, Gianutsos and Lal (1977) demonstrated that both morphine and neuroleptics reduced this type of aggressive behavior. Dexetimide reversed the effects of the neuroleptics, but not that of morphine.

Rolinski (1977) examined the effects of elevating cerebral serotonin levels, using L-tryptophan or DL-5-hydroxytryptophan, on amphetamine-induced aggression in mice. Increasing serotonin levels suppressed aggression whilst increasing muscarinic cholinergic activity potentiated aggressive behavior.

Rolinski has also subsequently demonstrated a cholinergic-dopaminergic-serotonergic interaction in apomorphine-induced aggression in rats (Rolinski and Herbut, 1979).

Further investigations by Rolinski and Herbut (1981) have indicated a muscarinic cholinergic interaction with catecholamines during shock-induced fighting in mice.

5.   EVIDENCE FOR ROLE OF CHOLINERGIC MECHANISMS IN HUMAN AGGRESSION

In a study carried out by Cherek (1981) the effects of smoking cigarettes, containing either 0.42 mg or 2.19 mg nicotine, were investigated with respect to aggressive responses. Nicotine produced a dose dependent decrease in the frequency of aggressive responses in subjects.

Bonnet et al. (1980) indicated that administration of the anti-muscarinic drug artane (trihexyphenidyl hydrochloride) reduced aggression in a patient suffering from an organic brain syndrome. The improvement noted occurred without any reduction in positive social behavior.

In his smoking motives survey, McKennell (1979) asked smokers about mood states which lead them to light up a cigarette. The answers were factor analyzed to extract the major factors which would initiate smoking. One of these factors was "nervous irritation" smoking which included "smokes when angry." As an extension of this finding using her "habits of nervous tension" questionnaire, Thomas (1973) discovered that cigarette smokers and former smokers had higher levels of irritability and anger in comparison with lifetime non-smokers. When the smokers were divided into light (less than 20 a day) and heavy groups (more than 20 per day), the heavy smokers had greater anger responses under stress than the light smokers. In two studies of smokers at a stop-smoking clinic and non-clinic smokers (Russell et al., 1974) and student smokers (Warburton and Wesnes 1978), "smoking when angry" was one of the "top 10" reasons given for smoking by smokers attending a stop-smoking clinic (83 percent), non-clinic smokers (47 percent) and student smokers (65 percent). It appears from this consistency that feelings of anger is a major motive for smoking in a proportion of smokers.

Aggression is a difficult area in which to conduct human experiments and no really satisfactory studies on nicotine and aggression in people have been done. Schachter (1978) reports a study by Perlick which compared "irritability" in groups of unrestrained smokers and smokers who were trying to cut down their smoking and were smoking fewer cigarettes. Each group was then exposed to aircraft noise and asked to rate the annoyance caused by noise, after smoking either a 1.3 mg nicotine cigarette, a 0.3 mg cigarette or not smoking. It was found that unrestrained smokers, when deprived or smoking the low nicotine cigarette, were more annoyed than when smoking the medium nicotine cigarette. However, unrestrained smokers, when smoking the medium nicotine cigarette, were no better than non-smokers. The restrained group were just as irritated in all three conditions as the deprived or low nicotine, unrestrained smokers. There are at least two explanations for these results; either irritability is an abstinence sympton which is the consequence of nicotine dependence, or smoking helps to reduce this feeling.

Inferences about the effects of a nicotine on aggression can also be made from the abstinence symptoms that occur when smokers give up smoking. Studies of these symptoms that follow smoking cessation have shown that hostility and aggressive behavior increase markedly during abstinence (Mausner, 1980; Schechter and Rand, 1974; Shiffman and Jarvik, 1976). In studies of relapse, anger and interpersonal conflict are commonly reported as factors triggering relapse among ex-smokers, and these relapses occurred in the absence of smoking-related cues, such as "people around were smoking" (Shiffman, 1979; Marlatt, 1979). Clearly, the smoker who is deprived of nicotine is more prone to aggression and less calm. Evidence from a study by Thomas (1973), which showed that smokers and ex-smokers had similar scores for anger when stressed, suggests that smokers are constitutionally more angry and irritable and not that the increased aggression after cessation is due to the biochemical effects of nicotine withdrawal. From these data it follows that smoking may be being used as a form of self-medication by smokers for lowering aggression, but the important question is whether smoking is acting on a nicotinic system in the smoker's brain.

Experimental studies on smoking and aggression have provided no evidence of nicotine absorption from cigarettes, and therefore it is not usually possible to separate out the sedative effects of nicotine from the calming effects of the smoking ritual of cigarette manipulation. In a cigarette there is about 10 to 20 mg of nicotine and 14 to 20 percent is transferred into the mainstream smoke; so a 35 ml puff

on a 1.2 mg cigarette will give a mouth level of 150 to 250 μm of
nicotine (Armitage, 1973). Smoke inhalation results in very efficient
absorption of nicotine and over 80 to 90 percent of smokers say that
they inhale (Doll and Hill, 1964); in them nicotine absorption will
occur.

It is estimated that more than 90 to 95 percent of inhaled nicotine is absorbed (Artho and Grob, 1964). On the basis of the previous
estimates of 150 to 250 μm mouth level of nicotine from each puff,
over 100 μm would be taken up during each inhalation after each puff
from a medium delivery cigarette (Armitage et al., 1974) giving over
1.0 mg of nicotine per cigarette. After absorption, the nicotineload-
ed blood leaves the lungs and passes into the heart. From there the
nicotine is pumped out into the aorta from which the large arteries
branch off. The significant branch, from the point of view of smoking
and aggression is the carotid artery to the brain. About a fifth of
the blood from the heart ascends in the carotid artery so that a fifth
of the absorbed nicotine passes to the brain (Oldendorf, 1977) i.e.,
a dose of over 200 μm from a medium delivery cigarette. Studies in
the rat have found that well over 90 percent of the nicotine is taken
up on the first pass through the brain (Oldendorf, 1977) to give brain
levels of over 200 μm nicotine per cigarette, at a conservative
estimate.

Whole body autoradiograms of mice given intravenous doses of
14C-nicotine reveal a high accumulation of nicotine in cortical cells,
the hippocampus, hypothalamic nuclei, cerebellum and the brain stem
(Schmiterlow et al., 1967). This pattern of distribution throughout
the brain allows for neurochemical interaction of nicotine with the
regions that have been implicated in aggression earlier.

6.   CONCLUDING COMMENTS

The studies reviewed in this chapter strongly indicate a central
muscarinic cholinergic system which mediates aggressive behavior.
Similarly, investigations have provided evidence for the concept of a
nicotinic cholinergic mechanism which may inhibit aggression. It
should be noted, however, that the evidence for the role of muscarinic
and nicotinic cholinergic systems in the control of aggressive behavior cannot with certainty be generalized across all species. On the
other hand there is a slight evidence for the involvement of nicotinic
and muscarinic cholinergic systems in human aggression.

As noted by Rodgers (1979b), manipulating one neurotransmitter
may alter activity in a related system. Certainly, investigations
have implicated cholinergic interactions with dopamine and serotonin,
though the functional significance may be restricted to the particular
model of aggressive behavior being tested.

It is important to appreciate that, just as neurotransmitters interact, so it appears that limbic system structures also interact to produce a behavioral response (Siegel and Edinger, 1981). Thus the neuropharmacology of aggression seems to be a complex series of inter- actions between excitatory and inhibitory neurotransmitters conveying influences via interacting limbic structures.

ACKNOWLEDGEMENT

The authors would like to thank Professor David Warburton for his helpful comments and for contributing some useful additional material, and also Heather Johnston and Pamela Bell for their help in preparing this chapter.

REFERENCES

Abood, L. G., Reynolds, D. T., Booth, H., and Bidlack, J. M., 1981, Sites and mechanisms for nicotine's action in the brain, Neurosci. Biobehav. Rev. 5:479-486.

Albert, D. J., 1980, Suppression of mouse killing by lateral hypo- thalamic infusion of atropine sulfate in the rat: a general behavioral suppression, Pharmacol. Biochem. Behav. 12:681-688.

Alberts, J. R., and Freedman, M. I., 1972, Olfactory bulb removal but not anosmia increases emotionally and mouse-killing, Nature 238:434-435.

Allikmets, L. H., 1974, Cholinergic mechanisms in aggressive behavior Med. Biol. 52:19-30.

Armitage, A. K., 1973, Some recent observations relating to the ab- sorption of nicotine from tobacco smoke, in "Smoking Behavior," W. L. Dunn, ed., pp. 83-91, Winston J. Wiley, Washington, D.C.

Armitage, A. K., Dollery, C. T., George, C. F., Houseman, T. H., Lewis P. J., and Turner, D. M., 1974, Absorption and metabolism of nico- tine by man during cigarette smoking, Br. J. Clin. Pharmacol. 1:180P-181P.

Artho, A. J., and Grob, K., 1964, Nicotinabsorption aus dem Cigarettenrauch, Z. Praventiv. Med. 9:14-25.

Avis, H. H., and Peeke, H. V. S., 1973, Scopolamine and intraspecific aggression in cichlasoma nigrofasciatum: evidence for cholinergic mechanism in fish aggression. Paper presented at the meeting of the Western Psychological Association, Anaheim, California.

Azrin, N. H., Hutchinson, R. R., and Hake, D. F., 1967, Attach avoid- ance and escape reactions to aversive shock, J. Exp. Anal. Behav. 10:131-148.

Azrin, N. H., Ulrich, R. E., Hutchinson, R. R., and Norman, D. G., 1964, Effect of shock duration on shock-induced fighting, J. Exp. Anal. Behav. 7:9-11.

Balfour, D. J. K., 1973, Effects of nicotine on the uptake and reten- tion of 14C-noradrenaline and 14C-5-hydroxytryptamine by rat brain homogenates, Eur. J. Pharmacol. 23:19-26.

Bandler, R. J., 1971b, Chemical stimulation of the rat midbrain and aggressive behavior, Nature 229:222-223.

Bandler, R. J., 1970, Cholinergic synapses in the lateral hypothalamus for the control of predatory aggression in the rat, Brain Res. 20:409-424.

Bandler, R. J., 1971a, Direct chemical stimulation of the thalamus: effects on aggressive behavior in the rat, Brain Res. 26:81-93.

Bandler, R. J., 1969, Facilitation of aggressive behavior in the rat by direct cholinergic stimulation of the hypothalamus, Nature 224:1035-1036.

Bandler, R. J., 1975, Predatory aggression: midbrain-pontine junction rather than hypothalamus as the critical structure? Aggress. Behav. 1:261-266.

Barclay, A. M., and Haber, R. N., 1965, The relation of aggressive to sexual motivation, J. Pers. 3:462-475.

Baxter, B. L., 1967, Comparison of the behavioral effects of electrical or chemical stimulation applied at the same loci, Exp. Neurol. 19:412-432.

Beleslin, D. B., and Samardzic, R., 1979b, Comparative study of aggressive behavior after injection of cholinomimetics, anticholinesterases, nicotinic and muscarinic ganglionic stimulants into the cerebral ventricles of conscious cats: failure of nicotinic drugs to evoke aggression, Psychopharmacology 60:147-153.

Beleslin, D. B., and Samardzic, R., 1979d, Effects of 6-hydroxydopamine and reserpine on aggressive behavior induced by cholinomimetic and anticholinesterase injections into cerebral ventricles of conscious cats: dissociation of biting attack from snarling and hissing, Psychopharmacology 61:149-153.

Beleslin, D. B., and Samardzic, R., 1979a, Effects of paracholorophenylalanine and 5, 6-dihydroxytryptamine on aggressive behavior evoked by cholinomimetics and anticholinesterases injected into the cerebral ventricles of conscious cats, Neuropharmacology 18:251-257.

Beleslin, D. B., and Samardzic, R., 1979e, Evidence of central cholinergic mechanisms in the appearance of affective aggressive behavior: dissociation of aggression from autonomic and motor phenomena, Psychopharmacology 62:163-167.

Beleslin, D. B., and Samardzic, R., 1977, Muscarine- and carbachol-induced aggressions: fear and irritable kinds of aggression, Psychopharmacology 55:233-236.

Beleslin, D. B., and Samardzic, R., 1979c, The pharmacology of aggressive behavioral phenonema elicited by muscarine injected into the cerebral ventricles of conscious cats, Psychopharmacology 60:155-158.

Bell, R., and Brown, K., 1980, Shock induced defensive fighting in the rat: evidence for cholinergic mediation in the lateral hypothalamus, Pharmacol. Biochem. Behav. 12:487-491.

Bernstein, H., and Moyer, K. E., 1970, Aggressive behavior in the rat: effects of isolation and olfactory bulb lesions, Brain Res. 20:75-84.

Bernston, G. G., Beattie, M. S., Walker, J. M., 1976, Effects of nicotinic and muscarinic compounds on biting attack in the cat, Pharmacol. Biochem. Behav. 5:235-239.

Blanchard, R. J., Blanchard, D. C., and Takahashi, L. K., 1977, Reflexive fighting in the albino rat: aggressive or defensive behavior, Aggress. Behav. 3:145-155.

Blanchard, R. J., Fukunaga, K. K., Blanchard, D. C., and Kelley, M. J., 1975, Conspecific aggression in the rat, J. Comp. Physiol. Psychol. 89:1204-1209.

Bonnet, K. A., Freidhoff, A. J., Anderson, L. T., Green, W. H., 1980, Anticholinergic remediation of human aggression resulting from an organic brain syndrome, Prog. Clin. Biol. Res. 39:462.

Brudzynski, S. M., 1981a, Carbachol-induced agonistic behavior in cats: aggressive or defensive response? Acta Neurobiol. Exp. 41:15-32.

Brudzynski, S. M., 1981b, Growling component of vocalization as a quantitative index of carbachol-induced emotional-defensive response in cats, Acta. Neurobiol. Exp. 41:33-52.

Brudzynski, S. M., Kielczykowska, E., Romaniuk, A., 1982, The effects of external stimuli on the emotional-aversive response evoked by intrahypothalamic carbachol injections, Behav. Brain Res. 4:33-43.

Cain, D. P., 1974, Olfactory bulbectomy: neural structures involved in irritability and aggression in the male rat, J. Comp. Physiol. Psychol. 86:213-220.

Cain, D. P., and Paxinos, G., 1974, Olfactory bulbectomy and mucosal damage: effects on copulation, irritability and interspecific aggression in male rats, J. Comp. Physiol. Psychol. 86:202-212.

Charpentier, J., 1969, Analysis and measurement of aggressive behavior in mice, in "Aggressive Behavior," S. Garattini and E. B. Sigg, eds., pp. 86-100, Wiley, New York.

Chaurand, J. P., and Karli, P., 1970, Effects of lesions of the central gray matter of the mesencephalon on the interspecific aggressive behavior and the feeding habits of the rat, C. R. Soc. Biol. 164:1345-1380.

Chaurand, J. P., Schmitt, P., Karli, P., 1972, Substance grise central du mesencephale et le comportement d'agression interspecifique du rat, Physiol. Behav. 9:475-481.

Chaurdan, J. P., Vergnes, M., Karli, P., 1973, Effets du lesions du tegmentum ventral du mesencephale sur le comportement d'agression rat-souris, Physiol. Behav. 10:507-517.

Cherek, D. R., 1981, Effects of smoking different doses of nicotine on human aggression behavior, Psychopharmacology 75:339-345.

Colpaert, F. C., 1975, The ventromedial hypothalamus and the control of avoidance behavior and aggression: fear hypothesis versus response-suppression theory of limbic system function, Behav. Biol. 15:27-44.

Consolo, S., and Valzelli, L., 1970, Brain choline acetylase and monoamine oxidase activity in normal and aggressive mice, Eur. J. Pharmac. 13:129-130.

Creer, T. L., and Powell, D. A., 1971, The effect of repeated shock presentations and different stimulus intensities on shock-induced aggression, Psychon. Sci. 24:133-134.

DaVanzo, J. P., 1969, Observations related to drug-induced alterations in aggressive behavior, in "Aggressive Behavior," S. Garattini and E. B. Sig, eds., pp. 263-272, Wiley, New York.

Decsi, L., and Nagy, J., 1974, Chemical stimulation of the amygdala with special regard to influence on the hypothalamus, Neuropharmacology 13:1153-1162.

De Souza, H., and Palermo-Neto, J., 1982, A quantitative study of cholinergic-dopaminergic interactions in the CNS, Pharmacology 24:222-229.

Didiergeorges, F., and Karli, P., 1967, Hormones steroides et maturation d'un comportement d'agression interspécifique du rat, C. R. Soc. Biol. 161:179-181.

Didiergeoroges, F., and Karli, P., 1966, Stimulation "sociales" et inhibition de l'agressivité interspécifique chez le rat privé de ses afférences olfactives, C. R. Soc. Biol. 160:2445-2447.

Didiergeorges, F., Vergnes, M., Karli, P., 1966, Privation des afférences olfactives et aggressivite interspecifique du rat, C. R. Soc. Biol. 160:866-868.

Doll, R., and Hill, A. B., 1964, Mortality in relation to smoking: ten years' observations of British doctors, Br. Med. J. 1:1339-1410 and 1460-1467.

Dreyer, P. I., and Church, R., 1968, Shock-induced fighting as a function of the intensity and duration of the aversive stimulus, Psychon. Sci. 10:271-272.

Driscoll, P., and Beattig, K., 1981, Selective inhibition by nicotine of shock-induced fighting in the rat, Pharmacol. Biochem. Behav. 14:175-179.

Eclancher, F., and Karli, P., 1971, Comportement d'agression interspécifique et comportement alimentaire du rat: effets de lésions des noyaux ventromédians de l'hypothalamus, Brain Res. 21:57-70.

Eclancher, F., and Karli, P., 1969, Comportement d'agression interspécifique rat-souris: effets de lésions du noyau dorso-médian du thalamus et des structures epithalamiques, J. Physiol. (Paris) 61:283.

Eclancher, F., and Karli, P., 1968, Lésion du noyan dorso-médian du thalamus et comportement d'agression interspécifique rat-souris, C. R. Soc. Biol. 162:2273-2276.

Edwards, A. E., and Adams, D. B., 1974, Role of midbrain central gray in pain induced defensive boxing of rats, Physiol. Behav. 13:113-121.

Egbe, P. C., 1982, The involvement of the catecholaminergic system in physostigmine-induced hyperactivity in rats, Arzneim-Forsch 32:27-29.

Eleftheriou, B. E., ed., 1972, "The Neurobiology of the Amygdala, Vol. 2 Adv. Behav. Biol.," Plenum Press, New York.

Emley, G. S., Hutchinson, R. R., Hunter, N. A., 1971, Selective actions of morphine, chlorpromazine, chlordiazepoxide, nicotine and d'amphetamine on shock-produced aggressive and motor responses in the squirrel monkey, Fed. Proc. 30:390.

Essman, W. B., 1971, Changes in cholinergic activity and avoidance behavior by nicotine in differentially housed mice, Int. J. Neurosci. 2:199-205.

Garattini, S., and Sigg, E. B., 1969, "Aggressive Behavior," Wiley, New York.

Gianutsos, G., and Lal, H., 1976, Blockade of apomorphine-induced aggression by morphine or neuroleptics: differential alteration by antimuscarinics and naloxone, Pharmacol. Biochem. Behav. 4:639-642.

Gianutsos, G., and Lal, H., 1977, Modification of apomorphine induced aggression by changing central cholinergic activity in rats, Neuropharmacology 16:7-10.

Grossman, S. P., 1972b, Aggression, avoidance and reaction to novel environments in female rats with VMH lesions, J. Comp. Physiol. Psychol. 78:274-283.

Grossman, S. P., 1970, Intracranial administration of drugs and emotional behavior, in "The Physiology of Emotion," P. Black, ed., pp. 73-79, Academic Press, New York.

Grossman, S. P., 1972a, The ventromedial hypothalamus and aggressive behaviors, Physiol. Behav. 9:721-725.

Hernandez-Peon, R., Chavez-Ibarra, G., Morgane, P. J., Timo-Iaria, C., 1963, Limbic cholinergic pathways involved in sleep and emotional behavior, Exp. Neurol. 8:93-111.

Horovitz, Z. P., Piala, J. J., High, J. P., Burke, J. C., and Leaf, R. C., 1966, Effects of drugs on the mouse-killing (muricide) test and its relationship to amygdaloid function, Int. J. Neuropharmacol. 5:405-411.

Hull, C. D., Buchwald, N. A., Ling, G. M., 1967, Effects of direct cholingeric stimulation of forebrain structures, Brain Res. 6:22-35.

Hutchinson, R. R., and Emley, G. S., 1973, Effects of nicotine on avoidance conditioned suppression and aggression response measures in animals, and man, in "Smoking Behavior," W. L. Dunn, ed., pp. 171-196, Winston (J. Wiley), Washington, D.C.

Hutchinson, R. R., and Emley, G. S., 1981, Nicotine ingestion reduces elevated blood pressures in rats and squirrel monkeys, Life Sci. 28:801-809.

Igic, R., Stern, P., Basagic, E., 1970, Changes in emotional behavior after application of cholinesterase inhibitor in the septal and amygdala regions, Neuropharmacology 9:73-75.

Jacobs, B. L., and Cohen, A., 1976, Differential behavioral effects of lesions of the median or dorsal raphe nuclei in rats: open field and pain elicited aggression, J. Comp. Physiol. Psychol. 90:102-108.

Karczmar, A. G., and Scudder, C. L., 1969, Aggression and neurochemical changes in different strains and genera of mice, in "Aggressive Behavior," S. Garattini, and S. B. Sigg, eds., pp. 209-227, Wiley, New York.

Karli, P., 1960, Septum, hypothalamus posterieur et agressivité interspécifique rat-souris, J. Physiol. (Paris) 52:135-136.

Karli, P., 1956, The Norway rat's killing response to the white mouse: an experimental analysis, Behavior 10:81-103.

Karli, P., and Vergnes, M., 1964, Dissociation expérimentale du comportement d'agression interspécifique rat-souris et du comportement alimentaire, C. R. Soc. Biol. 158:650-653.

Karli, P., and Vergnes, M., 1965, Role des différentes composantes du complexe nucléaire amygdalien dans la facilitation de l'agressivité interspécifique du rat, C. R. Soc. Biol. 159:754-756.

Karli, P., Vergnes, M., Didiergeorges, F., 1969, Rat-mouse aggressive behavior and its manipulation by brain ablation and brain stimulation, in "Aggressive Behavior," S. Garattini and S. B. Sigg, eds., pp. 47-55, Wiley, New York.

Karli, P., Vergnes, M., Eclancher, F., Schmitt, P., Chaurand, J. P., 1972, Role of amygdala in the control of mouse-killing behavior in the rat, in "The Neurobiology of the Amygdala, Vol. 2," B. E. Eleftheriou, ed., pp. 553-480, Plenum Press, New York.

Katz, R. J., 1981, Possible muscarinic-cholinergic mediation of patterned aggressive reflexes in the cat, Prog. Neuropsychopharmacol. 5:49-56.

Kesner, R. P., and Keiser, G., 1973, Effects of midbrain reticular lesions upon aggression in the rat, J. Comp. Physiol. Psychol. 84:194-206.

Kimbrell, G. M. A., 1969, Relationship of upright posture in foot-shock situation to dominance-submission in male C57BL/6 mice, Psychon. Sci. 16:167-168.

King, M. B., and Hoebel, B. G., 1968, Killing elicited by brain stimulation in rats, Commun. Behav. Biol. 2:173-177.

Knutson, J. R., and Hynan, M. T., 1972, Influence of upright posture on shock-elicited aggression in rats, J. Comp. Physiol. Psychol. 81:297-306.

Kostowski, W., 1968, A note on the effects of some cholinergic and anticholinergic drugs on the aggressive behavior and spontaneous electrical activity of central nervous system in the ant, formica rufa, J. Pharm. Pharmacol. 20:381-384.

Krsiak, M. and Tomasikova, Z., 1980, Effects of scopolamine on agonistic behavior in mice, Act. Nerv. Super. 22:201-203.

Krsiak, M., Sulcova, A., Tomasikova, Z., 1981, Drug effects on attack, defense and escape in mice, Pharmacol. Biochem. Behav. 14 (Suppl. 1):49-52.

Ladinsky, H., Consolo, S., Tierelli, A. S., Forloni, G. L., Segal, M., 1981, Regulation of cholinergic activity in the rat hippocampus: in vivo effects of oxotremrine and fenfluramine, Adv. Behav. Biol. 25:781-793.

Leaf, R. C., Lerner, L., and Horovitz, Z. P., 1969, The role of the amygdala in the pharmacological and endocrinological manipulation of aggression, in "Aggressive Behavior," S. Garattini and E. B. Sigg, eds., pp. 120-131, Wiley, New York.

Legrand, R. and Fielder, R., 1973, Role of dominance-submission relationships in shock induced fighting in mice, J. Comp. Physiol. Psychol. 82:501-506.

Leroux, A. G., and Myers, R. D., 1975, Action of serotonin microinjected into hypothalamus sites at which electrical stimulation produced aversive responses in the rat, Physiol. Behav. 14:501-505.

Malick, J. B., 1970, A behavioral comparison of three lesion-induced models of aggression in the rat, Physiol. Behav. 5:679-681.

Malick, J. B., and Barnett, A., 1976, The role of serotonergic pathways in isolation induced aggression in mice, Pharmacol. Biochem. Behav. 5:55-61.

Mandel, P., Mack, G., and Kempf, E., 1979, Molecular basis of some models of aggressive behavior in "Psychopharmacology of Aggression," M. Sandler, ed., pp. 95-110, Raven Press, New York.

Marlatt, A., 1979, A cognitive-behavioral model of the relapse process, in "Behavioral Analysis and Treatment of Substance Abuse," J. Krasnegor, Ed., pp. 191-199, National Institute for Drug Abuse, Washington, D.C.

Mausner, J. S., 1980, Cigarette smoking among patients with respiratory disease, Ann. Rev. Respir. Dis. 102:704-706.

McCarthy, D., 1966, Mouse-killing in rats treated with pilocarpine, Fed. Proc. 15:293-298.

McKennell, A. C., 1970, Smoking motivation factors, Br. J. Soc. Clin. Psychol. 9:8-22.

Meierl, G., and Schmidt, W. J., 1982, No evidence for cholinergic mechanisms in the control of spontaneous predatory behavior of the ferret, Pharmacol. Biochem. Behav. 16:677-681.

Mollenauer, S., White, M., Plotnik, R., Tiffany, P. B., 1979, Physostigmine: effects on fear or defense responses in the rat, Pharmacol. Biochem. Behav. 11:189-195.

Moyer, K. E., 1968, Kinds of aggression and their physiological basis, Commun. Behav. Biol. 2:65-87.

Moyer, K. E., 1976, "The Psychobiology of Aggression," Harper and Row, New York.

Myers, R. D., 1964, Emotional and autonomic responses following hypothalamic chemical stimulation, Can. J. Psychol. 18:6-14.

Nordberg, A., and Larsson, C., 1981, Search for nicotine-like receptor binding sites in brain, Adv. Behav. Biol. 25:639-646.

O'Kelly, L. W., and Steckle, L. C., 1939, A note on long-enduring emotional responses in the rat, J. Psychol. 8:125-131.

Oldendorf, W. H., 1977, Distribution of drugs in the brain, in "Psychopharmacology in the Practice of Medicine," M. E. Jarvik, ed., pp. 167-175, Appleton-Century-Crofts, New York.

Panksepp, J., 1971, Effects of hypothalamic lesions on mouse-killing and shock-induced fighting in rats, Physiol. Behav. 6:311-316.

Panksepp, J., and Trowill, J., 1969, Electrically-induced affective attack from hypothalamus of the albino rat, Psychon. Sci. 16:118-119.

Plotnik, R., Mollenauer, S., Gore, W., Popov, A., 1975, Comparing the effects of scopolamine on operant and aggressive responses in squirrel monkeys, Pharmacol. Biochem. Behav. 3:739-748.

Reynierse, J. H., 1971, Submissive postures during shock-elicited aggression, Anim. Behav. 19:102-107.

Rodgers, R. J., 1979a, Effects of nicotine, mecamylamine and hexameth-
    onium on shock-induced fighting, pain reactivity and locomotor
    behavior in rats, Psychopharmacology 66:93-98.
Rodgers, R. J., 1979b, Neurochemical correlates of aggressive behav-
    ior: some relations to emotion and pain sensitivity, in "Chemical
    Influences on Behavior," K. Brown and S. J. Cooper, eds., pp. 373-
    419, Academic Press, New York.
Rodgers, R. J., 1977, The medical amygdala: serotonergic inhibition
    of shock-induced aggression and pain sensitivity in rats, Aggress.
    Behav. 3:277-288.
Rodgers, R. J., 1975, The role of central cholinergic mechanisms in
    shock-induced aggression in rats, Unpublished PhD Thesis, Queen's
    University of Belfast.
Rodgers, R. J., and Brown, K., 1976, Amygdaloid function in the cen-
    tral cholinergic mediation of shock-induced aggression in the rat,
    Aggress. Behav. 2:131-152.
Rodgers, R. J., and Brown, K., 1973b, Increased shock-induced attack
    in rats by physostigmine, IRCS Med. Sci. 75-79.
Rodgers, R. J., and Brown, K., 1973a, The inhibition of shock-induced
    attack in rats by scopolamine, IRCS Med. Sci. 73-75.
Rodgers, R. J., Semple, J. M., Cooper, S. J., Brown, K., 1976, Shock-
    induced aggression and pain sensitivity in the rat: catecholamine
    involvement in the corticomedial amygdala, Aggress. Behav.
    2:193-204.
Rolinski, 1977, The role of serotonergic and cholinergic systems in
    the aggression stereotype complex produced by amphetamine in mice,
    Pol. J. Pharmacol. Pharm. 29:591-602.
Rolinski, Z., and Herbut, M., 1979, Determination of the role of sero-
    tonergic and cholinergic systems in apomorphine induced aggres-
    siveness in rats, Pol. J. Pharmacol. Pharm. 31:97-106.
Rolinski, Z., and Herbut, M., 1981, The importance of central nico-
    tinic receptors in foot-shock-induced aggression in mice, Pol. J.
    Pharmacol. Pharm. 33:569-576.
Romaniuk, A., Brudzynski,S., Gronska, J., 1974, The effects of intra-
    hypothalamic injections of cholinergic and adrenergic agents on
    defensive behavior in cats, Acta Physiol. Pol. 25:297-305.
Romaniuk, A., Golebiewski, H., 1977, Midbrain interaction with the
    hypothalamus in expression of aggressive behavior in cats, Acta.
    Neurobiol. Exp. 37:83-97.
Russell, M. A. H., Peto, J., and Patel, U. A., 1974, The classifica-
    tion of smoking by factorial structure of motives, Roy. Stat.
    Soc. J. (A) 137:313-333.
Schachter, S., 1978, Pharmacological and psychological determinants of
    smoking, in "Smoking Behavior," R. E. Thornton, ed., pp. 208-228,
    Churchill-Livingstone, Edinburgh.
Schechter, M.D., and Rand, M. J., 1974, Effect of acute deprivation of
    smoking on aggression and hostility, Psychopharmacology 35:19-28.
Schmiterlow, C. G., Hansson, E., Andersson, G., Appelgren, L. E., and
    Hoffman, P. C., 1967, Distribution of nicotine in the central
    nervous system, Ann. N. Y. Acad. Sci. 142:2-14.

Scott, J. P., 1958, "Aggression," University of Chicago Press, Chicago.

Scott, J. P., 1966, Agonistic behavior in mice and rats: a review, Am. Zool. 6:683-701.

Shiffman, S. M., 1979, Analysis of relapse episodes following smoking cessation. Paper presented at the 4th World Congress on Smoking and Health.

Shiffman, S. M., and Jarvik, M. E., 1976, Smoking withdrawal symptoms in two weeks of abstinence, Psychopharmacology 50:35-39.

Siegel, A., and Edinger, H., 1981, Neural control of aggression and rage behavior, in "Handbook of the Hypothalamus, Vol. 3., Part B," P. J. Morgane and J. Panksepp, eds., pp. 203-240, Dekker, New York.

Silverman, A. P., 1979, Aggression in a social context: what can drugs do? In "Psychopharmacology of Aggression," Merton Sandler, ed., Raven Press, New York.

Silverman, A. P., 1971, Behavior of rats given a smoking dose of nicotine, Anim. Behav. 19:67-72.

Smith, D. E., King, M. B., Hoebel, B. G., 1970, Lateral hypothalamic control of killing: evidence for a cholinoceptive mechanism, Science 167:900-901.

Spector, S. A., and Hull, E. M., 1972, Anosmia and mouse-killing by rats: a non-olfactory role for the olfactory bulbs, J. Comp. Physiol. Psychol. 80:354-356.

Stern, P., Igić, R., and Muftić, R., 1975, Cholinergic mechanisms and aggressivity, in "Cholinergic Mechanisms," P. G. Waser, ed., pp. 477-482, Raven Press, New York.

Stokman, C. L. J., and Glusman, M., 1981, Directional interaction of midbrain in hypothalamus in the control of carbachol-induced aggression, Aggress. Behav. 7:131-144.

Thomas, C. B., 1973, The relationship of smoking and habits of nervous tension, in "Smoking Behavior," W. L. Dunn, ed., pp. 157-170, Winston (Wiley), New York.

Thor, D. H., Ghiselli, W. B., Lambelet, D. C., 1974, Sensory control of shock-elicited fighting in rats, Physiol. Behav. 13:683-686.

Thorne, B. M., Aaron, M., Latham, E. E., 1973, Effects of olfactory bulb ablation upon emotionally and muricidal behavior in four rat strains, J. Comp. Physiol. Psychol. 84:339-344.

Thorne, B. M., Aaron, M., Latham, E. E., 1974, Olfactory system damage in rats and emotional, muricidal and rat pup-killing behavior, Physiol. Psychol. 2:157-163.

Ulrich, R. E., and Azrin, N. H., 1962, Reflexive fighting in response to aversive stimulation, J. Exp. Anal. Behav. 5:511-520.

Ulrich, R., Wolfe, M., Dulaney, S., 1969, Punishment of shock-induced aggression, J. Exp. Anal. Behav. 12:1009-1015.

Uyeno, E. T., and White, M., 1967, Social isolation and dominance behavior, J. Comp. Physiol. Psychol. 63:157-159.

Valzelli, L., 1967, Drugs and Aggressiveness, Adv. Pharmacol. 5:79-108.

Vergnes, M., 1976, Contrôle amygdalien de comportements d'aggression
    chez le rat, Physiol. Behav. 17:439-444.
Vergnes, M., and Chaurand, J. P., 1973, Effets comportement aux de
    lesions de la partie posterieure de la substance grise periacque-
    ductale, C. R. Soc. Biol. 167:351-356.
Vergnes, M., and Karli, P., 1963a, Declenchment du comportement
    d'agression interspecifique rat-souris par ablation bilaterale
    des bulbs olfactifs. Acetion de 1;hydroxyzine sur cette
    aggressivite provoquee, C. R. Soc. Biol. 157:1061-1063.
Vergnes, M., and Karli, P., 1969, Effects of stimulation of lateral
    hypothalamus, amygdala and hippocampus on interspecific rat-mouse
    aggressive behavior, Physiol. Behav. 4:889-894.
Vergnes, M., and Karli, P., 1963b, Effets de lesions experimentales du
    neocortex frontal et du noyau caude sur l'agressivite interspeci-
    fique rat-souris, C. R. Soc. Biol. 157:176-177.
Vergnes, M., and Karli, P., 1970, Elicitation of mouse-killing behav-
    ior by electrical stimulation of the medial hypothalamus in the
    rat, Physiol Behav. 5:1427-1430.
Vergnes, M., and Karli, P., 1972, Stimulation electrique du thalamus
    dorsomedian et comportement d'agression interspecifique du rat,
    Physiol. Behav. 9:889-892.
Vergnes, M., Mack, G., and Kempf, E., 1973, Lesions due raphe et
    reaction d'agression interspecifique rat-souris. Effets comporte-
    ment aux et biochemiques, Brain Res. 57:67-74.
Vogel, J. R., and Leaf, R. C., 1972, Initiation of mouse-killing in
    non-killer rats by repeated pilocarpine treatment, Physiol. Behav.
    8:421-424.
Waldbillig, R. J., 1980, Suppressive effects of intraperitoneal and
    intraventricular injections of nicotine on muricide and shock-
    induced attack on conspecifics Pharmacol. Biochem. Behav.
    12:619-623.
Warburton, D. M., and Wesnes, K., 1978, Individual differences in
    smoking and attentional performance, in "Smoking Behavior," R. E.
    Thornton, ed., pp. 19-43, Churchill-Livingstone, Edinburgh.
Waser, P. G., ed., 1975, "Cholinergic mechanisms," Raven Press, New
    York.
Westfall, T. C., 1974, Effect of nicotine and other drugs on the
    release of 3H-norepinephrine and 3H-dopamine from rat brain
    slices, Neuropharmacology 13:693-700.
Wnek, D. J., and Leaf, R. C., 1973, Effects of cholinergic drugs on
    prey-killing by rodents, Physiol. Behav. 10:1107-1113.
Woodworth, C. H., 1971, Attack elicited in rats by electrical stimula-
    tion of lateral hypothalamus, Physiol. Behav. 6:345-353.
Yoburn, B. C., Glusman, M., Potegal, M., Skaredoff, L., 1981, Facili-
    tation of muricide in rats by cholinergic stimulation of the
    lateral hypothalamus, Pharmacol. Biochem. Behav. 15:747-753.
Yoshimura, H., and Ogawa, N., Pharmaco-ethological analysis of agonis-
    tic behavior between resident and intrude mice: effect of anti-
    cholinergic drugs, Jap. J. Pharmacol. 32:1111-1116.

Chapter 7

CHOLINERGIC MECHANISMS, SCHIZOPHRENIA, AND NEUROPSYCHIATRIC ADAPTIVE DYSFUNCTIONS

Alexander G. Karczmar and Daniel L. Richardson

Department of Pharmacology and
Institute for Neuropharmacology
Loyola University Medical Center
Maywood, Illinois 60153, U.S.A.

Department of Pharmacology
Chicago College of Osteopathic Medicine
Chicago, Illinois 60615, U.S.A.

---

1. INTRODUCTION

This paper deals with central and, to a lesser extent, peripheral cholinergic mechanisms which may be involved in some basic functional

193

defects characterizing schizophrenia. To make these mechanisms
intelligible it will be necessary, first, to describe the central
cholinergic pathways, particularly those that may be pertinent for
schizophrenia. Then, behavioral and functional correlates of these
pathways that may be relevant for schizophrenia will be discussed.
Finally, schizophrenic processes that may be dependent on behavioral
correlates of cholinergic function will be emphasized, and an attempt
will be made to explain these processes in terms of cholinergic deficits. The cholinergic functions that will be especially evaluated
concern the arousal (reticular) and the limbic systems and their role
in mentation as well as adaptive processes.

While we shall focus on the importance of the cholinergic system
in schizophrenia, it must be stressed that there is no general accep-
tance today of the hypothesis that the cholinergic system or the imbalance between the cholinergic and other transmitter systems constitute the primary etiology of schizophrenia; nor is this the belief of
the present authors.

2.   CENTRAL CHOLINERGIC PATHWAYS

As will be emphasized subsequently (Section 5), several brain
systems appear to be of particular significance for schizophrenia (see
Flor-Henry, 1979; Singh and Lal, 1979, 1982); in fact, no particular
insight is required to predict such a significance for the limbic system or mesodiencephalic reticular formation and its thalamic and cortical projection; perhaps less obviously, the extrapyramidal system
may be important as well (Haase, 1965; Singh and Lal, 1979, 1982;
Flor-Henry, 1979). At this time, it is important to note that these
and related systems exhibit a high density of cholinergic synapses and
nuclei. Indeed, the sites in question exhibit high concentrations of
cholinergic markers such as cholineacetyl transferase (choline acetylase; CAT) and acetylcholinesterases (AChE), and high values of acetylcholine (ACh) turnover. ACh levels may not be, necessarily, predictive of high density and activity of cholinergic synapses; on the
other hand, these areas contain also cholinoceptive sites (Krnjevic,
1976; Kimura et al., 1981) and cholinergic receptors (Morley et al.,
1977; for general review, see Karczmar, 1981a,b, 1976, 1979a,b and
Robinson, Chapter 2).

On the basis of these markers, cholinergic - i.e., containing CAT
and, presumably, releasing ACh - and cholinoceptive cells were identified rather definitely (Kimura et al., 1981). Cholinergic neurons
abound throughout the brain stem, being particularly dense within several pontine and medullary nuclei such as nuclei pontis parabrachialis,
reticularis, lemniscus lateralis and brachium conjunctivum, and
giganto cellular (FTG), magnocellular and lateral tegmental fields;
all these cell clusters contain also cholinoceptive cells. It is of
interest that catecholaminergic and peptidergic neurons are also

located in these general areas; such serotonergic areas as raphe nuclei contain few if any cholinergic, although many cholinoceptive, cells. The basal forebrain contains additional cholinergic cell clusters present for instance in the striatum, several limbic sites such as the diagonal band of Broca and substantia innominata, these two last loci exhibiting particularly high densities of CAT containing cells (Robinson, Chapter 2; Kimura et al., 1981).

The described cell clusters project their cholinergic axons to multiple cell formations that contain cholinoceptive receptors and may or may not contain cholinergic neurons; for example, most of the cortex receives ascending projections from several forebrain sites without presumably containing cholinergic neurons (Kimura et al., 1981; see however, Robinson, this book). It is not easy at this time to define, except for a few cases, the actual layouts of cholinergic pathways. However, the 1960's conceptualizations of Shute and Lewis (see Shute and Lewis, 1975) based essentially on histochemically (see Koelle, 1963) determined distribution of AChE, may be still tenable, particularly if amended to accommodate the new findings. It must be realized that thus described, the cholinergic pathways are not to be understood as purely cholinergic, i.e., as consisting of cholinergic long-axon projections or as containing only cholinergic synapses – alternate junctions activated by other transmitters may be also present within these pathways.

The pathways in question originate in the midbrain reticular formation (MRF), FTG and tegmental areas abutting upon but not comprising nigral neurons (Kimura et al., 1981), and branch into ventral and dorsal components. The ventral tegmental pathway constitutes an ascending tegmental-mesencephalic-cortical cholinergic system corresponding essentially to the diffuse mesodiencephalic activating system of Rinaldi and Himwich (1955) which is an expanded version of Magoun's (1952) ascending reticular activating system of the midbrain, ARAS (see also Krnjevic, 1976; Cheney et al., 1976; Fibiger and Lehmann, 1981; Kimura et al., 1980; McGeer and McGeer, 1979; Karczmar, 1979a,b). This pathway projects to the cerebellum and basal ganglia, several hypothalamic nuclei and thalamus, and it radiates via the diagonal band and septum to the hippocampus and "cholinergic limbic system" (Shute and Lewis, 1975). In fact, McGeer and McGeer (1979) and Kimura et al. (1980, 1981) feel that the septo-hippocampal and habenulo-interpeduncular (cf. Robinson, Chapter 2) connections constitute the most reliably demonstrated cholinergic pathway of the brain. Additional cell clusters contribute to these projections, e.g., neurons of substantia innominata (Robinson, Chapter 2).

The dorsal tegmental pathway originates, again, in the MRF and ascends to the midbrain tectum and diencephalon, innervating corpora guadrigemina, pretectal area, anterior and medial thalamus with its non-specific nuclei and medial and geniculate bodies, and subcortical visual centers.

Several areas, such as the cortex, striatum, the retinal plexi-
form layer, the trabecullar meshwork, and the olivocochlear bundle,
may contain localized cholinergic networks or fibers. Finally, descending mesencephalic (cf. Myers, 1974) and spinal pathways (besides
those involving the Renshaw cells and the motor nuclei) contain cholinergic synapses. These systems contribute to the cholinergic input
to sensory and motor phenomena, including spinal reflexes and spinal
modulation of sensory afferent stimulation (Nishi et al., 1974;
Nicoll, 1975).

3.   RELEASE OF ACETYLCHOLINE, CHOLINERGIC DRUGS, AND THE LIMBIC
      SYSTEM AND RETICULAR FORMATION

If the relation between functions of such brain circuits as the
limbic system and reticular formation and schizophrenia is to be cholinergic in nature, the stimulation of these sites should cause release of ACh as well as certain functional phenomena. This appears,
indeed, to be the case. For example, electric stimulation of several
sites within the ARAS (or the Rinaldi-Himwich system, see above,
Section 2) causes EEG and behavioral effects as well as liberation of
ACh from the cerebral cortex and also from certain subcortical sites
(Pepeu, 1974). The cortical release is spread out over visual, auditory and somatosensory areas. Release of ACh release may also be activated by peripheral stimulation or by the stimulation of auditory
and visual pathways; in turn, the release may be blocked or attenuated
by transection of the reticular formation.

Similarly, ACh release and/or change in ACh metabolism result
from the stimulation of the limbic system (cf. Pepeu, 1974 and
Karczmar, 1979a); such a stimulation may lead, again, to EEG or behavioral arousal and/or to emotional behavior (See Karczmar, 1979a,b;
Myers, 1974).

The cholinergic nature of certain functions and behaviors served
by these two systems, i.e., the limbic and ascending midbrain pathways, is also reflected in the effect of cholinergic and anticholinergic drugs, both on behavior and on ACh kinetics or release. Thus,
nicotinic and muscarinic agonists arouse the EEG (see below; cf.
Domino, 1968; Domino et al., 1977) and this is consistent with the
finding that nicotine increases ACh release. Other types of chemical
stimulation of the MRF - as, e.g., by amphetamine - also cause ACh
release (Pepeu, 1974; Saelens and Simke, 1976). The relationship between EEG activation, cholinergic agonists and ACh release breaks
down, however, when muscarinic agents such as oxotremorine or anti-
AChE's on the one hand, and atropinics on the other, are considered.
Thus, while oxotremorine and anti-AChE's activate EEG, they decrease
ACh release, although the effects of oxotremorine are controversial
(Karczmar, 1979a; Guggenheimer and Levinger, 1975). Similarly, atro-

pinics which deactivate and hypersynchronize the EEG (see below)
increase, similarly to nicotine, release of ACh both in situ and in
vitro, and deplete brain ACh.

Some of these inconsistencies may be explained by the fact that
we deal here with complex systems that include several feed-back reg-
ulations. For instance, atropine-induced release of ACh may not deal
with the blockade of postsynaptic muscarinic receptors leading via
this mechanism to EEG hypersynchrony, in other words to an effect
which is diametrically opposite of that of cholinergic muscarinic agonists, but with the atropine block of presynaptic cholinergic receptors. As the activation of these receptors inhibits ACh release
(Szerb, 1979), this effect of atropine increases ACh release (and
ultimately depletes, brain ACh; Schmidt and Wecker, 1981). Furthermore, while at most central synapses (not all, see Randic et al.,
1964; Phillis and York, 1968; and Krnjevic, 1976) ACh acts as an
excitatory neurotransmitter, certain cholinergic pathways are inhibitory in terms of their functional or behavioral significance; when
acting at these sites atropine produces functional disinhibition.
Thus, atropine may block inhibitory cholinergic septo-hippocampal
pathways to the cortex (Marczynski, 1971). Jointly with the arousal
system the septo-hippocampal pathways form a dipole which controls the
EEG patterns; as both areas of this dipole are affected by atropine
this biphasic nature of atropine action may explain its complex EEG
effects that include in man the induction of both slow and fast wave
forms (Itil and Fink, 1966).

As will be described later (Section 4), both atropinics and cholinergic agonists produce many behavioral and functional effects that
may be pertinent to the schizophrenic processes. However, as the effects of these substances on the arousal and limbic systems are, as
described above, most complex, it is difficult to pinpoint the specific mechanisms which may be involved. In other words, is a specific
behavioral or functional effect of atropine dependent on its block of
the inhibitory septo-hippocampal pathways? Is it related to increase
of ACh relase due to the presynaptic action of atropine? Is it related to the subsequent depletion of brain ACh? Or, finally, is it
related to atropinic block of cholinoceptive, limbic or cortical
sites?

4.   CHOLINERGIC CORRELATES OF THE EEG INCLUDING EVOKED POTENTIALS,
      AND SOME OF THEIR BEHAVIORAL CONCOMITANTS

As will be seen later (Section 5), the EEG and the evoked potentials appear to be affected in the course of the schizophrenic process.
In view of this, it is of interest to discuss the cholinergic actions
of these phenomena.

4.1 EEG AND Pertinent Behavioral Effects of Cholinergic and Anti-
     cholinergic Drugs

     Cholinergic agonists and anti-AChE's exert similar EEG effects
in several animal species and in man (see Karczmar, 1979a; Pfefferbaum
et al., 1979; Duffy and Birchfiel, 1980). It is useful to initiate
the description of these effects with the description of the effects
induced by a reversible anti-AChE, physostigmine (eserine), given via
an in-dwelling catheter to an non-anesthetized animal protected
against peripheral effects of physostigmine by means of a quaternary
atropinic. Following the i.v. administration of physostigmine, 0.05
to 0.10 mg/kg, the resting EEG which usually exhibits waves of mixed
frequencies and voltages, is shifted within a minute of the administration towards slower frequencies and increased voltage (Van Meter,
1969; Karczmar, 1977, 1979a). These slow frequency and high voltage
patterns appear in all leads including motor, cortical, thalamic and
hippocampal derivations. Within two minutes of this initial state,
EEG desynchronization and fast-wave, 10 to 20 Hz, patterns of decreased voltage are noticed in cortical and sub-cortical leads; furthermore, a prominent theta rhythm appears in the hippocampus (see
Fig. 1 in Karczmar, 1979a).

     It should be emphasized that these effects are induced by doses
of physostigmine which do not induce in unanesthetized animals any
marked motor activity. The animals may appear to be asleep during the
first two minutes following the administration of physostigmine while
subsequently, without showing overt motor activity, they tend to exhibit some signs of behavior alertness such as sniffing or head motion.
However, with large doses (0.7 to 1.0 mg/kg of physostigmine or other
anti-AChE's the EEG ultimately exhibits patterns of intermittent convulsive activity (Van Meter at al., 1978).

     It is important to note that essentially similar effects can be
obtained in animals with intracerebral localized injections of ACh,
physostigmine and other anti-AChE's, and cholinomimetics (for references, see Myers, 1974 and Karczmar, 1976, 1979a). Of additional interest is that these substances may produce EEG arousal when injected
into the brain sites either outside of the components of the ARAS
(Myers, 1974) or following sectioning of the reticular formation on
the midbrain level (Domino, 1968; Karczmar, 1967). Thus, cholinergic
drugs seem to be able to cause desynchronization of electrical activities (such as those represented by excitatory and inhibitory potentials) of neuronal populations of many brain areas via mechanisms independent of the control of reticular formation (Karczmar, 1974).

     The behavioral concomitants of the EEG effect of cholinergic ago-
nists and antagonists are of interest. Originally, it was expected
that atropinic hypersynchrony (Longo, 1966) and cholinergic EEG a-
rousal should correlate with sleep and behavioral arousal phenomena,
respectively. Actually, the reverse, if anything, is true as the cholinergic agonists generally induce arrest of on-going motor behavior

while atropinics, including scopolamine, may produce excitement and hypermotility. Indeed, in 1952 Wikler coined the term "divorce" to describe the apparent dissociation between the EEG and behavioral effects of cholinergic agonists and antagonists. Subsequent work (Montplaisir, 1975; McKenna et al., 1974; Steriade and Hobson, 1976; Karczmar et al., 1970) demonstrated that cholinergic EEG arousal is distinct from EEG alerting that accompanies behavioral arousal and motor activity (Montplaisir, 1975). In fact, cholinergic agonists and antagonists produce behavioral changes which reflect certain unique behavioral states that do not correspond to classically expected consequences of EEG alerting and EEG hypersynchrony, respectively. Specifically, the behavior induced by cholinergic agonists was referred to by Karczmar (1977, 1979a,b, 1981a,b) as cholinergic alert non-mobile behavior (CANMB); this behavior corresponds also to Klemm's (1976) immobility reflex. As the term indicates, besides being accompanied by fast (10 to 20 Hz) corticogram and hippocampal theta rhythm, this cholinergic motor immobility is coupled with several signs of alertness such as head motion, sniffing, face washing, scratching and chewing, while the eyes remain wide open.

It is of interest that CANMB may be related to REM sleep. Originally it was proposed that the locus coeruleus and its catecholamines are particularly concerned about REM sleep (Jouvet, 1961, 1967). However, Jouvet also stressed the fact that REM sleep is blocked by atropine. Subsequent investigations (Karczmar et al., 1970; Myers, 1974; Steriade and Hobson, 1976; Karczmar, 1979a) have demonstrated that REM sleep includes an important cholinergic component. In fact, catecholamines may not constitute an obligatory substance for the production of REM sleep, since even a marked depletion of brain norepinephrine does not prevent cholinergic induction of REM sleep in animals (Karczmar et al., 1970). It is important to stress that similarly to what happens in animals, atropine attenuates while physostigmine and cholinergic agonists facilitate the occurrence of man's REM sleep (see, for instance Sitaram et al., 1976). Interesting areas of similarity that characterize both REM sleep and CANMB include active mentation and motor inactivity which is accompanied by marked muscular relaxation in the case of REM sleep (Steriade and Hobson, 1976) and by some decrease of muscle tonus in that of CANMB (Van Meter and Karczmar. 1973).

Several other behaviors that exhibit cholinergic correlates are important in the context of CANMB.

One of these is the cholinergic analgesia. Cholinergic agonists are potent inducers of analgesia; in fact, on a dose basis, they are more potent in this respect than morphine (see for instance Koehn and Karczmar, 1978).

Even more important for behavioral significance of CANMB and for the general understanding of the effects of cholinergic activation on mentation, is the relation between the cholinergic activation, learning, the habituation or stereotypic behavior. It appears that, at least in the case of moderate doses of cholinergic agonists, the activation of the cholinergic system facilitates learning and speeds up habituation. Indeed, there seems to be an attenuation of responsiveness to stimuli that never have or, after some repetition, cease to have a vital meaning to the organism, so that stereotypic behavior is reduced and habituation is increased. The opposite effects are exhibited by atropinic drugs, including scopolamine and atropine.

These important correlates of the cholinergic activation warrant a few additional remarks. The theoretical basis for the pro-habituation and the related pro-learning effects of cholinergic agonists was laid down first by Carlton (1968). Carlton proposed that cholinergic agonists inhibit responsiveness to stimuli that are trivial or whose importance diminished during their repetition; the converse effect is exerted by atropine as well as by amphetamines. As a result, cholinergics facilitate and amphetamines inhibit learning, although state-dependent learning occurs with amphetamines. Subsequently, Stein (1968) referred to Olds' (1958) concept of anatomical substrates for punishment and reward that may be represented by a dipole consisting of periventricular gray and median forebrain bundle or related ascending catecholaminergic projections, and adduced evidence indicating that the reward system may be activated by amphetamine and related drugs, while the punishment centers are activated by cholinergic agonists. Habituation may then depend on the activation via cholinergic systems of the punishment pathways while undue attention to trivial stimuli may result from activation of the reward component of the dipole.

It must be stressed that the results of animal experiments concerning learning, responses to trivial stimuli, etc., are sometimes controversial and depend on the dose and on the paradigm employed (see for instance, Bignami and Rosic, 1971; Bignami, 1976; Karczmar, 1976); however, the generalization that cholinergic drugs facilitate habituation and learning and antagonize stereotypic behavior while atropinics exhibit opposite effects, seems to be supported by much evidence. Thus, cholinergic agonists, in fact, of both muscarinic and nicotinic types, facilitate learning and memory, perhaps even in man (Drachman, 1978; Bovet et al., 1966; Karczmar, 1976, 1981b: Warburton and Wesnes, Chapter 8). Also, this generalization is consistent with some of the EEG phenomena attributed to cholinergic agonists and antagonists. For instance, the theta rhythm and hippocampal activation engendered by cholinergic agonists accompanies learning and memory processes (see Drachman, 1978; and Longo and Loizzo, 1973), and these phenomena are in agreement with the evidence indicating the importance of the hippocampus for the memory processes (Drachman, 1978); conversely atropinics which cause amnesia, also disrupt the hippocampal theta activity (for references. see Karczmar, 1979a). Furthermore, cholinergic antagonism of stereotypic behavior and facilitation of habituation was demonstrated by means of paradigms involving both operant behavior and

natural habitats (Karczmar, 1981b) while atropinics exert opposite
effects. The prostereotypic effect of these latter drugs can be dramatically illustrated using "novelty seeking" behavior as the paradigm.
This paradigm tests the activity of rodents in a Y-shaped runout. In
this situation, the animal is statistically more likely to explore the
left-arm rather than the right arm of the Y-shaped maze if in the earlier trial it selected the right arm of the maze. This novelty seeking behavior is blocked by atropinics (Hughes, 1982), as atropinized
animals show perseveration as they tend to revisit the arm of the Y-
shaped maze that they visited previously. It should be emphasized
that novelty-seeking behavior is related to habituation; in other
words, unless habituation develops with respect to responses to repeated environmental cues, the animal or man will not follow new cues,
since in this case the old signals would not have lost the quality of
novelty. Indeed, atropine blocks both novelty-seeking behavior as
well as habituation.

The meaning, with respect to schizophrenia, of this anti-stereotypic effect of cholinergic agonists and anti-habituation action of
atropinics will be adduced subsequently (Section 5). At this time,
let it be emphasized that the activation of cholinergic systems and
the employment of cholinergic agonists induce a unique pattern of behavior that exhibits many aspects of facilitated mentation including
alerting and improved learning. It must be stressed that the behavior
in question includes also certain inhibitory or "depressive" phenomena
such as analgesia and attenuation of motor activity. These inhibitory
phenomena may not be construed as antagonistc to learning; to the contrary, they may contribute to the development by the organism of a new
strategy for an effective encounter with a novel environment (Pribram
and McGuiness, 1975; Pribram and Isaacson, 1975).

Finally, it must be added in the context of the CANMB that the
cholinergic activation of subcortical sites that include pontine and
limbic loci, may induce slow-sleep phenomenon (Hernández-Peón, 1965;
Marczynski, 1967). This phenomena may be reflected in the early effects of physostigmine on behavior and on the EEG (see above).

4.2 Evoked Potentials and Cholinergic Drugs

The effects of cholinergic and anticholinergic drugs on evoked
potentials are complex and controversial. Evoked potentials include
environmentally- or electronically-induced changes in on-going EEG
such as post-reinforcement synchronization (PRS), (Clemente et al.,
1964; Buchwald et al., 1964; Marczynski et al., 1968) and thalamo-cortical recruitment (Andersen and Andersson, 1968), or evoked potentials
(EP's) induced at several brain sites by appropriate sensory and/or
brain stimulation, such as somatosensory, auditory or visual EP's.
In either case, complex response result; EP's for instance consist of
a series of components (early and late) that overlap in time (Shagass,
1977)

Unfortunately, the action of cholinergic agonists and antagonists on these phenomena has not been investigated systematically. Available results suggest that they depend on the potential, the drug, or on the pattern and phase of evoked potential, and both depressant and facilitatory effect of cholinergic agonists and antagonists have been reported (see Borbely, 1973; Karczmar, 1979a). It is tempting, however, to generalize as follows: It may be considered that the amplitude of evoked potentials and certain related synchronizing processes form a dipole with the activity of the reticular formation. This may be illustrated by the fact that on-going synchronization phenomena such as PRS (Marczynski, 1969) or recruitment (Monnier et al., 1960) are blocked by the stimulation of reticular formation. Accordingly, it could be expected that desynchronizing drugs such as amphetamine as well as anti-AChE's, attenuate various forms of EP's. Frequently, this is the case. Thus, both recruitment and PRS appear to be blocked by anti-AChE's and/or cholinergic agonists (Marczynski and Burns, 1976; Longo and Silvestrini, 1957; Karczmar, 1974, 1975). Similarly, cortical potentials evoked by sensory or peripherally applied stimulation may be attenuated by anti-AChE's and/or cholinergic agonists (Karczmar, 1979a). Speculatively, this effect of cholinergic agonists may depend on their capacity to throw out of phase synchronous electrical activity of neurons perhaps by affecting the balance between inhibitory and facilitatory circuitry. This cholinergic phenomenon may occur with respect to all or most neuronal populations, i.e., not necessarily via the activation of the cholinergic EEG arousal system (see Section 4.1, and Karczmar, 1974). This desynchronizing or "dysrhythmic" (Karczmar, 1974) effect would, of course, tend to attenuate EP's as their occurrence depends on synchronized neuronal activity and processes provided for the latter (Andersen and Andersson, 1968). However, as already indicated, the pertinent data are controversial (Karczmar, 1974, 1979a; Borbely, 1973) and the complexity of the matter is well illustrated by the fact that while physostigmine or nicotine repress PRS as they induce EEG desynchronization, yet PRS is also blocked by antimuscarinic substances (Marczynski and Burns, 1976).

5.   CERTAIN ASPECTS OF SCHIZOPHRENIA AND THE CHOLINERGIC SYSTEM

That the cholinergic system may be involved in schizophrenia seems reasonable in view of the presence of cholinergic pathways and synapses at sites that appear to be important for this condition. These sites were described above (see Section 2., and Robinson, Chapter 2); cholinergically rich pathways that should be stressed in the present context are the ARAS and its diffuse projections, the mesodiencephalic limbic system, its septo-hippocampal pathway and related pathways between the entorhinal cortex and the hippocampus, and finally, the extrapyramidal system including nigro-striatopallidal pathways. Indeed, ablations studies and analysis of behavior resulting from brain damage have implicated limbic sites in schizophrenia-related dysfunctions such as non-habituation, perseveration, impaired cognitive-emotional coupling, and hallucinations (for references, see Flor-Henry, 1979; Singh and Kay, 1975, 1979; Singh and Lal, 1979 and 1982). Similarly, malfunctioning of the reticular formation and the resulting abnormalities of evoked potentials and their correlates, perception and the reaction times, were speculatively related to schizophrenia; the pertinent cholinergic phenomena will be discussed subsequently.

The importance of the nigro-striato-pallidal system may be less evident. It may be that appropriate psychokinetic conation and effective operant behavior require the adjustment of the extrapyramidal threshold; this elevation of threshold which is believed to be beneficial in schizophrenia may result from the action of antipsychotic drugs (Haase, 1965; Singh and Kay, 1979). Second, there may be anatomical connections, between the extrapyramidal system and basal ganglia on the one hand, and the olfactory and limbic systems on the other (Lidsky et al., 1979) and these connections may underlie the importance of the extrapyramidal system for schizophrenia.

5.1 EEG Alerting, EEG Phenomena and Their Behavioral Concomitants, and the Schizophrenic Process

That one of the characteristics of schizophrenics is their poor environmental response was stressed by classical investigators of schizophrenia including Kraepelin (1919) and Bleuler (1924, 1937). This poor linkage with the environment is reflected in a number of phenomena pertinent for schizophrenia. One of these phenomena is non-habituation and perseveration, as the schizophrenic tends to disregard the triviality of certain stimuli and continues to respond to these stimuli; or, the schizophrenic loses the capacity to cease reacting to stimuli that may have originated as novel and vital but ceased to be so after a while (Shakow, 1967). Another aspect of weak relationship to the environment consists of poor attention and the linked process of slow reaction time. Furthermore, the reaction time of the schizophenic may not improve when the signal is repeated at regular intervals (Garmezy, 1977). Altogether, the schizophrenic has problems in responding to, focusing on, and following environmental cues.

Several investigators feel that the processes that underlie the poor environment-response coupling of the schizophrenic consist of hyperarousal and break-down in filtering the environmental signals (Garmezy, 1977), and it seems reasonable that this phenomenology is related to high incidence of beta-2 EEG frequency of above 27 Hz (see for example Kornetsky and Hecht-Orzack, 1978; Itil, 1977). The phenomenon that may be related to this high incidence of disorganized fast activity EEG, is the absence in schizophrenics of slow-wave sleep (see Kornetsky and Hecht-Orzack, 1978). This does not necessarily mean that REM sleep dominates in schizophrenics, although in certain other forms of mental disease, such as affective depressive illness, REM sleep latency is short and the nightly frequency of REM sleep high (Kupfer and Edwards, 1978; Sitaram et al., 1981).

5.2. Autonomic Responsiveness and Schizophrenia

An interesting aspect of schizophrenia concerns its autonomic
responsivity to arousal and/or stress situations. There are two parameters of this phenomenology, the response itself and the recovery
following its occurrence, i.e., maintenance of autonomic homeostasis.

Considerable literature indicates that schizophrenics exhibit autonomic hyper-responsiveness as measured in terms of, e.g., galvanic skin
response (GSR) and cardiac rate change (Shakow, 1962, 1970; Mednick
and Schulsinger, 1970; Singh and Kay, 1979; Zahn, 1975). However,
there is also past (Shakow, 1962) and recent (Kornetsky and Hecht-
Orzack, 1978) evidence of the occurrence of autonomic hypoarousal in
schizophrenics. What we may deal here with actually, is not so much
increased or decreased but an improper autonomic response of schizophrenics to stress and environmental stimuli. For instance, normals
exhibit a characteristic sequence of pupillary dilatation and constriction upon reception and processing of sensory information, respectively (Buchsbaum, 1977), whereas the phase of pupillary constriction may be diminished in the schizophrenic (Buchsbaum, 1977). Similarly, in the normal the processing of sensory information or sensory
rejection may be associated with vasodilatation; this response again
may be faulty or indeed converted into vasoconstriction in the schizophrenic (Williams et al., 1973, 1975; Buchsbaum, 1977; see also
Funkenstein et al., 1949). It was also proposed that abnormalities of
autonomic reactivity in schizophrenics (that may extend to the remission period) depend on "non-integrative autonomic activity," i.e., on
autonomic cholinergic-adrenergic imbalance (Rubin and Barry, 1970).

General hyperarousal of the schizophrenic patients discussed previously may be causally related to improper autonomic responses to
environmental sensory stimuli. Indeed, the general hyperarousal may
lead to improper autonomic responses via either the cortico- and
sub-cortico-spinal connections that may involve the limbic system
(Shinnick-Gallagher et al., 1982), or the hypothalamico-pituitary
axis. In fact, there is a notion that at least some forms of mental
illness are characterized by instability of the hypothalamico-
pituitary axis and malfunction of the steroid and adrenal response to
stress. Older literature is replete with descriptions of exaggerated
or malfunctioning autonomic and steroid response of schizophrenics to
stress (see for instance Michaels, 1959; Arieti, 1959; Lidz, 1959;
Arnold, 1960; Shattock, 1950); recent information is also consistent
with this concept (e.g., Carroll, 1980; Tamminga, 1976).

The other aspect of autonomic response, that is, its homeostasis
may also be affected in schizophrenia. For instance, Funkenstein et
al. (1949) claimed that schizophrenics not only exhibit an exaggerated
vasodilator response to intravenous administration of mecholyl, but
also show reduced habituation to the response and deficient capacity
of recovery. Similarly, Horvath (1978) observed the failure of the

habituation of the GSR responses to stimuli. In other words, the
schizophrenic has problems with autonomic habituation and with return
to autonomic homeostasis following single or repeated outside stimuli.
Altogether, it may be argued that the autonomic hyper-responsiveness,
particularly failure in maintaining autonomic homeostasis, may be related in schizophrenics to the hyperactivity of the reticular formation and/or the limbic system.

5.3 Evoked Potentials and Schizophrenia

As stated above, EEG hyperarousal may constitute a dipole with
respect to evoked potentials; thus, it may be expected that beta-2 EEG
activity which is characteristic of schizophrenics should be correlated with attenuation of potentials evoked by auditory, visual and related stimulation. This expectation was borne out by experiments of
Shagass (1977) which indicate that particularly the early components
of the evoked potentials (those occurring at 10 to 100 milliseconds
following the presentation of the stimulus) are attenuated and variable in schizophrenics. Other abnormalities of evoked potentials,
such as diminution of facilitation normally noticed upon employment
of repeated stimuli, may also be present in schizophrenics (Shagass,
1968; Szelenberg, 1979). Furthermore, instability of evoked potentials seems to characterize systems (such as the left hemisphere) that
are pertinent to schizophrenic malfunction (Roemer et al., 1978, 1979).
Related interesting studies (Callaway et al., 1969) indicated that
schizophrenics show not only the attenuation of auditory evoked potentials (AEP's) but also exhibit dissimilar AEP's with response to two-
tone signals, different in frequency but both trivial, while normals
do not discriminate, AEP-wise, such two stimuli.

5.4. Schizophrenic Process and its Putative Cholinergic Concomitants

All this information leads to conceptualization that takes off
from earlier postulates of uncoupling in schizophrenics between environment and the responsiveness (Bleuler, 1924; Kraepelin, 1919) as it
relates this uncoupling to hyperactivity of the reticular formation,
abnormality of reaction times and learning, poor adaptation and habituation, and abnormalities of sleep patterns particularly as regards the
slow-wave sleep and, possibly, hyperactivity of REM sleep. Altogether,
there appears to be in schizophrenics a break-down in filtering and
appropriate evaluation of the environmental sensory information
(Garmezy, 1977).

How do these conceptualizations relate to the cholinergic system?
The fact that the pertinent central sites such as the limbic system and
the ARAS are rich in cholinergic synapses was already emphasized. Furthermore, the central cholinergic activity as related in the CANMB and
related behavioral changes, seems to be diametrically opposed to the
hyperarousal and motor activity that are encountered in at least some
forms of schizophrenia. It must be added here that while schizophrenic
EEG which reflects hyperarousal is characterized by high frequency

beta-2 waveform as well as delta epochs thus resembling the dual EEG
effects of atropinics (see above, 5.1 and Itil and Fink, 1966), the
EEG characteristic for CANMB exhibits theta waves and slower (10 to
20 Hz) than beta-2 fast components (see Fig. 1 in Karczmar, 1979a).

It is relevant in the present context that the activation of the
cholinergic system promotes adaptive behavior and habituation as well
as antagonizes stereotypic behavior; this anti-stereotypic quality of
the cholinergic activation was described at some length in the past
by Singh and his associates (see for instance Singh and Lal, 1979,
1982), while an analogy between CANMB and adaptive and non-stereotypic
behavior was noticed some time ago in our laboratory. In the experiment in question footshock was applied to mice repeatedly in a non-
escape situation; while early response to this stress consisted of
hyperactivity, stereotypic motor acts and non-teleological aggression,
subsequently cessation of stereotypy and adaptation to this paradigm
occurred as reflected in immobility response to this inescapable situation. Furthermore, following the stress paradigm and the development
of the immobility "reflex," the mice performed better as compared to
controls in learning test (Fig. 1). Finally, at the peak of the
stress, the ACh content of the mesencephalon of the animals was significantly increased (Fig. 2). It may then be speculated that the
adaptation and habituation observed with this paradigm as well as improved learning were due to the increased ACh level that resulted in
increased cholinergic stimulation, constituting an analogy with CANMB.
It should be added, however, that it was our experience (Kindel and
Karczmar, 1981; Magistrelli and Karczmar, 1984) and that of others,
that increased levels of brain ACh correlate with decreased ACh synthesis and turnover; in other words, with decreased activity of cholinergic neurons. Further it should be emphasized that the paradigm
in question also led to decrease in concentration of dopamine in
mesencephalon, a finding which is pertinent to the hypothesis that
relates dopamine to schizophrenia (see below, Section 5). It is of
interest in this context that antipsychotic neuroleptics increase
striatal release of ACh (Stadler et al., 1973).

A far reaching speculation that relates the cholinergic system
to adaptive behavior and to meaningful assessment of environmental
stimulation was advanced by Marczynski (1978; see also Karczmar,
1981b). Marczynski employed as the paradigm the evocation of post-
reinforcement EEG synchronization (PRS); as PRS arises upon the animal
receiving positive reinforcement, such as food or liquid, this response was termed "hedonistic" response. It was found (Marczynski,
1969, 1971; Marczynski and Burns, 1976; Marczynski et al., 1968) that
during the occurrence of slow surface potentials and the PRS, the
organism responds to novel stimuli by increased evoked potentials.
Accordingly, Marczynski speculated that this augmentation reflects the
adaptability of the animal, its habituation, and its capacity for
facilitated response to the environment; this renders the animal--
including man--capable of selection of response to the environment

from the effector repertory that would be appropriate for developing adequate perception. The actual mechanism described by Marczynski concerns both facilitatory and inhibitory (such as the septo-hippocampal pathway) cholinergic systems; it involves complex interactions between ARAS and brain stem reticular formation (BSRF), relay systems such as median forebrain bundle (MFB) and periventricular gray (PVG) which constitute reward-punishment axis, ARAS and BSRF radiation to the limbic system, and the loop consisting of the thalamocortical pathway, perforant pathway of Cajal, and limbic system. EEG-wise this interaction is reflected in slow surface potential (SP's), such as compound EP's, contingent negative variation (CNV) or anticipatory wave (Bereitschafft potential), PRS, as well as synchronization-desynchronization dipole. Marczynski speculated further that this dipole depends on the interaction between cholinergic ARAS which induces muscarinic depolarization of apical pyramidal dendrites as well as activation of inhibitory GABAergic interneurons in the nucleus reticularis thalami and in the cortex on the one hand, and dopaminergic ARAS and BSRF which inhibit the interneurons in question causing disinhibition (arousal) on the other (see Fig. 1 in Karczmar, 1981b). Slackening of the dopaminergic tonus increases inhibition, and relates to positive SP's and synchronization. In schizophrenics, changes in SP's slowing of their recovery upon repeated stimulation, lower CNV amplitude, etc., result from imbalance between these systems.

Besides these basic aspects of the putative cholinergic contribution to processes opposed to schizophrenia, certain clinical data seem to point out in the same direction. Indeed, the early observations of Pfeiffer and Jenney (1957) that muscarinic agonists such as arecoline may evoke a lucid moment in hebephrenic schizophrenics were subsequently confirmed by other investigators. For instance, oral physostigmine given with neuroleptics to chronic schizophrenics unresponsive to neuroleptics alone, produced a dramatic reduction in symptoms, although this amelioration was shortlived (Rosenthal and Bigelow, 1973). Furthermore, Davis et al. (1977) reported that intravenous physostigmine prevents exacerbation of schizophrenia induced by methylphenidate. Conversely, Singh and Kay (1979) demonstrated that atropinics administered to schizophrenics concomitantly with antipsychotic medication (in order to prevent the occurrence of Parkinsonian side-actions) attenuated the clinical effectiveness of the antipsychotic neuroleptics (see also Singh and Kay, Chapter 9); this evidence is consistent with that indicating the possible clinical effectiveness of cholinergic agonists. It is pertinent also that patients suffering from Huntington's chorea may show unduly high frequency of schizophrenic disease (Klawans et al., 1976); Klawans conceptualized that as there is evidence in Huntington's chorea of the imbalance in the extrapyramidal system of the cholinergic-catecholaminergic axis with the shift towards catecholaminergic hyperactivity, this imbalance may extend also to the limbic and cortical system with concomitant increased incidence of schizophrenic disease. Interestingly, schizophrenia encountered among patients suffering also from Huntington's chorea is of the choreathetoid type (Kraepelin, 1913, 1919) which presents very poor prognosis. Another consistent clinical observation is that while atropinics produce in normals some degree of schizoid or hallucinatory behavior and while they decrease the clinical effectiveness of neuroleptics (see above; Singh and Kay, 1975), they also worsen the schizoid symptomology when given without neuroleptics to psychotics as well as activate latent psychotic symptoms in schizophrenics (see Weiss et al., 1976).

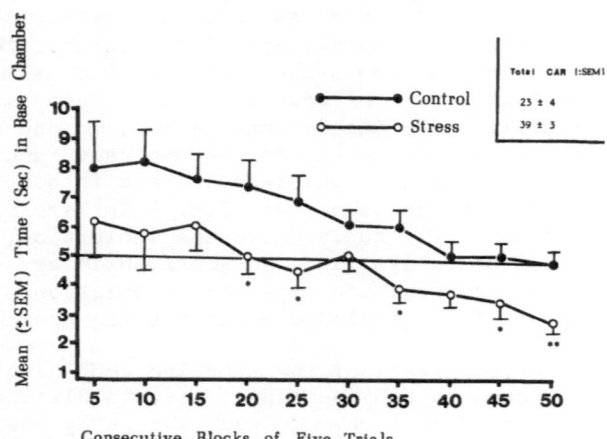

Consecutive Blocks of Five Trials

Fig. 1.   Learning of CF-1 Mice as Affected by Stress (Unavoidable Foot-shock). Penta-level (5 chambered) Climbing Screen was used to evaluate learning (Karczmar et al., 1973). In this test, punishing foot-shock was delivered if the mouse did not leave (avoid the shock) the chamber within 5 seconds of tone signal (see cross-hatched line in the middle of the figure). Each point represents mean time in the chambers for each block of five trials (N=50); standard errors are indicated by vertical lines. Full circles--controls; empty circles-- stressed mice. Abscissae: consecutive 50 trials in blocks of five; ordinates: time (in seconds) in chambers (base chambers; see Karczmar et al., 1973). Stressed mice were exposed, one hour prior to learning trials, to 60 unavoidable shocks. Note that stressed mice reached learning criterion (and differed from the controls significantly in their avoidance time) after 20 trials, whereas controls reached criterion only after 50 trials. In the offset, total number of conditioned avoidance responses (out of 50 trials) for controls and stressed mice; note that the latter avoided almost twice as often as the controls. From Richardson and Karczmar, 1981.

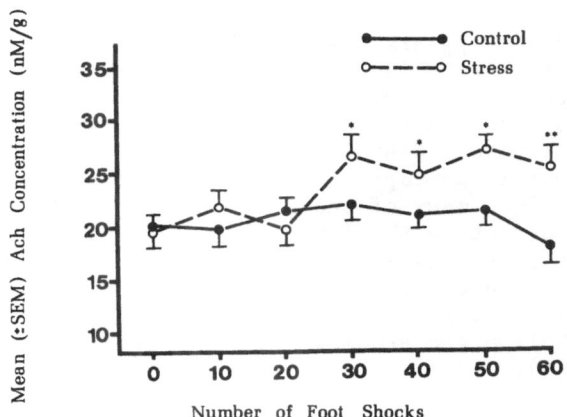

Fig. 2. Levels of Acetylcholine in Midbrain-diencephalon of CF-1
Stressed (unavoidable foot-shock) Mice. Mice were sacrificed
by means of microradiation; acetylcholine was measured by
means of high-voltage paper chromatography method (Kindel and
Karczmar, 1981). Each point represents an average of 10 to
12 determinations, 4 to 6 mice were used to pool brain parts
for each determination; standard errors are shown by vertical
lines. Footshock, 0.05 MV for 2 seconds, was applied every
60 seconds, in Lehigh Valley Electronics Model 1002 Shock
Chambers. Full circles - controls, empty circles - stressed
(foot-shocked) mice. Abscissae: consecutive number of foot-
shocks; ordinates: acetylcholine (ACh) concentration of
midbrain-diencephalon (in nN/g). Note that significant differences from controls appeared at 30 shocks. *:P >0.05,
*:P >0.002. From Richardson and Karczmar, 1981.

On the other hand, it may be surprising that while the case may
be made with respect to amelioration of schizophrenia following treatment with cholinergic agonists, yet cholinergic agonists produce also
hallucinatory and delusional behavior, thought disorganization and
sleep disturbances in normals accompanied by marked depressive reactions (Karczmar, 1982; see also next Section). It is of further
interest that schizoid reactions and related effects including EEG
changes induced in normals by organophosphorus anti-AChE's may be
long-lasting and extend for a number of years (Metcalf and Holmes,
1969; Duffy and Burchfiel, 1980). What complicates the matter even
further is the claim of Neubauer et al. (1975) that the treatment of
a small number of selected schizophrenics with an alpha adrenergic
blocker combined with atropine was as successful as the treatment of
the same subjects with neuroleptics; this finding has not yet been
replicated by other investigators.

6.   CONCLUSIONS

To summarize, it appears that cholinergic activity, strategically
localized in the midbrain, limbic and extrapyramidal system, is related to a unique, complex behavioral pattern that includes both inhibitory and excitatory phenomena and consists of special type of EEG and
behavioral arousal (i.e., CANMB), the facilitation of habituation and
adaptation, changes in perception and reaction time, and changes in
sleep patterns. Since many of these phenomena seem to be impaired in
schizophrenia, a defect in the functioning of central cholinergic
mechanisms may be suspected in this condition. Furthermore, many,
although not all, clinical results may be consistent with this speculation as generally atropinics seem to exacerbate or unmask schizophrenia, while cholinergic agonists may have opposite effects (Singh
and Kay, Chapter 9).

Several warning remarks are necessary at this time.

First of all, while it was the aim of this paper to emphasize the
role of the cholinergic system in schizophrenia, it may be more appropriate to ascribe the latter to an imbalance that involves the cholinergic and another neurotransmitter system or systems, rather than to
the malfunction of the cholinergic system alone. Thus, Marczynski's
(1978) speculation (5.4) that concerns the possible malfunction in
schizophrenia of perceptive processes involves imbalance of the cholinergic and several other transmitter systems, including GABA and
dopamine. Similarly, Klawans et al. (1976) refers to cholinergic-
catecholaminergic imbalance as the underlying cause of schizophrenia.
It should be emphasized also that a shift toward dopamine in the dopaminergic-cholinergic balance seems to lead to stereotypy and "hyper-
viligance" (Bell, 1965; Weiss et al., 1976; Hingtgen and Aprison,
1976), a behavior pattern which resembles schizophrenic phenomenology
(5.1). In this context, it should also be emphasized that cholinergic
hypo- or hyper-activity induces changes in other neurotransmitters
and hormonal systems. This interaction extends from catecholamines
(Glisson et al., 1974) to GABA and such peptides as endorphins and
enkephalins, peptide pituitary hormones such as prolactin, and ster-
oids (for references; Roth and Bunney 1976; Van Woert, 1976; Glowinski
and Karczmar, 1979; and Karczmar, 1981a,b). In fact, it should be
stressed that the activation of the cholinergic system alone may not
relate strictly to the amelioration of schizophrenia. Indeed, alone,
this hyperactivity may be depressant in nature, and it was already
pointed out that cholinergic agonists and anti-AChE's induce, particularly in normal subjects, a syndrome that includes marked depressive
components (Janowsky et al., 1980; Harris et al., 1979). It may be
that the CANMB which is so characteristic for the cholinergic hyperactivity of animals may induce depression in man because its marked
negative psychomotor component may have a dysphoric effect on man.

Still another pertinent factor concerns the site of the cholinergic effect. The effect of the activation of endogenous cholinergic systems and of cholinergic agonists on behavior and mood may depend on the brain site that may be particularly involved. For example, effects on ACh levels and synthesis of the administration of choline or of anti-AChE's vary from one brain site to another (Kindel and Karczmar, 1981), and the resulting behavioral effect may depend on the site at which the major change in the ACh level or turnover has occurred. Furthermore, it may be speculated that the discrete site of the major cholinergic involvement may depend on the environmental situation, environmental stimuli, perceptual factors, changes in hormonal levels, etc. Thus, if two different environmental situations were to engender changes in the afferent cerebellar pathway and in the septo-hippocampal system, respectively, the resultant mood and behavior would be very different in these two situations.

Finally, it must be emphasized that the hypothesis that relates schizophrenia to the cholinergic system and/or imbalance between the cholinergic and other neurotransmitter systems is just one among many hypotheses or speculations that have been posited to explain schizophrenia. In fact, the cholinergic hypothesis of schizophrenia is a newcomer. Not only older (Arieti, 1959) but also many recent texts of psychiatry (Arieti, 1981) do not refer at all to the cholinergic abnormalities or to the imbalance that may involve the cholinergic system as constituting possible etiology of schizophrenia; also, while the earliest research results indicating that the cholinergic system plays a role in schizophrenia are those of Pfeiffer and Jenney (1957) and of H. E. Himwich (Karczmar, 1967), the earliest reviews that present a systematic approach to the cholinergic system as a factor of schizophrenia are those of Singh and his associates (Singh and Kay, 1976; see also Weiss et al., 1976). The older speculations in this field which continue to be vigorously proposed, experimented upon, or opposed, are many; they range from hypotheses that refer to the malfunction of a single transmitter (other than ACh) such as, for instance, dopamine, histamine or GABA, to those implicating abnormal plasma proteins (Heath, 1963), schizogenic molecules present in the plasma or in the brain such as phenylethylamine, neuroendocrine imbalance, and, finally, abnormal metabolism as in the case of the transmethylation hypothesis of schizophrenia (Berger and Barchas, 1981). In fact, while dopaminergic hypothesis of schizophrenia may be most widely accepted at this time, fashion plays a part in the game of explaining schizophrenia; this is illustrated by the fact that recent newcomers into the list of putative or authentic neurotransmitters such as GABA and endorphins are currently being implicated in schizophrenia (Berger and Barchas, 1981; Barchas et al., 1977). It should also be emphasized that while in this presentation schizophrenia has been considered as a single unit for the sake of presenting this complex subject with some degree of simplicity and clarity, schizophrenia probably is not a homogeneous unitary process, as stressed elsewhere in this book (Singh and Kay, Chapter 9); it may be that different mechanisms underlie various schizophrenia processes and schizophrenias that differ with regard to their outcome and prognosis.

ACKNOWLEDGEMENTS

     Published and unpublished investigations carried out in these laboratories and referred to in this paper were supported in part by USPHS NIH grant NS-06455, BRSG grant 4830 and a grant from the M. E. Ballweber Foundation.

REFERENCES

Andersen, P., and Andersson, S. A., 1968, "Physiological basis of alpha rhythm," Appleton-Century-Crafts, New York.
Arieti, S., ed., 1959, "American Handbook of Psychiatry, Vols. 1-2," Basic Books, Inc., New York.
Arieti, S., ed., 1981, "American Handbook of Psychiatry, Vols. 7, Advances and New Directions," Basic Books, Inc., New York.
Arieti, S., 1974,"Interpretation of Schizophrenia," 2nd ed., Basic Books, Inc., New York.
Arieti, S., 1959, Schizophrenia-other aspects; psychotherapy, in "American Handbook of Psychiatry, Vol. 1," S. Arieti, ed., pp. 485-507, Basic Books, Inc., New York.
Arnold, M. B., 1960, "Emotion and Personality," Columbia University Press, New York.
Barchas, J. D., Berger, P. A., Ciavanello, R. D., and Elliott, J. R., Jr., 1977, "Psychopharmacology," pp. 197, Oxford University Press, New York.
Bell, D. S., 1965, Comparison of amphetamine psychosis and schizophrenia, Br. J. Psychiatry 3:701-707.
Berger, P. A., and Barchas, J. D., 1981, Biochemical hypothesis of schizophrenia, in "Basic Neurochemistry," G. J. Siegel, R. Wayne Albers, B. W. Agranoff and R. Katzman, eds., pp. 759-774, Little, Brown and Co., Boston.
Bignami, G., 1976, Behavioral pharmacology and toxicology, Ann. Rev. Pharmacol. Toxicol. 16:329-366.
Bignami, G., and Rosic, N., 1976, The nature of disinhibitory phenomena caused by central cholinergic (muscarinic) blockade, in "Advances in Neuro-Psychopharmacology," O. Vinar, Z. Votava and P. B. Bradley, eds., pp. 481-495, North Holland Publishing Co., Amsterdam.
Bleuler, E., 1924, "Textbook of Psychiatry," MacMillan, New York.
Bleuler, E., 1937, "Lehrbuch der Psychiatrie," Springer-Verlag, Berlin.
Borbely, A. A., 1973, "Pharmacological modifications of evoked brain potentials," Hans Huber Publs., Bern.

Bovet, D., Bovet-Nitti, F., and Oliverio, A., 1966, Effects of nico-
    tine on avoidance conditioning of inbred mice strains of mice,
    Psychopharmacologia 101:1-5.
Buchsbaum, M. S., 1977, Psychophysiology and schizophrenia, Schizophr.
    Bull. 3:7-14.
Buchwald, N. A., Horvath, F. E., Wyers, E. J., and Wakefield, C.,
    1964, Electroencephalogram rhythm correlated with milk reinforce-
    ment in cats, Nature 201:830-831.
Callaway, E., and Jones, R. T., 1969, Evoked responses to schizophren-
    ic thinking, in "Neurophysiological and Behavioral Aspects of
    Psychotropic Drugs," A. G. Karczmar and W. P. Koelle, eds., pp.
    105-112, C. C. Thomas, Springfield, Illinois.
Carlton, P. L., 1968, Brain acetylcholine and habituation, Brain Res.
    24:48-60.
Carroll, B. J., 1980, Neuroendocrine aspects of depression: theoreti-
    cal and practical significance, in "Psychobiology of Affective
    Disorders," J. Mendels and J. D. Amsterdam, eds., pp. 83-98,
    Karger, Basel.
Cheney, D. L., Racagni, E., and Costa, E., Appendix II: Distribution
    of acetylcholine and choline acetyltransferase in specific nuclei
    and tracts of rat brain, in "Biology of Cholinergic Function," A.
    M. Goldberg and I. Hanin, eds., pp. 655-660, Raven Press, New
    York.
Clemente, D. C., Sterman, M. B., and Wyrwicka, W., 1964, Post-rein-
    forcement EEG synchronization during alimentary behavior,
    Electroencephalogr. Clin. Neurophysiol. 16:355-365.
Davis, J. M., Janowsky, D., and Casper, R. L., 1977, Acetylcholine and
    mental disease, in "Neuro Regulators and Psychiatric Disorders,"
    E. Usdin, D. Hamburg and J. Barchas, eds., pp. 434-441, Oxford
    University Press, New York.
Domino, E. F., 1968, Cholinergic mechansism and the EEG, Electroen-
    cephalogr. Clin. Neurophysiol. 124:292-293.
Domino, E. F., Bartolini, A., and Kawamura, H., 1977, Effects of
    reticular stimulation, d-amphetamine and scopolamine on acetylcho-
    line release from the hippocampus of brainstem transected cats,
    Arch. Int. Pharmacodyn. Ther. 225:294-302
Drachman, D. A., 1978, Central cholinergic system and memory, in
    "Psychopharmacology: A Generation of Progress," M. A. Lipton, A.
    DiMascio and K. F. Killam, eds., pp. 651-662, Raven Press, New
    York.
Duffy, F. H., and Burchfiel, J. L., 1980, Long term effects of the
    organophosphate sarin on EEG in monkeys and humans, Neurotoxicol.
    1:667-689.
Fibiger, H. G., and Lehmann, J., 1981, Anatomical organization of some
    cholinergic systems in the mammalian forebrain, in "Cholinergic
    Mechanisms," G. Pepeu and H. Ladinsky, eds., pp. 663-672, Plenum
    Press, New York.
Flor-Henry, P., 1979, On certain aspects of the localization of the
    cerebral systems regulating and determining emotion, Biol.
    Psychiatry 14:667-698.

Funkenstein, D. H., Greenblatt, M., and Solomon, H. C., 1949,
    Psychophysiology study of mentally ill patients, Part I - The
    status of the peripheral autonomic nervous sytem as determined by
    the reaction to epinephrine and mecholyl, Am. J. Psychiatry
    106:16-28.
Garmezy, N., 1977, The psychology and psychopathology of attention,
    Schizophr. Bull. 3:360-369.
Glisson, S. N., Karczmar, A. G., Barnes, L., 1974, Effects of DFP on
    acetylcholine, cholinesterase and catecholamines of several rabbit
    brain parts, Neuropharmacology 13:623-632.
Glowinski, J., and Karczmar, A. G., 1979, Interdependence of neuro-
    transmitter system in the CNS, in "Neurotransmitters. Adv. Proc.
    VII Internatl. Congr. Pharmacol.," P. Simon, ed., pp. 145-158,
    Pergamon Press, Oxford.
Guggenheimer, E. H., and Leringer, I. M., 1975, The effect of
    oxotremorine on the acetylcholine output from the CSF containing
    spaces, Experientia 31:88-89.
Haase, H. J., 1965, Clinical observations on the action of neuro-
    leptics, in "Actions of Neuroleptics, A Psychiatric, Neurologic
    and Pharmacological Investigation," H. J. Haase and P. A. J.
    Janssen, eds., pp. 1-118, North Holland Publ. Co., Amsterdam.
Harris, C. M., Davis, J. M., and Janowsky, D. S., 1979, The use of
    cholinergic drugs in mental illness, in "Nutrition and the Brain,
    Vol. 5," A. Barbeau, J. H. Growdon and R. J. Wurtman, eds.,
    pp. 397-414, Raven Press, New York.
Heath, R. G., 1963, "Serological Fractions in Schizophrenia," Hoeber,
    New York.
Hernández-Peón, R., 1965, Central neurohumoral transmission in sleep
    and wakefulness, in "Progress in Brain Research Sleep Mechanisms,"
    K. Akert, C. Bally, and J. P. Schade, eds., pp. 96-116, Elsevier
    Publ., Amsterdam.
Hingtgen, J. N., and Aprison, M. H., 1976, Behavioral environmental
    aspects of the cholinergic system, in "Biology of Cholinergic
    Function," A. M. Goldberg and I. Hanin, eds., pp. 515-566, Raven
    Press, New York.
Horvath, F., 1979, An experimental comparison of the psychological
    stress evaluation and the galvanic skin response in detection of
    deception, J. Appl. Psychol. 63:338-344
Hughes, R. N., 1982, A review of atropinic drug effects on explora-
    tory choice behavior in laboratory rodents, Behav. Neural Biol.
    35:5-41.
Itil, T., 1977, Qualitative and quantitative EEG findings in schizo-
    phrenia, Schizophr. Bull. 3:610-679.
Itil, T., and Fink, M., 1966, Anticholinergic drug-induced delirium:
    experimental modification, quantitative EEG and behavioral corre-
    lations, J. Nerv. Ment. Dis. 143:492-507.
Janowksy, D. S., Risch, C., Huey, L., Parker, D., Davis, J., and
    Judd, L., 1980, The cholinergic nervous system and depression, in
    "Psychobiology of Affective Disorders," J. Mendels and J. D.,
    Amsterdam, eds., pp. 83-98, Karger, Basel.

Jouvet, M., 1967, Neurophysiology of the states of sleep, in "The Neurosciences, A. Study Program," G. C. Quarton, T. Melnechuk and F. U. Schmidt, eds., pp. 529-544, University Press, New York.

Jouvet, M., 1961, Telencephalic and rhombencephalic sleep in the cat, n "The Nature of Sleep," G. E. W. Wolstenholme and M. O'Conner, eds., pp. 188-208, Churchill, London.

Karczmar, A. G., 1981b, Basic phenomena underlying novel use of cholinergic agents, anticholinesterases and precursors in neurological including peripheral and psychiatric disease, in "Cholinergic Synapses, Adv. in Behav. Biol., Vol. 25," G. Pepeu and H. Ladinsky, eds., pp. 853-869, Plenum Press, New York.

Karczmar, A. G., 1979a, Brain acetylcholine and animal electrophysiology, in "Brain Acetylcholine and Neuropsychiatric Disease," K. L. Davis and P. A. Berger, eds., pp. 265-310, Plenum Press, New York.

Karczmar, A. G., 1974, Brain acetylcholine and seizures, in "Psychobiology of Convulsive Therapy," M. Fink, S. Kety, J. McGaugh and T. A. Williams, eds., pp. 251-270, V. H. Winston, Washington, D.C.

Karczmar, A. G., 1976, Central actions of acetylcholine, cholinomimetics and related drugs, in "Biology of Cholinergic Function," A. M. Goldberg and I. Hanin, eds., pp. 395-449, Raven Press, New York.

Karczmar, A. G., 1982, Central effects of anticholinesterases with emphasis on behavior, sleep phenomena and psyche. Report for NAS Committee on Toxicology, National Research Council Anticholinesterase Panel, Washington, D.C.

Karczmar, A. G., 1975, Cholinergic influences on behavior, in "Cholinergic Mechanisms," P. G. Waser, ed., pp. 501-529, Raven Press, New York.

Karczmar, A. G., 1977, Exploitable aspects of central cholinergic function, particularly with respect to the EEG, motor, analgesic and mental functions, in "Cholinergic Mechanisms and Psychopharmacology," D. J. Jenden, ed., pp. 679-708, Plenum Press, New York.

Karczmar, A. G., 1981a, Multifactorial and multitransmitter basis of behaviors, and their cholinergic concomitants, Psychopharmacol. Bull. 17:68-70.

Karczmar, A. G., 1979b, Overview: Cholinergic drugs and behavior - what effects may be expected from a "cholinergic diet"? in "Nutrition and the Brain, Vol. 5," A. Barbeau, J. H. Growdon and R. J. Wurtman, eds., pp. 141-175, Raven Press, New York.

Karczmar, A. G., 1967, Pharmacologic, toxicologic and therapeutic properties of anticholinesterase agents, in "Physiological Pharmacology, Vol. 3," W. S. Root and F. G. Hofman, eds., pp. 163-322, Academic Press, New York.

Karczmar, A. G., Longo, V. G., and Scotti de Carolis, A., 1970, Pharmacological model of paradoxical sleep: the role of cholinergic and monoamine systems, Physiol. Behav. 5:175-182.

Karczmar, A. G., Scudder, C. L., and Richardson, D. L., 1973, Interdisciplinary approach to the study of behavior in related mice types, "Neuroscience Research, Vol. 5," I. Kopin, ed., pp. 159-224, Academic Press, New York.

Kimura, H., McGeer, P. L., Peng, F., and McGeer, E. G., 1980, Choline acetyltransferase-containing neurons in rodent brain demonstrated by immunohistochemistry, Science 208:1057-1059.

Kimura, N., McGeer, P. L., Peng, J. H., and McGeer, E. G., 1981, The central cholinergic system studied by choline acetyltransferase immunohistochemistry in the cat. J. Comp. Neurol. 200:151-201.

Kindel, G., and Karczmar, A. G., 1981, Effect of single and repeated choline administration on brain choline, acetylcholine and acetyl-choline turnover of CF-1 mice. Fed. Proc. 40-269.

Klawans, H. A., Jr., Westheimer, R., and Goetz, C. G., 1976, A pharma-cological model of the pathophysiology of schizophrenia, Dis. Nerv. System 36:267-275.

Klemm, W. R., 1976, Physiological and behavioral significance of hippocampal rhythmic slow actrivity (Theta Rhythm), Prog. Neuro-psychopharmacol. 6:23-47.

Koehn, G. L., and Karczmar, A. G., 1978, Effect of dispropylphospho-fluoridate on analgesia and motor behavior in the rat, Prog. Neuropsychopharmacol. 2:169.

Koelle, G. B., 1963, Cytological distributions and physiological func-tions of cholinesterases, in "Cholinesterases and Anticholines-terase Agents, Hndbch. D. Exper. Pharmakol., Ereganzangswk, Vol. 15," G. B. Koelle, ed., 187-298, Springer-Verlag, Berlin.

Kornetsky, C., and Hecht-Orzack, M., 1978, Physiological and behav-ioral correlates of attention dysfunction in schizophrenic patients, J. Psychiatr. Res. 4:69-79.

Kraepelin, E., 1913. "Psychiatrie, 8th Ed.," V. J. Ambrosius Barth Verlag, Leipzig.

Kraepelin, E., 1919, (Transl. by R. M. Barclay), "Dementia Praecox and Paraphrenia," E. S. Livingston, Edinburgh.

Krnjevic, K., 1976, Acetylcholine receptors in vertebrae CNS, in "Handbook of Psychopharmacology," L. L. Iversen, S. D. Iversen and S. H. Snyder, eds., pp. 97-125, Plenum Press, New York.

Kupfer, D. J., and Edwards, D. J., 1978, Multitransmitter mechanisms and treatment of affective disease, in "Interrelationship Between Various Neurotransmitter Systems, Neuro-Psychopharmacology, Vol. 1," A. G. Karczmar and J. Glowinski, eds., pp. 609-623, Pergamon Press, Oxford.

Lidsky, T. I., Weinhold, P. M., and Levin, F. M., 1979, Implications of basal ganglionic dysfunction for schizophrenia, Biol. Psychiatry 14:3-12.

Lidz, T., 1959, General concepts of psychosomatic medicine, in "American Handbook of Psychiatry, Vol. 1," S. Arieti, ed., pp. 647-658, Basic Books, Inc., New York.

Longo, V. G., 1966, Mechanisms of the behavioral and electroencephal-ographic effects of atropine and related compounds, Pharmacol. Rev. 18:965-996.

Longo, V. G., and Loizzo, A., 1973, Effects of drugs on hippocampal 0-rhythm. Possible relationships to learning and memory processes in "Brain, Nerves and Synapses," F. E. Bloom and G. H. Acheson, eds., pp. 46-54, Karger, Basel.

Longo, V. G., and Silvestrini, G., 1957, Action of eserine and amphet-
    amine on the electrical activity of rabbit brain, J. Pharmacol.
    Exp. Ther. 120:160-170.

Magistrelli, G., and Karczmar, A. G., 1984, Effect of aggression
    versus losing fights on brain acetylcholine levels and turnover
    of CF-1 mice, Prog. Neuropsychopharmacol. (in press).

Magoun, H. W., 1952, An ascending reticular activating system in the
    brain stem, Arch. Neurol. Psychiat. 67:145-154.

Marczynski, T. J., 1971, Cholinergic mechanisms determines the occur-
    rence of reward contingent positive variation (RCPV) in cat.
    Brain Res. 28:71-83.

Marczynski, T. J., 1969, Invited discussion: Post-reinforcement syn-
    chronization and the cholinergic system, in "Symposium on Central
    Cholinergic Transmission and Its Behavioral Aspects," A. G.
    Karczmar, ed., Fed. Proc. 28:132-134.

Marczynski, T. J., 1978, Neurochemical mechanisms in the genesis of
    slow potentials: A review and some clinical implications, in
    "Multidisciplinary Perspectives in Events Related to Brain
    Potential Research," D. Otto, ed., pp. 25-35, U.S, Environmental
    Protection Agency, Washington, D.C.

Marczynski, T. J., 1967, Topical application of drugs to subcortical
    brain structures and selected aspects of electrical stimulation,
    Ergebn. d. Physiol. Biol. Chem. Exo,. Pharmacol. 59:86-159.

Marczynski, T. J., and Burns, L. L., 1976, Reward contingent positive
    variation (RCPV) and post-reinforcement EEG synchronization (PRS)
    in the cat: physiological aspects, the effects of morphine and
    LSD-25, and a new interpretation of cholinergic mechanisms, Gen.
    Pharmacol. 7:211-228.

Marczynski, T. J., Rosen, A. J., and Hackett, J. T., 1968, Reinforce-
    ment, electrocortical synchronization and facilitation of cortical
    auditory evoked potentials in appetitive instrumental condition-
    ing, Electroencephalogr. Clin. Neurophysiol. 24:227-241.

McGeer, P. L., and McGeer, E. G., 1979, Central cholinergic pathways,
    in "Choline and Lecithin in Brain Disorders, Nutrition and Brain,
    Vol. 5," A. Barbeau, J. H. Growdon, and R. J. Wurtman, eds.,
    pp. 177-198, Raven Press, New York.

McKenna, T., McCarley, R. W., Amatruda, T., Black, D., and Hobson,
    J. A., 1974, Effects of carbachol at pontine sites yielding long
    duration desynchronized sleep episodes, in "Sleep Research, Vol.
    3," M. H. Chase, W. C. Stern and P. L Walter, eds., p. 35,
    BIS/BRI, Los Angeles.

Mednick, S. A., and Schulsinger, F., 1970, Factors related to break-
    down in children at high risk in schizophrenia, in "Life History
    Research in Psychopathology," M. Roff and D. F. Ricks, eds.,
    pp. 51-93, University of Minnesota Press, Minneapolis.

Metcalf, D. R., and Holmes, J. H., 1969, EEG, psychological, and
    neurological alterations in humans with or without organophosphate
    exposure, Ann. N.Y. Acad. Sci. 160:357-365.

Michaels, J. J., 1959, Character structure and character disorders,
    in "American Handbook of Psychiatry, Vol. 1," S. Arieti, ed.,
    pp. 353-377, Basic Books, New York.

Monnier, M., Kalberer, M., and Krupp, P., 1960, Functional antagonism between diffuse reticular and intralaminary recruiting projections in the medial thalamus, Exp. Neurol. 2:271-289.

Montplaisir, J. Y., 1975, Cholinergic mechanisms involved in cortical activation during arousal, Electroencephalogr. and Clin. Neurophysiol. 38:263-272.

Morley, B. J., Robinson, G. R., Brown, G. B., Kemp, G. E., and Bradley, R. J., 1977 Effects of dietary choline on nicotinic acetylcholine receptors in the brain, Nature 266:848-850.

Myers, R. S., 1974, "Handbook of Drug and Chemical Stimulation of the Brain," Reinhold, New York.

Neubauer, H., Adams, M., and Redfrom, P., 1975, The role of central cholinergic mechanisms in schizophrenia, Med. Hypotheses 1:32-34.

Nicoll, R. A., 1975, The action of acetylcholine antagonists on amino acid responses in the frog spinal cord, Br. J. Pharmacol. 55:449-458.

Nishi, S., Minota, S., and Karczmar, A. G., 1974, Primary afferent neurons: the ionic mechanism of GABA-mediated depolarization, Neuropharmacology 13:215-220.

Olds, J., 1958, Self-stimulation on the brain. Its use to study local effects of hunger, sex and drugs, Science 127:315-324.

Pepeu, G., 1973, The release of acetylcholine from the brain: an approach to the study of the central cholinergic mechanisms, Prog. Neurobiol. 2:259-288.

Pfefferbaum, A., Davis, K. L., Coulter, C. L., Mohr, R. C., and Kopell, B. S., 1979, Electrophysiological effects of physostigmine in humans, in "Brain Acetylcholine and Neuropsychiatric Disease," K. L. Davis and P. A. Berger, eds., pp. 345-360, Plenum Press, New York.

Pfeiffer, C. C., and Jenney, E. H., 1957, The inhibition of the conditioned response and the counteraction of schizophrenia by muscarinic stimulation of the brain, Ann. N.Y. Acad. Sci. 66:753-764.

Phillis, J. W., and York, D. H., 1968, Pharmacological studies on a cholinergic inhibition in the cerebral cortex, Brain Res. 10:297-306.

Pribram, K. H., and Isaacson, R. L., 1975, "The Hippocampus, Vol. 2," pp. 429-441, Plenum Press, New York.

Pribram, K. H., and McGuiness, D., 1975, Arousal, activation and effort in the control of attention, Psychol. Rev. 82:116-140.

Randic, M., Siminoff, R., and Straughan, D. W., 1964, Acetylcholine depression of the cortical neurons, Exp. Neurol. 9:236-242.

Richardson, D. L., and Karczmar, A. G., 1981, Effect of stress on avoidance conditioning and neurotransmitters, J. Amer. Osteo. Assoc. 62:68.

Rinaldi, R., and Himwich, H., 1955, Cholinergic mechanisms involved in function of mesodiencephalic activating system, Arch. Neurol. Psychiatry 73:394-402.

Roemer, R. A., Shagass, C., Straumanis, J. J., and Amadeo, M., 1978, Pattern evoked potential measurements suggesting lateralized hemispheric dysfunction in chronic schizophrenics, Biol. Psychiatry 13:185-202.

Roemer, R. A., Shagass, C., Straumanis, J. J., and Amadeo, M., 1979, Somatosensory and auditory evoked potential studies of functional differences between the cerebral hemispheres in psychosis, Biol. Psychiatry 14:357-373.

Rosenthal, R., and Bigelow, L. G., 1973, The effects of physostigmine in phenothiazine resistant chronic schizophrenic patients: preliminary observations, Compr. Psychiatry 14:489-495.

Roth, R. H., and Bunney, B. S., 1976, Interaction of cholinergic neurons, with other chemically defined neuronal systems in CNS, in "Biology of Cholinergic Function," A. M. Goldberg and I. Hanin, eds. pp.379-394, Raven Press, New York.

Rubin, L. S., and Barry, T. J., 1970, Disautonomia in schizophrenic remission, Psychosomatics 11:506-512.

Sachar, E. J., 1981, Psychobiology of schizophrenia, in "Principles of Neural Science," E. R. Kandel and J. H. Schwartz, eds., pp. 599-610, Elsevier-North Holland, Amsterdam.

Saelens, J. K., and Simke, J. P., 1976, Appendix IV: Effects of various drugs on acetylcholine and choline concentrations in various biological tissues, in "Biology of Cholinergic Functions," A. M. Goldberg and I. Hanin, eds., pp. 683-706, Raven Press, New York.

Schmidt, D. W., and Wecker, L., 1981, CNS effects of choline administration: evidence for temporal dependence, Neuropharmacology 20:535-539.

Shagass, C., 1968, Averaged somatosensory evoked responses in various psychiatric disorders, in "Recent Advances in Biological Psychiatry, Vol. 10," J. Wortis, ed., pp. 205-219, Plenum Press, New York.

Shagass, C., 1977, Early evoked potentials, Schizophr. Bull. 3:80-92.

Shakow, D., 1962, Segmental set, Arch. Gen. Psychiatry 6:1-17.

Shakow, D., 1967, Understanding normal psychological function, contributions from schizophrenia, Arch. Gen. Psychiatry 17:306-319.

Shattock, M. F., 1950, The somatic manifestations of schizophrenia. A clinical study of their significance, J. Ment. Sci. 96:32-142.

Shinnick-Gallagher, P., Gallagher, J. P., and Yoshimura, M., 1984, The pharmacology of sympathetic preganglionic neurons, in "Ganglionic Transmission in Vertebrates," A. G. Karczmar, K. Koketsu and S. Nishi, eds., Karger Publs., Basel, (in press).

Shute, C. C. D., and Lewis, P. R., 1975, Cholinergic pathways 1. Histochemical localization, Pharmacol. Ther. 1:79-87.

Singh, M. M., and Kay, S. R., 1979, Therapeutic antagonism between anticholinergic anti-Parkinsonism agents and neuroleptics in schizophrenia. Implications for a neuropharmacological model. Neuropsychobiol. 5:74-78.

Singh, M. M., and Kay, S. R., 1975, Therapeutic reversal with benztropine in schizophrenics - practical and theoretical significance, J. Nerv. Ment. Dis. 160:258-266.

Singh, M. M., and Lal, 1982, Central cholinergic mechanisms, neuro-
    leptic actions and schizophrenia, in "Clinical Application in
    Neuropharmacology," W. B. Essman and L. Valzelli, eds.,
    pp. 337-389, Spectrum Publications, New York.
Singh, M. M., and Lal, H., 1979, Dysfunctions of cholinergic processes
    in schizophrenia, in "Biological Psychiatry Today Vol. 2A,"
    pp. 434-438, Proc. 2nd World Congress Biological Psychiatry.
Sitaram, N., Moore, A. M., Varskiver, C., Blendy, J., Nurnberger,
    J. I., Jr., Gershon, E. S., and Gillin, J.C., 1981, Hypersensitive
    cholinergic functioning in primary affective illnesses, in
    "Cholinergic Mechanisms," G. Pepeu and H. Ladinsky, eds.,
    pp. 947-962, Plenum Press, New York.
Sitaram, N., Wyatt, R. J., Dawson, S., and Gillin, J. C., 1976, REM
    sleep induction by physostigmine infusion during sleep, Science
    191:1281-1282.
Stadler, H., Lloyd, K. G., Gadea-Ciria, M., and Bartolini, G., 1973,
    Enhanced striatal acetylcholine release by chlorpromazine and its
    reversal by apomorphine, Brain Res. 55:476-480.
Stein, L., 1968, Chemistry of reward and punishment, in "Psychopharm-
    acology: A Review of Progress 1957-1967," D. H. Efron, J. O.
    Cole, J. Levine, and J. R. Wittenborn, eds., pp. 105-123, U.S.
    Govt. Printing Office, Washington, D.C.
Steriade, M., and Hobson, J. A., 1976, A neuronal activity during the
    sleep-waking cycle, Prog. Neurobiol. 6:155-376.
Szelenberger, W., 1979, Visual evoked response modified recovery cycle
    and personality dimensions in healthy schizophrenia subjects,
    Biol. Psychiatry 14:141-153.
Szerb, J. C., 1979, in "Presynaptic Receptors," S. Z. Langer,
    K. Starke and M. L. Dubcovich, eds., pp. 293-398, Pergamon Press,
    Oxford.
Tamminga, C., Smith, R. C., Chang, S., Haraszti, J. S., and Davis,
    J. M., 1976, Depression associated with choline, Lancet p.905.
Van Meter, W. G., 1969, Central nervous system responses to anticho-
    linesterases in rabbits: evidence for a non-inhibitory action
    and for an adrenergic link, Ph.D. Thesis, Loyola University,
    Chicago.
Van Meter, W. G., and Karczmar, A. G., 1973, Unpublished data.
Van Meter, W. G., and Fiscus, R. R., 1978, CNS effects of anticholin-
    esterases, Arch. Int. Pharmacodyn. Ther. 23:249-260.
Van Woert, M. H., 1976, Myasthenia Gravis, Eaton Lambert Syndrome
    and Familial Dysautonomia, in "Biology of Cholinergic Function,"
    A. M. Goldberg and I. Hanin, eds., pp. 567-577, Raven Press, New
    York.
Weiss, B. L., Foster, F. G., and Kupper, D. J., 1976, Cholinergic
    involvement in neuropsychiatric disorders, in "Biology of
    Cholinergic Function," A. M. Goldberg and I. Hanin eds.,
    pp. 603-617, Raven Press, New York.
Wikler, A., 1952, Pharmacologic dissociation of behavior and EEG sleep
    patterns in dogs: Morphine n-allyl normorphine and atropine,
    Proc. Soc. Exp. Biol. Med. 79:261-265.

Williams, R. B., Frankel, B. L., Gillin, J.C., and Weiss, J. L., 1973, Cardiovascular response during a word association test and an interview, Psychophysiology 1:571-577.

Williams, R. B., Bittker, T. E., Buchsbaum, M. S., and Wynne, L. C., 1975, Cardiovascular and neurophysiological correlates of sensory intake and rejection. I. Effect of cognitive tasks, Psychophysiology 12:427-433.

Zahn, T. P., 1975 Psychophysiological concomitants of task performance in schizophrenia, in "Experimental Approaches to Psychopathology," 12:427-433.

Chapter 8

ACETYLCHOLINE AND ATTENTIONAL DISORDER

David M. Warburton and Keith Wesnes

Department of Psychology
University of Reading
Reading, RG62AL, U.K.

---

1. INTRODUCTION

In this paper we will be considering the pattern of cognitive changes that are produced by cholinergic blocking drugs (cholinolytics) as a model of some types of schizophrenia. One major problem of developing a drug model of some aspects of schizophrenias is the bewildering number of symptoms that have been listed as schizophrenic. However the major symptoms on which there is general agreement are cognitive and include the processes of sensation, perception, attention, thought, memory, association, decision-making and language. The major dispute is whether an impairment of one of these cognitive processes is the fundamental disturbance from which all other schizophrenic symptoms arise.

223

As a result of clinical work with both young, acute schizophrenics (McGhie and Chapman, 1961) and older, chronic schizophrenics (Freeman, Cameron and McGhie, 1958), McGhie and Chapman noted that some schizophrenics not only had problems filtering out internal information like associations, but also suffered from interference by external information. Accordingly they proposed a broader deficit in information processing in which some schizophrenics have problems in selecting the relevant information from both the external and internal environments while filtering out the irrelevant information. As a result of this loss of selective-inhibitory control of information processing, some schizophrenics are bombarded by a mass of disconnected sensations, thoughts and associations which they cannot sort out. Thus the deficits of information processing, such as bizarre language, memory, thought disturbances like delusions, and disturbances of perception like hallucinations, are argued to be secondary to this inability to concentrate on relevant inputs and ignore irrelevant ones.

This theorizing was supported by other eminent researchers· Shakow (1962) proposed that there is a deficit in the stimuli scanning process so that some schizophrenics are unable to select information relevant for an optimal response. As they cannot select out the irrelevant possibilities there are intrusions into their thinking of chance distractors from the environment, irrelevant stimuli from the immediate situation, and irrelevancies from past experience. In a similar vein, Lehmann (1966) commented that some schizophrenics are receiving a higher number of discrete sensory stimuli per unit time of experience than non-schizophrenic individuals and because they cannot process this information effectively then psychotic patterns of behavior develop.

From his work on perception Weckowicz (1980; Weckowicz and Blewett, 1959) postulated a deficit in perceptual selectivity in which there was a lowered ability to reduce redundancy of information input by suppressing some information. Consequently as Weckowicz and Blewett picturesquely phase it "the floodgates are open wide, the cortex is flooded with irrelevant stimuli...." Payne (1964) came to much the same conclusions from his work on schizophrenic thinking. He hypothesized that a defective attentional mechanism no longer excludes the irrelevant information and so thinking becomes distracted by external events and irrelevant personal thoughts. As a result irrelevancies are considered rather than the essentials of a problem.

McDonald (1960) who suffered an acute schizophrenic episode has summarized her own experience of this shift in attention and has interpreted in it the same way as these research psychiatrists.

"At first it was as if parts of my brain 'awoke' which had been dormant, and I became interested in a wide assortment of people, events, places, and ideas which normally would make no impression on me. Not knowing that I was ill, I made no attempt to

understand what was happening, but felt that there was some over-
whelming significance in all this, produced either by God or
Satan, and I felt that I was duty-bound to ponder on each of
these new interests, and the more I pondered the worse it became.
The walk of a stranger on the street could be a 'sign' to me
which I must interpret. Every face in the windows of a passing
streetcar would be engraved on my mind, all of them concentrating
on me and trying to pass me some sort of message.Now, many years
later, I can appreciate what had happened. Each of us is capable
of coping with a large number of stimuli, invading our being
through any one of the senses. We could hear every sound within
earshot and see every object, line, and color within the field
of vision, and so on. It's obvious that we would be incapable
of carrying on any of our daily activities if even one-hundredth
of all these available stimuli invaded us at once. So the mind
must have a filter which functions without our conscious thought,
sorting stimuli and allowing only those which are relevant to the
situation in hand to disturb consciousness. And this filter must
be working at maximum efficiency at all times, particularly when
we require a high degree of concentration. What had happened to
me in Toronto was a breakdown in the filter, and a hodge-podge
of unrelated stimuli were distracting me from things which should
have had my undivided attention." (McDonald, 1960, pp 219-220).

2.   ATTENTIONAL DISORDER IN SCHIZOPHRENIC SUBGROUPS

Kraepelin (1899; translated 1919) subdivided schizophrenic disorder into paranoid, hebephrenic and catatonic and while other groups,
like simple schizophrenia have been added, these categories remain.
Although it is not always too easy to classify individuals, one of the
easiest decisions is between paranoid and nonparanoid. Shakow (1963)
reviewed 58 studies and found that paranoids seemed consistently to
deal with situations in different ways from nonparanoid patients.
From the point of view of attention, paranoids show over-selective
type of attention whereas the lack of filtering that was described
above is found mainly among the nonparanoids (McGhie, 1969). Thus on
tests of attention span nonparanoids were clearly worse than paranoids (Kay and Singh, 1974). In later work (Kay and Singh, 1979) it
was found that within the acute nonparanoid groups disturbance of
attention was most clearly associated with patients who were diagnosed
as catatonic rather than hebephrenic.

Prospective and retrospective studies have tried to obtain criteria, both patterns of symptoms and social factors, which could be
related to treatment and to prognosis. A synthesis of these studies
has led to distinctions between two subgroups of schizophrenia which
are differentiated with respect to their premorbid history, the onset
of the illness and, of course, their potential for recovery. The two
subgroups have been given various names: nuclear-schizophreniform,
typical-atypical, process-reactive.

The premorbid history of a process-nuclear-typical schizophrenic patient has many of the following features. Frequently other siblings were pathological. There was often early prolonged psychological trauma. The child showed "odd" behavior and was very often withdrawn, introverted, and passive. Problems at school were common, with respect to relationships with teachers, and normal adolescent interests in the opposite sex were not exhibited and in general social relationships were minimal. The work pattern of the patient was usually poor with a discrepancy between ability and achievement and there was repeated failure in the face of adversity. There was evidence of a general breakdown of social and mental function from early life in the patient's life so that the onset of the psychosis was gradual and insidious without any obvious precipitating factor. By the time he was hospitalized, there was usually a fully developed delusional system, often with ideas of external forces influencing his mind and body. There was blunted affect and loss of reality. The reaction to any form of therapy was poor and there was rarely a favorable outcome.

Patients diagnosed as examples of the reactive-schizophreniform-atypical schizophrenics showed an almost opposite set of features. There were no early traumas. The child tended to react forcefully in the face of adversity and fulfilled his intellectual potential. He was usually heterosexual and had a wide circle of friends. He was often a leader and aggressively successful in his job. The onset of the psychosis was suddenly precipitated by a set of events that could not be solved by action. The result was a state of tremendous anxiety and emotional disorganization with delusions and hallucinations.

In the acute set of patients of Kay and Singh (1979) attentional dysfunction was most evident in the reactive-schizophreniform-atypical subgroup, i.e., the group with the best prognosis. When a set of chronic patients was tested a somewhat different picture emerged. Claridge (1967) found that process-nuclear-atypical patients had much poorer performance in an auditory vigilance test than reactive-schizophreniform-atypical patients. Surveys of reactive and process patients have shown that the process-nuclear-atypical patients were most frequently diagnosed as hebephrenic on admission. Thus in the more chronic patients most attentional disturbance is found among the hebephrenic category.

In summary, paranoid patients appear to have an over-selective attentional mechanism while nonparanoid patients have problems filtering out irrelevant information. The severest problem in acute cases are found among the catatonic patients and hebephrenics are less impaired as a group but the hebephrenics were predominant among the chronic patients and have been most studied. In our studies we are concerned with the disruption of the attentional process and so our data apply directly to nonparanoid groups. However we believe that our finding can be extrapolated to apply to paranoid patients who seem to have an over-reactive attentional mechanism.

3.   AN ATTENTIONAL MECHANISM

Attention is used to refer to the process by which information is selected for analysis. It is important to remember that attention cannot be observed but can only be inferred from behavioral changes. It is defined by excluding processes that we would not wish to call attentional such as muscular fatigue, motivation and learning. Exclusion is complicated by the fact that both motivation and learning modify the attentional process. Motivational shifts can influence stimulus selection e.g., changes in sexual motivation are correlated with changes in the selection of sexual stimuli. The pattern of stimuli that are selected are also modified by experience e.g., repeated stimuli are filtered out as the result of habituation while stimuli associated with significant events continue to be selected. As a consequence, attentional studies with people use well-trained subjects and aim to maintain motivation constant during the test. These tests always take the form of selecting classes of stimuli in a situation where there are other sources of information competing for attention. The problem of measurement is that changes in attention may not always be manifested in overt behavior and so performance is not always a certain index of attention. However subjects can usually report attentional shifts and provide a reasonable subjective assessment of their level of attention, and so it is useful to use both subjective as well as objective data as indices of variation in the processing of information.

We believe that processing of both external and internal information is modulated directly by a system with its origin in the midbrain reticular formation. There are marked changes in sensory evoked potentials through the continuum from slow wave sleep, relaxed awakefulness to extreme alertness and there are neurons in the reticular formation whose functioning is inversely correlated with the size of the potential. It has been believed for many years that the level of electrocortical arousal is directly controlled by the midbrain reticular neurons and so it is argued that the reticular system modulates the sensory input by controlling the level of cortical activity. Neuropharmacological studies have produced evidence which is consistent with this pattern. Drugs that modify cortical desynchronization, change the size of the sensory evoked potential in comparison with the undrugged control group (see review Warburton, 1981). These changes occur in evoked potentials for all sensory modalities and so it must be concluded that the midbrain reticular system is a non-specific, sensory modulated system which acts by controlling the level of cortical activity.

There is strong evidence (Warburton, 1981) that electrocortical arousal is controlled by a cholinergic neural network. There are two pathways that ascend to the cortex that stain for actylcholinesterase and they both have their origins in the ventral tegmental areas of the reticular formation. Part of the neocortex is innervated by axons

whose cell bodies are located in the globus pallidus and terminate in
the lateral cortex above the rhinal or limbic fissure, which includes
regions such as the temporal and occipital cortices that are involved
in sensory functions. The input to this sytem comes from the external
sensory pathways, the internal sensory systems, like chemoreceptors,
and the visceral sensory system. Changes in attention result from the
variations in electrocortical activation which in turn result in cortical desynchronization from the level of activity in the pathways
ascending from the tegmental area of the reticular formation (Shute
and Lewis, 1967).

In addition to the cortical pathway, the system has a branch to
the hippocampus and there is a non-cholinergic pathway which returns
from the hippocampus to the tegmental region. The spontaneous hippocampal activity of the unanesthetized animal is characterized by
large amplitude, fast and slow waves which are irregularly distributed. This irregular activity is unstable and is interrupted at times
by brief periods of synchronization, which is termed theta activity.
Drowsiness is correlated with hippocampal desynchronization in contrast to cortical synchronization while alertness is correlated with
theta activity. Theta activity is elicited by reticular stimulation
(Green and Arduini, 1954) and novel sensory stimuli in the resting
animal.

The non-cholinergic pathway from hippocampus to the tegmental
regions is suitable for a feedback loop to control electrocortical
arousal, and certainly stimulation of the hippocampus produces changes
in electrocortical arousal (see Warburton, 1972). A negative feedback
loop prevents unnecessary activation of the cortex (i.e., superfluous
electrocortical arousal) by repeated and therefore predictable stimuli.
Thus the amount of electrocortical arousal is related to the uncertainty of the stimulus input.

People establish expectancies about the certainties in the world
around them and the increase in electrocortical arousal will be a
function of size of the mismatch between expectancy and input (see
Pribram, 1967). Electrocortical arousal is elicited by high information inputs, i.e., those with a low probability of occurrence for the
individual like novel stimuli. It seems likely that the hippocampus
is responsible for differentiating simple, low information stimuli
from simple, high information stimuli and then blocking electrocortical arousal via the feedback pathway to the tegmental region for
low information inputs. More complex events must be analyzed at the
cortex first to identify any mismatch between input and expectancy and
then the cortex will excite the hippocampus. Thus simple expectancies
depend on cortical analysis. In this way electrocortical arousal, and
so attention, varies with the information of the inputs.

Subjective and objective shifts in attention are correlated with
changes in cortical desynchronization and changes in the sensory

evoked potential. There is an increase in early components of the averaged cortical response that is evoked by sensory stimuli, so that the amplitudes of these initial sensory potentials are proportional to the degree of attention. At the same time, the later components of the evoked responses are increased in duration. Both these changes can be related to desynchronization in the following way. Desynchronization is an increase in the random spontaneous activity of some cells at the sensory cortex and is produced by the release of acetylcholine from excitatory neurons (Krnjevic and Phillis, 1963). The increased excitability of the cells would result in a greater number being activated when there is sensory input and consequently the evoked potential will be larger. The later components of the sensory evoked potential were prolonged after acetylcholine was applied to the sensory cortex or when the mesencephalic reticular pathways were stimulated (Spehlman, 1969; Krnjevic et al., 1971).

If the probability of a response is proportional to the size of the evoked potentials at the cortex, then behavior will be variable when there are many evoked potentials of similar magnitude and stable when there is one dominant potential. Selective activation of one of the sensory cortices will produce dominant potential at that area, i.e., concentration on one modality. Brown (1974) has shown that people differ with respect to the form, location and appearance of electrocortical activity. These differences may give an explanation of differences in perception and thought among individuals in terms of differences in attention.

During lapses in concentration the cortex becomes more synchronized and there is a reduction in the overall evoked potential size, which results in fewer dominant potentials so that stimuli from external and internal sources of information will intrude, producing distraction. The consequences of distraction will be impaired concentration and vigilance and selective attention performance will suffer. When the external sensory input is decreased to a low level, previously stored information may be released into awareness to produce fantasies, images and hallucinations. Creative thought consists of establishing connections between previously unconnected information. This process will be facilitated by a synchronized cortical activity of relaxed wakefulness. This critical point will be the relative sizes of the externally-evoked and the internally-activated potentials. The occurrence of hallucinations has been reported for many types of sensory deprivation in the laboratory, in prison, in the Arctic, and at sea (see La Barre, 1975), i.e., when external input is low.

The importance of the duration of cortical activity for awareness was demonstrated by studies in which very weak electric pulses were applied to the somaesthetic cortex of conscious subjects (Libet, 1966). At threshold intensities no conscious experience of touch was elicited until 0.5 seconds of stimulation had been given, and the

just detectable somaesthetic sensation did not increase, but remained
at the same subjective intensity when stimulation was continued. This
idea of a minimum activation period is supported by a study which
demonstrated that awareness of a near-threshold visual stimulus did
not occur until at least 0.2 seconds after the input reached the
cortex (Crawford, 1947). From these two studies prolongation of the
evoked potential by a minimum activation period is essential for
awareness of the stimulus.

     Eccles (1970) has calculated that there would be a serial activ-
ation of as many as 200 synapses before even the simplest conscious
experience is produced at 0.2 seconds. Once that experience is related to past experiences and given meaning, many thousands of cells
are activated in waves as a whole series of cells is excited simultaneously. Of course conscious experience only involves a small proportion of all the neuronal patterns at the cortex at any one moment
and so the direction of attention to one pattern of activity is probably achieved by activation of specific cortical areas. Altogether
the whole selection system is extremely important, because total
awareness is chaotic, as the evidence from studies of the schizophrenias has shown.

4.   A CHOLINERGIC MODEL PSYCHOSIS

     In the first sections we have outlined evidence for the hypothe-
sis that the fundamental symptom of many schizophrenics is an attentional dysfunction and in the last section we presented evidence that
a cholinergic system in the brain was at least part of the mechanism
that controlled attentional processes. In this section we will discuss the possibility of using cholinergic drugs to induce cognitive
changes which are characteristic of some nonparanoid types of schizophrenia, i.e., a model psychosis. This idea is based on one of the
fundamental principles of psychopharmacology that was stated by
Seymour Kety. "That principle is simply that no drug ever introduces
a new function into an organism; it merely accentuates or inhibits or
otherwise modifies a function which already exists. We cannot expect
drugs to introduce anything new into the mind or behavior, but merely
to accentuate or to suppress functions in behavior which are already
present." (Kety 1961, p. 79). It follows from this principle that
drugs can be used as tools (Russell, 1960) to produce a model psychosis, i.e., behavioral changes that are identical to some or all symptoms of the psychosis. It must be remembered that a model in science
is an approximation to reality and need not correspond exactly to it.
In the same way drug-induced, model psychosis need not match exactly
the pattern of symptoms of the natural psychosis. A drug will act on
many parts of the brain while psychotic symptoms are probably the result of changes in a discrete set of pathways. The real psychosis
will have developed over a period of time in a person who was not
aware that changes were occurring, at least initially, while the
model psychosis is an acute phenomenon in an informed volunteer.

It would be very surprising if there were a one-to-one match between the behavior in the two states. However, this problem is not of major importance provided the model psychosis provides a framework for experimentation and acts as an aid for seeing new relationships.

A model psychosis must be seen initially as an analogy for the naturally-occuring psychosis and tested to see if the behavioral changes in the two states are more than superficially analogous but are similar and result from changes in the same brain systems. Similarity is established by the enumeration of the set behavioral patterns, cognitive processes and electrophysiological patterns which are common to the two states, and those which are characteristic of one state not the other. The success of the model will be judged not on the absolute size of the relevant resemblances but on the magnitude of relative resemblances and differences compared with other models of the schizophrenic state.

The major competitors to the cholinergic model psychosis are the states that are induced by the hallucinogens. In fact the term "model psychosis" was first used by Mayer-Gross (1951) who translated the German term which Beringer (1927) used to refer to the effects of mescaline. The term became widely used during the extensive research on lysergic acid diethylamide (LSD) in the 1950's and 1960's. Indeed the rationale for much of this work was that the LSD-induced behavioral state was similar to, or even identical with, schizophrenic dysfunction. The strength of this assumption has been the subject of considerable dispute; some groups of researchers reported a one-to-one match between the states (Rinkel et al., 1952) while others deny any resemblance at all (Bleuler, 1965). In general it has been concluded that some features of the acute reaction to LSD and mescaline are remarkably similar to the acute schizophrenic breakdown but that the typical LSD model psychosis and the typical acute schizophrenic syndrome are dissimilar.

5.   SIMILARITY OF THE CHOLINERGIC MODEL PSYCHOSIS

In this section we will discuss some evidence for the resemblance between drug-induced cognitive changes and those occurring in schizophrenia. Similarity is discussed in terms of rapid information processing, distraction, sustained attention, hallucinations and thinking. Within each of these five subsections we will briefly summarize some relevant research with schizophrenic patients, some previous psychological studies using cholinergic blocking drugs, like scopolamine and atropine, and then some relevant research from our laboratory.

5.1. Rapid Information Processing

During each day there are many occasions when we are receiving a rapid input of related or partly related information. The most common example of this sort of input is speech, where meaningfully related words occurring at around 150 per minute must be associated and processed rapidly to obtain the meaning. Assimilation is aided by the fact that there are some redundant words in speech which can be filtered out so that every word need not be processed. The subjective reports of schizophrenics clearly highlight the difficulty that schizophrenics have with the rapid information processing that is required for comprehension. For example: "When people talk to me now its like a different kind of language. It's too much to hold at once. My head is over-loaded and I can't understand what they say." (McGhie and Chapman, 1961).

From this sort of statement it seems that speech comprehension of some schizophrenics is impaired as a consequence of their inability to filter the redundancy of the rapid verbal input. A similar phenomenon occurs after doses of cholinergic blocking drugs given to normal subjects. These studies found that decreased clarity of thought occurred after 15 mg/kg doses of atropine and 24 mg/kg doses of scopolamine (Crowell and Ketchum, 1967). Subjects complained of difficulty in following a train of thought which was manifested both in an inability to explain proverbs and in an inability to identify word similarities and word differences (Ketchum et al., 1973). As a result they could answer simple questions (Ostfeld et al., 1960) but had difficulty in following complex conversations and carrying out instructions (White et al, 1956; Ketchum et al., 1973).

Speech processing not only requires attention but involves a short memory component of storing speech units for the complex information analysis that is involved in comprehension. However, schizophrenics have been compared with non-pathological subjects on a less complex rapid information processing task. The subjects listened to random numbers presented at a rate of 60 per minute for 30 minutes and were asked to respond whenever they heard three consecutive odd numbers. As a group the psychotics performed worse than normals (a mean 45 percent compared with a mean 68 percent correct detections). Particularly poor were the hebephrenic nonparanoid patients while the paranoid schizophrenics performed as well as the non-pathological subjects (Claridge, 1967). This study is important because it suggests that it may be only a subgroup of the schizophrenic population, the hebephrenics, who have an attentional impairment.

In our laboratory we used a similar rapid information processing test to examine the effect of scopolamine. The task was the detection of either three consecutive odd numbers or three consecutive even numbers in a sequence of digits that were presented at a rate of 100 per minute. Scopolamine given after the 10 minute baseline and one hour before testing produced significantly fewer correct decisions than after a placebo dose, but there was no change in decision time. As a control for the possibly distracting peripheral effects of scopolamine, e.g., dryness of the mouth, an equivalent dose of methscopolamine, which passes into the brain poorly but acts in the same way as scopolamine on the rest of the body, was also tested. Its effect on performance was not different from placebo which indicated that the attentional improvement was due to scopolamine's action on the brain. One possible hypothesis of the mechanism is that these effects were due to a reduction of electrocortical arousal by reducing functional acetylcholine at cortical synapses.

This hypothesis was tested by using nicotine which releases acetylcholine at the cortex and increases electrocortical arousal (Warburton and Wesnes, 1979). Oral doses of 0, 0.5, 1.0 and 1.5 mg of nicotine were given to non-smokers who were then tested with the rapid information processing test described previously. In comparison with baseline that day and the other doses, the highest dose of nicotine increased the number of correct detections and decreased decision time indicating faster and more accurate processing of information. A similar pattern of enhanced performance had previously been found with smokers smoking nicotine-containing cigarettes (Wesnes and Warburton, 1978). The effects of nicotine were in the opposite direction from the effects of scopolamine, as one would expect if two drugs of opposite cholinergic action were acting on the same neural system. Further evidence for this notion was found when subjects were given both drugs together during the same session and the two drugs were antagonistic.

In summary cholinolytic drugs produce a deficit in rapid information processing which is similar to that seen in some types of schizophrenia.

5.2. Distraction

Another distinctive feature of schizophrenic cognitive functioning is a greater than normal susceptibility to distraction in some patients. One patient's description makes this clear - "Everything seems to grip my attention although I am not particularly interested in anything. I'm speaking to you just now but I can hear noises going on next door and in the corridor. I find it difficult to shut these out and it makes it more difficult for me to concentrate on what I am saying to you." (McGhie and Chapman, 1961).

In an experimental study on selection with distraction, Wechowicz (1960) compared the performance of patients with different psychiatric diagnoses on simple figure identification and on an embedded figures test. He found that simple perception of figures was the same for all patients but the schizophrenic group's performance was inferior when it had to identify figures hidden in an irrelevant background. In an earlier study Chapman (1956) used a card sorting test in which subjects had to use only the picture in one corner in sorting and disregard the remainder. The response cards featured irrelevant pictures as well as the relevant ones. The schizophrenics were distracted by the irrelevant pictures on the cards and so performed worse than control subjects. Thus the schizophrenic group was less able to ignore

irrelevant information and attend selectively to the relevant aspects
of the input. Another way of describing this difference is to say
that they have broader attention.

Two later studies of distraction (McGhie et al., 1964; Lawson et
al., 1967) studied the effect of either auditory or visual distracting
stimuli on the earlier stages of auditory or visual information processing (iconic and echoic memory). A large decrement was found when
distracting auditory or visual information was presented together with
an auditory main task. Unfortunately the performance of the schizophrenic group on the visual main task was so poor that it cannot be
concluded that there was no distraction effect because performance
could not have been much worse. In these studies of distraction there
was a large variance and there was clear evidence of bimodal distribution which gave evidence that the schizophrenic group was composed of
two homogenous populations. Consequently the subjects were divided
into hebephrenics and paranoid groups and it was found that only the
hebephrenic patients were markedly distracted while paranoid patients
performed as well as non-pathological controls or better. Once again
these studies also give evidence that attentional impairment is only
associated with the hebephrenic subgroup of chronic schizophrenics.

The effect of cholinergic blockers on distraction has been tested
in several ways by Callaway and Band (1958). In one test they used
an embedded figures type of test and found that scopolamine slowed the
discovery of figures hidden within a larger design. In a second test
they used the Stroop Test in which speed of naming color spots was
compared with speed of naming the print color of color names that were
printed in an incongruous ink (e.g., the word "red" printed in blue).
The difference between the two scores indicated the amount of distraction by semantic interference. Atropine slowed the speed of naming
in the distraction condition and in a similar study of Ostfeld and
Aruguete (1962) scopolamine impaired performance in the distraction.
However Callaway (Callaway and Dembo, 1958; Callaway and Band, 1958)
has argued that these changes represent "broadened attention." Broadened attention was defined as an increase in the influence of peripheral factors such as relatively current environmental events which are
removed from the central focus of attention by space, time, or by difference of meaning (Callaway and Dembo, 1958). In summary non-pathological subjects receiving scopolamine experience a broadening of attention and so greater susceptibility to distraction just like hebephrenic patients.

5.3. Sustained Attention Performance

We have already discussed in some detail the theorizing that ex-
plains the schizophrenic experience in terms of an attentional disorder. A common description of this experience is the following: "I
can't concentrate. It's diversion of attention that troubles me...
the sounds are coming through to me but I feel my mind cannot cope

ith everything. It is difficult to concentrate on any one sound...
it's like trying to do two or three different things at the one time."
(McGhie and Chapman, 1961).

In spite of this sort of subjective experience of some schizophrenics, there has been relatively little experimental work on sustained attentional performance in tasks lasting more than 10 minutes.
In a span of attention test lasting with a range up to 400 seconds,
Kay and Singh (1979) found a markedly shorter span in acute schizophrenic patients in comparison with non-pathological subjects. The
most disturbed were the catatonic patients, none of whom had attention
spans higher than 200 seconds, while the paranoid subjects were unimpaired.

After cholinolytics most subjects report loss of awareness or
alertness, difficulty in concentrating and shortened attention span
(White et al, 1956; Michelson, 1961; Ostfeld et al., 1960; Crowell and
Ketchum, 1967; Ketchum et al., 1973). It was difficult to attract the
subject's attention and the subject appeared to be in a "world of his
own" or "daydreamer" (Ketchum et al., 1973). Some subjects described
the condition as a sense of detachment from reality (Callaway and
Band, 1958).

Experimental evidence has given clear evidence that scopolamine
impairs sustained attention. Colquhoun (1962) tested subjects with a
checking test in which they had to check a list of numbers that were
presented over headphones with a printed list in front of them. Two
and a half hours after an oral dose of 1 mg, subjects were poorer at
detecting discrepancies between the two lists which is what we would
expect with a drug that impaired attention.

Accordingly we tested the effects of scopolamine on the sustained
attention task of Mackworth (1965). Subjects were required to detect
brief pauses in the second hand of a clock which occurred at the average rate of one every 48 seconds during a one hour session. Both
doses of scopolamine decreased the number of correct detections compared with placebo with the largest decreases occurring at the end of
the session. A 1.2 mg dose of methscopolamine had no greater effect
than the placebo, once again indicating that it was the action of scopolamine on the central nervous system which was important.

In order to obtain further support for the hypothesis that it was
the action of scopolamine on electrocortical arousal, nicotine was
tested. Subjects who took oral doses of 1 or 2 mg produced performance which was superior to that when they had a placebo dose, and the
scopolamine-induced decrement in correct detections and the rise in
incorrect detections across the session was partially prevented.
Tests of cigarettes in vigilance situations showed that nicotine-containing cigarettes produced performance that was better than non-nico-
tine cigarettes (Wesnes and Warburton, 1978). These opposite effects

of scopolamine and nicotine on sustained attention are consistent
with the hypothesized mechanism of a cholinergic system controlling
attention.

5.4. Hallucinations

An interesting aspect of the previous findings was the occurrence
of incorrect decisions and the fact that these were significantly increased by scopolamine. A percept in the absence of external stimulus
which is thought to be real is the classical definition of a hallucination (Siegal and West, 1975). According to Horowitz (1975) it is a
conscious awareness in which information is represented by means of
intense imagery from the inner realm of information (increased internal input), which is appraised as if it originated in the outside
world (impaired information processing). Hallucinations occur without
conscious interest and the person is not aware that the image has its
origins internally rather than externally (impaired control).

At one time or another hallucinations occur in acute cases of
schizophrenia. One of the earliest descriptions of a schizophrenic
breakdown includes a paragraph on the hallucinatory experience.

"During this year, also I heard very beautiful voices, singing
to me in the most touching manner - and on one occasion I heard
the sounds of cattle lowing and of other beasts in the fields,
conveying articulate sentences to me, as it is written of Balaam.
On another I was threatened terribly by the thunder from heaven -
in short, nearly all sounds that I heard were clothed with artic-
ulation. I saw also visions, and the same day that I heard the
cattle addressing me, on looking up into heaven, as I was leaving
Dr. Fox's premises, I saw a beautiful vision of the Lord descending with all his saints. During the same year, I also saw the
faces of persons who approached me, clothed with the features of
my nearest relations, and earliest acquaintance, so that I called
out their names, and could have sworn, but for the immediate
change of countenance, that my friends had been there."
(Perceval, 1838).

Auditory hallucinations are the most common type of hallucinatory
experience. These range from plain whistling noises, inarticulate
voices, and single words, to comments on the patient's actions, and
coherent instructions. Some patients describe them as thoughts that
come aloud which serves to make them real and important. These
'voices' interfere with the person's ideas and by repeating or contradicting what has been said or read they interfere with every action.
Tactile, gustatory and olfactory hallucinations are not uncommon but
visual hallucinations are rare.

Kraepelin (1919) believed that hallucinations were an essential
diagnostic sign of the schizophrenias and it was the occurrence of

this sympton that set schizophrenics apart from non-pathological
people. The consequence is that "the notion of the discreteness of
these symptoms encourages the conception of psychosis and schizophrenia as states that are also discrete and discontinuous and the further
conception that patients with these diagnoses are somehow different
from other people" (Strauss, 1969, p. 151). It is our view that hallucinations are not intrinsically different and so hallucinations can
occur in any person and not only in schizophrenics. All the evidence
(Savage and Wade, 1975) suggests that hallucinations are not in principle different from perceptions and that they are the outcome of cognitive processes. They can be interpreted as internal stimuli which
are normally filtered out, but as attention becomes broader they are
able to reach awareness and influence behavior (Warburton, 1979a).

    All normal people have hallucinatory experiences as they pass
through alpha and theta activity while relaxing and falling asleep.
A detailed study of these hypnagogic states correlated the subjective
experiences with electrocortical arousal (Vogel et al., 1966). The
early state, when alpha waves occur, was characterized by logical
thought processes and the subjects could distinguish easily between
internal images and external information. In the intermediate state,
when there was slow alpha activity, the subjects had lost contact completely with the external world and reported rather bizarre images and
thoughts. During the late hypnagogic state, when theta activity was
observed, the images became more plausible and realistic, and the subjects could not distinguish these internal images from reality. Thus
the hypnagogic states are exactly like hallucinations and very interestingly they are correlated with cortical synchronization.

    As we pointed out earlier, cortical synchronization with some
fast beta activity is induced by scopolamine and atropine. Atropine,
scopolamine and other belladonna alkaloids occur naturally in the
Solanaceae, a group of plants including nighshade (Atropos belladonna)
and thornapple (Datura stramonium). They have been used ceremonially
by the priests, magicians and witches of many cultures to produce hallucinations (Lewin, 1964; Warburton, 1979a). These hallucinatory experiences were culturally determined and were based on the beliefs and
attitudes of the individuals, i.e., set and setting of the user like
any other hallucinogenic drug (Warburton, 1975). The widespread occurrence of the Solanaceae has led to a large number of cases of accidental poisoning being recorded. These accounts describe auditory,
visual, gustatory, tactile and olfactory hallucinations as well as
disturbance of awareness and misperceptions (Warburton, 1979a). These
cases of poisoning are interesting because in many cases the doctors
have given a provisional diagnosis of acute schizophrenia until the
true facts become known.

    In the laboratory it has been found that high doses of cholinoly-
tics induce hallucinations (Crowell and Ketchum, 1967; Ketchum et al.,
1973) which were usually visual, but auditory, tactile, olfactory and
gustatory hallucinations have been reported (Abood and Biel, 1962).

The visual hallucinations were integrated and extremely realistic with familiar objects and faces (Ketchum et al., 1973). Some subjects smoked imaginary cigarettes (Crowell and Ketchum, 1967) and drank from non-existent glasses, making appropriate drinking movements and commenting on taste and smell (Abood and Biel, 1962; Ketchum et al., 1973). Subjects hear recognizable voices and music played by single instruments and whole orchestras (Abood and Biel, 1962). Even informed subjects were convinced by the intensity of the hallucinations and so they cannot be considered as pseudo-hallucinations like those produced by LSD.

In order to investigate the phenomenon of cholinolytic hallucinations in the laboratory we designed a sensory conditioning study in which a light and a faint two second tone were paired but the onset and offset of the tone were gradual so subjects believed that it was a test of auditory acuity. They were asked to press a key when they thought that they could hear a tone and press again when they could hear it no longer. After performance had stablized, a set of test trials were given in which the light was switched but no tone was presented until either the subject pressed the key or 30 seconds had elapsed. A "hallucination" was a response before the stimulus was presented and it was found that the percentage of subjects having any hallucinations increased from 30 percent with placebo to 85 percent with scopolamine and the mean number of hallucinations for the group increased significantly from 2.33 to 4.24. The latency for making a response was similar 11.2 (placebo) and 11.8 (scopolamine) which gives no indication of a loss of response inhibition which would have lowered the criterion for reporting detections. These data are in agreement with animal studies which have shown that cholinolytics do not disrupt response inhibition (Warburton, 1977).

In summary, clinical and laboratory studies have demonstrated that cholinolytics can produce hallucinations which are similar to those occurring in acute schizophrenia.

5.5. Thinking

As it is used in everyday speech the word "thinking" is applied to a number of different processes: remembering (I am thinking of my holiday last year), fantasizing (I am thinking about having my holiday with Miss World) and planning (I am thinking about my holidays next year). In this section we will be considering problem solving, a form of planning. Problem solving refers to internal events that use material from past experience but is usually triggered by external events. As we said earlier the same principles are involved in the control of thinking as sensations.

The reduced attentional selectivity for external stimuli in schizophrenics is paralleled by a lack of filtering of internal events and this is manifested as the characteristic thought disorder of schizophrenics as well as hallucinations. AS one of McGhie and

Chapman's patients expressed it "My trouble is that I've too many thoughts. You might think about something, let's say an ashtray and just think, oh yes, that's for putting my cigarette in, but then I would think of it and then I would think of a dozen different things connected with it at the same time" (McGhie and Chapman, 1961).

Cameron (1938, 1939) tested schizophrenics on category sorting tests of objects and colored blocks of various shapes. They performed worse than controls because they did not solve the problem in terms of the experiment's narrow set of categories but based their classifications on a wide range of their own concepts. Another way of describing these results is to say that the schizophrenic group was thinking more divergently than the control group but since test success depended on convergent thinking its performance was inferior.

It would be predicted that if cholinolytics produced broadened attention then they would improve problem solving where a solution depends on attending to peripheral clues (divergent thinking). We tested subjects in a problem solving task (Luchins Jar), in which subjects could solve the problems in the same way repeatedly for the first half of the test but in the second half a second simpler solution was also available. The undrugged discovered and used the appropriate solution in the first half (convergent thinking) and after the change they gradually discovered the easy solution (divergent (thinking) and used that one instead. However, fewer of the subjects given scopolamine used the correct solution repeatedly in the first half (poorer convergent thinking) but as a group they switched solutions more rapidly than the control group (better divergent thinking) giving evidence for broader attention after scopolamine.

Distraction in a boring vigilance task results from fantasies and task-irrelevant thoughts. If the improved performance by nicotine in vigilance tests is due to a reduction of this sort of irrelevant information, we would expect improved convergent thinking where irrelevant information would interfere with performance but disrupt performance in divergent thinking tests where irrelevant information might help problem solving. Once again we used the Luchins Jar Test and found that subjects who were given nicotine performed better on the first half of the test where subjects could use the same solution repeatedly (convergent thinking) but were slower to change to a simpler solution when it was available, i.e., think divergently.

Thus from this evidence subjects who receive cholinolytics and nonparanoid, acute (schizophreniform) and chronic (nuclear) schizophrenics, show divergent thinking patterns.

5.6. Electrocortical Arousal

An additional important piece of evidence for similarity between the cholinergic model psychosis and nonparanoid schizophrenia comes from studies of electrocortical arousal. Throughout this chapter it has been emphasized that the changes in information processing that are produced by cholinolytics are a consequence of their reduction of cortical desynchronization. It follows from this view that the electrocortical activity of a nonparanoid schizophrenic group should display a more synchronized pattern than a group of non-pathological subjects.

The problem of most electrophysiological studies of schizophrenic populations is that they have not divided them into diagnostic subgroups (see review by Mirsky, 1969) and so it is difficult to find relevant information. Lader (1975) reviewed in detail earlier studies which reported that the fundamental EEG patterns of their schizophrenic group were indistinguishable from control subjects although there were some unusual patterns in some subjects, i.e., presence of synchronized delta waves.

A quantitative analysis of the EEG in subgroups has proved more informative for our hypothesis. Kortchinskaia (1965) compared reactive, paranoid schizophrenics with process, nonparanoid schizophrenics which would include hebephrenics. The paranoid group displayed showed normal alpha activity at rest which was replaced by faster activity with a stimulus (alpha blocking). The nonparanoid subjects showed slow, diffuse electrocortical activity and poor alpha blocking. In another study also, young nonparanoid schizophrenics (mostly hebephrenic) showed more slow wave activity, delta and theta waves, and less fast beta activity than other psychotic groups (FInk et al., 1965).

In a recent review of this research Saletu (1980) found that most drug-free schizophrenic patients had less than normal alpha and slow beta activity and more than normal theta and fast beta activity than matched non-pathological subjects. It was interesting that those patients who responded to neuroleptic drugs had more fast beta activity while those patients who did not respond had a predominance of slow activity just like non-pathological subjects who had received doses of cholinolytics.

This evidence is consistent with the similarity argument that some nonparanoid schizophrenics have a slower less desynchronized pattern of electrocortical activity.

6.   CONCLUSIONS

In the previous sections we have presented evidence that cholinolytic drugs produce cognitive changes which are similar to those found in some types of schizophrenics. The subjective reports and the experimental studies of attentional phenomena are very similar to the experiences and performance of non-pathological subjects who had received cholinolytic drugs. Thus there is a similarity in the rapid

information processing, distractibility, sustained attention, hallucinations and thinking for both sets of subjects. These strong resemblances support the adequacy for some cholinergic model psychosis at
least as an analogy for some nonparanoid schizophrenic states. This
fact alone would justify the use of the model as a heuristic device
to generate experimentation.

Clinical evidence that the two states are more than analogous is
presented in the chapter by Singh and Kay in this book and shows that
cholinolytic drugs counteract the beneficial effects of antipsycotic
medication. Direct evidence for homology comes from studies of electrocortical activity after doses of scopolamine in schizophrenics.
In both states there is a slowing of electrocortical activity which
is consistent with the homology hypothesis that both states result
from similar changes in the same neurochemical pathways, the ascending
cholinergic pathways to the cortex.

Evidence against this simple cholinergic hypothesis of nonparanoid schizophrenia is the fact that the disorder can be treated with
drugs whose major mechanism of action is blockade of dopamine synapses.

One resolution of this dilemma is to combine the two sets of data
and propose a dopamine-acetylcholine balance hypothesis (Warburton,
1979b). According to this model there is a dynamic balance between
dopaminergic and cholinergic pathways, perhaps at the cortex. The
psychosis is a result of an imbalance between the two transmitter systems so that reduced activity in the cholinergic pathway which results
in dopaminergic predominance can be treated with dopamine antagonists.

ACKNOWLEDGEMENTS

We are grateful to Carreras-Rothmans Ltd., The Medical Research
Council and The Tobacco Research Council for financial support of the
research discussed in this chapter.

REFERENCES

Abood, L. G., and Biel, J. H., 1962, Anticholinergic psychomimetic
     agents, Int. Rev. Neurobiol. 6:218-273.
Beringer, K., 1927, "Mescaline Intoxication," Berlin - 363.
Bleuler, M., 1965, Conceptions of schizophrenia within the last fifty
     years and today, Int. J. Psychiat. 1:505-515.
Brown, B. B., 1974, "New Mind - New Body," Aldine-Atherton, Chicago.
Callaway, E., and Band, R. I., 1958, Some psychopharmacological effects
     of atropine, Arch. Neurol. Psychiat. (Chic.) 79:91-102.
Callaway, E., and Dembo, D., 1958, Narrowed attention: a psychological
     phenomenon that accompanies a certain physiological change, J.
     Neurol. Psychiat. 79:74-90.

Cameron, N., 1938, Reasoning, regression and communication in schizo-
    phrenics, Psychol. Mono. 50: No. 221:1-34.
Cameron, N., 1939, Deterioration and regression in schizophrenic think-
    ing, J. Abnorm. Soc. Psychol. 34:265-270.
Chapman, L. J., 1956, Distractibility in the conceptual performance of
    schizophrenics, J. Abnorm. Soc. Psychol. 53:286-291.
Claridge, G. S., 1967, "Personality and Arousal. A Psychophysiological
    Study of Psychiatric Disorder," Pergamon Press, London.
Colquhoun, W. P., 1962, Effects of hyoscine and meclozine on vigilance
    and short-term memory, Br. J. Ind. Med. 19:287-298.
Crawford, B. H., 1947, Visual adaptation in relation to brief condi-
    tioning stimuli, Proc. Roy. Soc. B. 134:283-302.
Crowell, E. B., and Ketchumn J. S., 1967, The treatment of scopolamine
    induced delirium with physostigmine, Clin. Pharmacol. Ther.
    8:409-414.
Eccles, J. C., 1970, "Facing Reality," Springer-Verlag, New York.
Fink, M., Itil, T., and Clyde, D., 1965, A contribution to the classi-
    fication of psychoses by quantitative E.E.G. measures, Proc. Soc.
    Biol. Psychiatry. 2:5-17.
Freeman, T., Cameron, J. L., and McGhie, A., 1958, "Chronic Schizo-
    phrenia," Tavistock Publications, London.
Green, J. W., and Arduini, H., 1954, Hippocampal electrical activity in
    arousal, J. Neurophysiol. 17:533-557.
Horowitz, M. J., 1975, Hallucinations: An information-processing ap-
    proach in "Hallucinations: Behavior, Experience and Theory," R. K.
    Siegal and L. J. West, eds., pp. 163-195, Wiley, New York.
Kay, S. R., and Singh, M. M., 1974, A temporal measure of attention in
    schizophrenia and its clinical significance, Br. J. Psychiatry.
    125:146-151.
Kay, S. R., and Singh, M. M., 1979, Cognitive abnormality in schizo-
    phrenia: a dual process model, Biol. Psychiatry. 14:155-176.
Ketchum, J. S., Sidell, F. R., Crowell, E. B., Aghajanian, G. K., and
    Hayes, A. H., 1973, Atropine, scopolamine and ditran: comparative
    pharmacology and antagonists in man, Psychopharmacologia
    28:121-133.
Kety, S. S., 1961, Chemical boundaries of psychopharmacology in "Con-
    trol of the Mind," S. M. Faber and R. H. L. Wilson, eds., pp.79-91,
    McGraw-Hill, New York.
Kortchinskaia, E. J., 1965, Etude électroencephalographique comparée de
    malades atteint de schizophrenie greffee et de malades atteint de
    schizophrenie non compliquee à évolutions maligne, Z. Nevropat.
    Psikhiat. 65:263-267.
Kraepelin, E., 1919, "Dementia Praecox and Paraphrenia," (trans. R. M.
    Barclay), Livingstone, Edinburgh.
Krnjevic K., and Phillis, J. W., 1963, Acetylcholine sensitive cells in
    the cerebral cortex, J. Physiol. Lond. 166:296-327.
Krnjevic, K., Pumain, R., and Renaud, L., 1971, The mechanism of exci-
    tation by acetylcholine in the cerebral cortex, J. Physiol.
    (Lond.) 215:247-268.

La Barre, W., 1975, Anthropological perspectives on hallucination and hallucinogens, in "Hallucinations," R. K. Siegal and L. J. West, eds., pp. 9-52, Wiley, New York.

Lader, M., 1975, "The Psychophysiology of Mental Illness," Routledge and Kegan Paul, London.

Lawson, J. S., McGhie, A., and Chapman, J., 1967, Distractibility in schizophrenic and organic cerebral disease, Br. J. Psychiatry. 113:527-535.

Lehmann, N., 1966, Pharmacotherapy of schizophrenia, in "Psychopathology of Schizophrenia," P. Hock and J. Zubin, eds., pp. 64-83, Grune and Stratton, New York.

Lewin, L., 1964, "Phantastica, narcotic and stimulating drugs," Routledge and Kegan Paul, London.

Libet, B., 1966, Brain stimulation and the threshold of conscious experience, in "Brain and Conscious Experience," J. C. Eccles, ed., pp. 165-181, Springer-Verlag, New York.

Mackworth, J. F., 1965, The effect of amphetamine on the detectability of signals in vigilance task, Can. J. Psychol. 19:104-109.

Mayer-Gross, W., 1951, Experimental psychoses and other mental abnormalities produced by drugs, Br. Med. J. 2:317-321.

McDonald, N., 1960, Living with schizophrenia, Can. Med. Assoc. J. 82:218-227.

McGhie, A., 1969, "Pathology of Attention," Penguin Books, London.

McGhie, A., and Chapman, J., 1961, Disorders of attention and perception in early schizophrenia, Br. J. Med. Psychol. 34:103-116.

McGhie, A., Chapman, J., and Lawson, J. S., 1964, Disturbances in selective attention in schizophrenia, Proc. Roy. Soc. Med. 57:419-422.

Michelson, M. J., 1961, Pharmacological evidences of the role of acetylcholine in the higher nervous activity of man and animals, Act. Nerv. Super. (Praha) 3:140-147.

Mirsky, A. F., 1969, Neurophysiological bases of schizophrenia, Ann. Rev. Psychol. 20:321-348.

Ostfeld, A. M., and Aruguete, A., 1962, Central nervous system effects of hyoscine in man, J. Pharmacol. 137:133-139.

Ostfeld, A. M., Machne, X., and Unna, K. R., 1960, The effects of atropine on the electroencephalogram and behavior in man, J. Pharmacol. 128:265-272.

Payne, R. W., 1964, The measurement and significance of overinclusive thinking and retardation in schizophrenic patients, paper presented to American Psychopathological Association.

Perceval, J., 1838, "A Narrative of the Treatment Experience by a Gentleman, During a State of Mental Derangement," Effingham Wilson, London.

Pribram, K. H., 1967, The new neurology and biology of emotion: a structural approach, Am. Psychol. 22:830-838.

Rinkel, M., Deshon, H. S., Hyde, R. W., and Solomon, H. C., 1952, Experimental schizophrenia-like symptoms, Am. J. Psychiatry. 108:572-578.

Russell, R. W., 1960, Drugs as tools in behavioral research in "Drugs and Behavior," L. Uhr and J. G. Miller, eds., pp. 19-40, Wiley, New York.

Saletu, B., 1980, Central measures of schizophrenia, in "Handbook of Biological Psychiatry," H. M. Van Praag, M. H. Lader, O. J. Rafaelsen and E. J. Sachar, pp. 97-144, Marcel Dekker, New York.

Savage, C., 1975, The continuity of perceptual and cognitive experiences, in "Hallucinations," R. K. Siegal and L. J. West, eds., pp. 257-286, Wiley, New York.

Siegal, R. K., and West, L. J., 1975, "Hallucinations," John Wiley, New York.

Shakow, D., 1962, Segmental set: A theory of the formal psychological deficit in schizophrenia, Arch. Gen. Psychiatry. 6:17-33.

Shakow, D., 1963, Psychological deficit in schizophrenia, Behav. Sci. 275-305.

Shute, C. C. D., and Lewis, P. R., 1967, The ascending cholinergic reticular systems in neocortical, olfactory, and subcortical projections, Brain. 90:497-520.

Spehlmann, R., 1969, Effect of acetylcholine and atropine upon excitation of cortical neurons by reticular stimulation, Fed. Proc. 28:795.

Strauss, J. S., 1969, Hallucinations and delusions as points on continua function, Arch. Gen. Psychiatry. 21:581-586.

Vogel, G., Foulkes, D., and Trosman, H., 1966, Ego functions and dreaming during sleep onset, Arch. Gen. Psychiatry. 14:238-248.

Warburton, D. M., 1972, The cholinergic control of internal inhibition in "Inhibition and Learning," R. Boakes and M. S. Halliday, eds., pp. 431-460, Academic Press, London.

Warburton, D. M., 1975, "Brain, Drugs and Behavior," Wiley, London.

Warburton, D. M., 1977, Stimulus selection and behavioral inhibition in "Handbook of Psychopharmacology," L. L. Iversen, S. D. Iversen and S. H. Snyder, eds., pp. 385-431, Plenum Press, New York.

Warburton, D. M., 1979a, Neurochemical bases of consciousness, in "Chemical Influences on Behavior," K. Brown and S. Cooper, eds., pp. 421-462, Academic Press, London.

Warburton, D. M., 1979b, Psychological aspects of information processing and stress, in "Human Stress and Cognition," V. Hamilton and D. M. Warburton, eds., pp. 33-66, John Wiley, London.

Warburton, D. M., 1981, Neurochemistry of behavior, Br. Med. Bull. 37:121-125.

Warburton, D. M., and Wesnes, K., 1979, The role of electrocortical arousal in the smoking habit in "Electrophysiological Effects of Nicotine," A. Remond and C. Izard, eds., pp. 183-200, Elsevier/North-Holland Biomedical Press, Amsterdam.

Weckowicz, T. E., 1960, Perception of hidden figures by schizophrenic patients, Arch. Gen. Psychiatry. 2:521-527.

Weckowicz, T. E., and Blewett, T. B., 1959, Size constancy and abstract thinking in schizophrenic patients, J. Ment. Sci. 105:909-934.

Wesnes K., and Warburton, D. M., 1978, The effect of cigarette smoking
    and nicotine tablets upon human attention in "Smoking Behavior:
    Physiological and Psychological Influences," R. E. Thornton, ed.,
    pp. 131-147, Churchill-Livingston, London.
White, R. P., Rinaldi, F., and Himwich, H. E., 1956, Central and peri-
    pheral nervous effects of atropine sulfate and mepiperphenidal
    bromide ('Darstine') on human subjects, J. Appl. Physiol.
    8:635-642.

Chapter 9

PHARMACOLOGY OF CENTRAL CHOLINERGIC MECHANISMS AND SCHIZOPHRENIC DISORDERS

Man Mohan Singh

Department of Psychiatry
Southern Illinois University
School of Medicine
P.O. Box 3926
Springfield, Illinois 62708, U.S.A.

Stanley R. Kay

Bronx Psychiatric Center
1500 Waters Place
Bronx, New York 10461, U.S.A.

---

1. INTRODUCTION

Although the first pharmacological experiments involving central cholinergic mechanisms in schizophrenia were conducted nearly four decades ago (Fiamberti, 1946), the work in this area has been neither extensive nor systematic. One reason for this, undoubtedly, has been the slow development of knowledge on the behavioral aspects of cholinergic transmission because, until recently, methodological difficulties prevented precise localization and manipulation of the cholinergic pathways in the brain, and the relationships between behavior and the cholinergic mechanisms could be studied only indirectly through the use of drugs as research tools (Russell, 1969). Another, perhaps even more powerful, reason has been the advent of neuroleptics as antipsychotic agents. Their powerful actions on the catecholaminergic, especially dopaminergic, neuronal systems of the brain, an apparent relationship between such actions and their therapeutic efficacy, as well as the elegant methodology available for the neuroanatomical, neurochemical, neurophysiological and neuropharmacological study of the catecholaminergic pathways have, quite understandably, promoted scientific attention on the possible role these brain systems may play in the pathophysiology of schizophrenia (Van Rossum, 1967; Randrup and Munkvad, 1972; Snyder et al., 1974; Meltzer and Stahl, 1976).

The relative neglect of brain cholinergic mechanisms in schizophrenia research has been encouraged by the belief that these mechanisms are relevant mainly to the undesirable extrapyramidal effects of neuroleptics rather than to their main antipsychotic effects (Cole and Clyde, 1961; Goldman, 1961; Ayd, 1961; NIHM Collaborative Study Group, 1964; Bishop et al., 1965). No apparent loss of antipsychotic efficacy from the common practice of combining anticholinergic anti-Parkinsonism drugs with neuroleptics, as well as the ability of drugs such as chlorpromazine and thioridazine to control psychosis despite built-in anticholinergic activity, have been taken to mean that cholinergic mechanisms are probably not important in the pathophysiology of schizophrenia (e.g., Davis et al., 1978). Yet there are good reasons to question this position. In nearly every behavioral pharmacological test in animals that predicts antipsychotic activity, the anticholinergic agents reverse the actions of neuroleptics in a dose-dependent fashion (Singh and Lal, 1982). Therefore, to the extent that behaviors such as amphetamine stereotypies and brain self-stimulation being examined in these tests are relevant to the schizophrenic process, and there are many reasons to believe they are (Randrup and Munkvad, 1972; Van Rossum, 1967; Snyder et al., 1974), these findings suggest that central cholinergic mechanisms may be implicated in at least those aspects of schizophrenia which are altered by neuroleptics. At the same time, the rapidly growing literature on the psychophysiological and behavioral roles of cholinergic transmission suggests that cholinergic mechanisms are involved in important ways in a number of the processes known to be deranged in schizophrenia. Included among these are disorders of arousal and attention as well as adaptational dysfunctions such as poor habituation, perseveration and poor autonomic control, in which ascending cholinergic projections from the brain-stem reticular formation to the cortex and the so-called cholinergic limbic circuit centered on the septal-hippocampal system seem to be important (Robinson, Chapter 2; Karczmar and Richardson, Chapter 7; Warburton and Wesnes, Chapters 1 and 8; Douglas, 1972, 1975; Shakow, 1977, Vanderwolf and Robinson, 1981, Singh, 1981; Singh and Kay, 1982; Singh and Lal, 1982).

Therefore, we review the available data on the pharmacology of cholinergic mechanisms in normal humans as well as in schizophrenics, both to try to assess the completeness and heuristic value of these data and to attempt an answer to the question, "Are central cholinergic mechanisms relevant to the pathophysiology of schizophrenia?"

However, in considering the cholinergic system pharmacology, four basic facts should be kept in mind from the outset. First, the cholinergic mechanisms involve at least two different types of receptors: the rapid action nicotinic receptors and the slow action muscarinic receptors (Lewis, 1964). Both are present in the brain and, when activated, may have opposite biochemical consequences, as for example in terms of the activity of catecholaminergic and serotonergic systems, and behavioral consequences, as for example in terms of brain self-stimulation (Frankenhaeuser et al., 1971; Pradhan, 1976; Hery et al., 1978). Thus, the nicotinic effects tend to resemble catecholaminergic actions in being facilitatory to behaviors such as brain self-stimulation, while the muscarinic actions are strongly inhibitory. Second, the cholinergic stimulation often has biphasic effects, so that high doses tend to produce effects opposite to those by low to moderate doses, and the gap between the optimal and the toxic doses can be very small (Feldberg, 1964; Russell, 1966; Warburton, 1972, 1975; Douglas, 1975; Van Meter et al., 1978). This is believed to be due to a depolarization block or a decreased receptor sensitivity produced by an excess of acetylcholine released by high level cholinergic stimulation or cholinesterase inhibition. Similarly, the consequences of low to moderate cholinergic blockade may be quite different from those with severe blockade. Third, the biological life of released acetylcholine is fairly short so that physiological effects of cholinergic manipulations are generally not long-lasting. However, pharmacological consequences of cholinergic stimulation or blockade may be delayed and prolonged (e.g., Duffy and Burchfiel, 1980). The reasons for these may be noncholinergic rather than cholinergic mechanisms, e.g., neurotoxicity and demyelination phenomena (Davis and Richardson, 1980; Petras, 1981), receptor damage and membrane changes through, for example, effects on phospholipids such as nucleotides (Greengard, 1978; Karczmar and Ohta, 1981), alteration of gluconeogenesis, oxygen uptake and dehydrogenases (Karczmar and Van Meter, 1963; Karczmar 1967), and changes in other neurotransmitters (Bowery et al., 1976) as well as neuropeptides (O'Neil, 1981). Fourth, the cholinergic systems do not function in isolation in the brain. They may be arranged in series or in parallel with other types of neurons, served by different neurotransmitters (Ladinsky et al., 1978), so that the consequences of their activity or inactivity will depend on what is happening to the neuronal systems with which they are connected. The effects may indeed be quite different in various situations because of variations in the dynamics of the neurobiological systems involved, due to reasons which may be internal or external to the organism.

Clearly, the interpretation of data from pharmacological manipulations of the central cholinergic mechanisms needs considerable circumspection.

2. CHOLINERGIC AGONISTS AND REVERSIBLE ANTICHOLINESTERASES

Cholinergic agonists such as arecoline, which act directly on the cholinergic receptors, or the reversible anticholinesterases such as physostigmine, which increase cholinergic activity indirectly by inhibiting cholinesterase and thus preventing inactivation of acetylcholine, are all relatively short-acting cholinergic agents. Studies with these compounds are, therefore, always of the nature of acute experiments, which may yield data quite different from the chronic experiments.

2.1. Early Clinical Trials

Cohen et al. (1944) and Fiamberti (1946) were probably the earliest investigators to try cholinergic stimulation in the treatment of schizophrenia; they claimed improvement in some schizophrenics with intravenous acetylcholine given in doses that often produced anoxia from cardiac arrest and seizures. A decade later, Pfeiffer and Jenney (1957) studied the effects of subcutaneous injections of arecoline (2 to 20 mg in 22 patients), pilocarpine (10 mg in one patient) and eserine or physostigmine (5 mg in two patients) in chronic institutionalized schizophrenics who had been protected against peripheral parasympathetic reactions with quaternary atropines (methylatropine, propantheline) which do not pass the blood-brain barrier. For brief periods (5 to 20 minutes), the patients showed varying degrees of lucidity and emotional responsiveness in the form of talking, laughing and exhibiting fearfulness. Many of these patients had been mute previously. Subsequently, the arecoline-induced lucid periods in chronic schizophrenics were noted to be similar to those produced by CO_2 and amobarbital (Fulcher et al., 1957).

Van Andel (1959) tried eserine in 18 chronic catatonic patients characterized by mutism, immobility and stupor. Fourteen patients had catatonic schizophrenia, three had encephalitic catatonia and one had hysterical catatonia. With peripheral effects prevented by probanthine, subcutaneously administered eserine in doses of 2 to 5 mg produced in all of the schizophrenic patients, a repeatable beneficial effect, which began about 30 minutes after injection and lasted for 45 minutes. The patients, some of whom had not talked for years, showed improved verbal and emotional communication; however, their speech showed obvious thought disorder. Neither the encephalitic patients, nor the lone hysterical patient showed any improvement, suggesting that the effect was limited to the schizophrenic group.

Collard et al. (1965) gave 0.05 to 5 mg of oxotremorine, a relatively long-acting cholinergic agonist, to five chronic schizophrenics. Of these, three were hebephrenic, one paranoid, and one catatonic. No improvement was noted in any case.

2.2. Recent Studies in Schizophrenic and Manic Depressive Patients

Interest in the possible use of cholinomimetics as therapeutic agents in schizophrenia was revived in the seventies by Rosenthal and Bigelow (1973). They gave physostigmine by mouth to five treatment-resistant chronic schizophrenics in increasing doses over a period of several weeks. Daily amounts of 4 to 12 mg were given in divided doses in two cases and in a single daily dose in three cases. Neuroleptics were continued in all cases. Two patients were diagnosed as hebephrenic, two undifferentiated and one paranoid. Marked clinical improvement was noted in all the cases. The most striking benefit was in terms of thought disorder, but hallucinations and delusions also improved. However, tolerance developed rapidly, especially on the divided dose schedule. In one case, a trial addition of atropine (centrally-active cholinolytic) to physostigmine antagonized its antipsychotic action. Few pheripheral parasympathetic or toxic effects were noted, although no peripheral anticholinergic drug had been used.

All of the above-noted studies were nonblind. Janowsky et al.,

(1973) conducted a very acute "blind" experiment with physostigmine.
The study involved schizophrenic and manic patients who were given a
consensus diagnosis by at least three psychiatrists according to DSM
II criteria. Using an infusion device, the patients were given two
or more doses of placebo every five minutes, then one of three active
drugs (methylphenidate, an adrenergic stimulant, 0.50 mg/kg in a
single dose; neostigmine, a peripheral cholinomimetic, 0.25 mg every
five minutes to reach a total dose of 1.25 mg; physostigmine, a
centrally-active cholinomimetic, 0.50 mg every five minutes to reach
a total dose of 2.50 mg), followed by placebo injections every five
minutes for at least 30 minutes. The whole experiment lasted an hour.
Every ten minutes throughout, a nurse "blind" to the protocol rated
patients for psychomotor activation-inhibition, dysphoria, irritability, unusual thought content, conceptual disorganization, blunted
affect and degree of psychosis. The study was designed particularly
to test the hypothesis that a catecholamine-acetylcholine reciprocity
within the brain may be the neurobiological substrate for the regulation of mood and activity along a continuum between an "excited-
activated-euphoric" state (catecholaminergic dominance) and an
"inhibited-retarded-depressed" state (cholinergic dominance).

     Of the schizophrenic patients, eight received physostigmine,
thirteen methylphenidate and six neostigmine. Pre-post-treatment comparisons showed no significant effects of neostigmine. Physostigmine
treatment decreased psychomotor activation, increased dysphoria and
psychomotor inhibition, but had no significant effect on ratings of
psychosis, unusual thought content or conceptual disorganization.
However, patients receiving this drug often felt sick with nausea and
vomiting, so that some of the dysphoria and psychomotor inhibition may
have been related to this. Methylphenidate treatment led to psychomotor activation and a significant increase in the level of psychosis,
unusual thought content and conceptual disorganization, suggesting a
worsening of the schizophrenic disorder. This exacerbation of psychosis was reversed by physostigmine. Correspondingly, the inhibitory
physostigmine effect was antagonized by methylphenidate. The manic
patients in the study showed a reduction in psychomotor activation and
elation and an increase in dysphoria ratings with physostigmine, while
methylphenidate generally had opposite and antagonistic effects. On
the basis of these data, the authors concluded that the disturbance of
adrenergic-cholinergic balance in the brain may be involved in mania
and depression but that the cholinergic mechanisms were probably not
involved in the primary psychotic process of schizophrenia. It should
be noted that the schizophrenic patients in the study were not subdivided into various diagnostic or prognostic types to determine if
the cholinergic or adrenergic effects were type-specific in any way,
nor was the chronicity or medication status of these patients considered in relation to the pharmacological response.

     Modestin et al. (1973a,b) studied the acute effects of physostig-
mine (0.75 mg to 1 mg) in comparison with neostigmine (0.75 mg to

1 mg) in a double-blind crossover study that involved 40 schizophrenics, 24 depressives, 4 manics and 40 patients with other diagnoses
such as neurosis, alcoholism and psychopathy. The treatment and
evaluation methods were essentially the same as in studies by Janowsky
et al. (1973). Both the cholinomimetics were given alone and also in
combination with a peripheral cholinergic blocker, methylscopolamine.
The schizophrenic group was comprised of chronic patients with long-
standing illness. No diagnostic or prognostic subgroups were recognized. The results suggested no "antischizophrenic" but a "depressiogenic" effect of physostigmine. The depressed patients showed a
worsening which took the form of agitated depression. There was no
unequivocal effect on symptomatology in manic patients. The remaining
patients who were emotionally stable before the test tended to develop
depressive features with physostigmine. The differences between physostigmine and neostigmine usually developed after the second dose,
which was given in the afternoon in each case.

Davis and Berger (1978) carried out a nonblind study of physostigmine in schizophrenic and manic patients. Only three schizophrenics, all of whom had a chronic type of illness, were studied with physostigmine, which was given in a larger amount (4.0 mg) through a slow
infusion lasting 60 minutes. Over the three hours of observations,
no significant reduction in schizophrenic pathology was noticed.
Eight manic patients were also studied with physostigmine. Euphoric
manics became less manic in mood and thought and more depressed, but
the irritable manics became more irritable. The authors concluded
that cholinergic mechanisms may be involved in mood disorders but not
in schizophrenia. Their exceedingly small schizophrenic sample was
not characterized in terms of diagnostic or prognostic subtypes.

Edelstein et al. (1981) reported on the effects of physostigmine
infusion in 11 patients meeting the Research Diagnostic Criteria (RDC)
for schizophrenia or schizoaffective disorder, who later underwent a
two-week course of treatment with lithium. The hypothesis was that a
subgroup of schizophrenics who show a therapeutic response to acute
physostigmine treatment may resemble manic patients in being responsive to lithium. The patients, all in their twenties and thirties,
had been recently admitted and maintained drug-free for two weeks
prior to the study. After pre-treatment with a peripheral anticholinergic (propantheline), 4 mg of physostigmine was infused over a one-
hour period. Using the Brief Psychiatric Rating Scale (BPRS), they
performed a baseline rating followed by a rating every 15 minutes during, and for 90 minutes after, physostigmine infusion. An attempt at
a double-blind procedure was made but abandoned because obvious somatic effects of physostigmine precluded a true double-blind. Following
the physostigmine test, all patients received lithium to maintain a
plasma level between 1.4 and 1.5 mEq/liter. Lithium response was
measured by repeated administration of The Serial Modified New Haven
Schizophrenia Index.

Four of the 11 patients responded to lithium treatment with a

mean improvement of 74 percent on the New Haven Index, while the seven
who did not respond showed a mean worsening of five percent. An ANOVA
for repeated measures revealed that the four lithium responders (two
diagnosed by RDC as schizophrenic and two as schizoaffective) also had
a significant improvement in the thinking disturbance factor of the
BPRS ($p < 0.05$) with physostigmine treatment, but the seven lithium-
resistant patients (five diagnosed by RDC as schizophrenic and two as
schizoaffective) showed no such improvement. The changes in thinking
disturbance were noted to be independent of any changes in withdrawal-
retardation scores, which failed to reach significance. The authors
concluded from this, admittedly preliminary, study that within the
syndrome of schizophrenia, there may be a subgroup of patients who
share with manic patients the property of showing temporary improvement in thinking disturbance with acute physostigmine treatment and
of being lithium responders. They hypothesized that such cases may
be suffering from an atypical affective disorder.

2.3. Summary

Acute behavioral effects of cholinergic stimulation in schizophrenia have been reported in four studies using cholinergic agonists
and in five studies using a reversible anticholinesterase, physostigmine. The studies were generally nonblind, and where double-blind
was attempted, it was vitiated by the obvious and unpleasant somatic
effects of cholinergic stimulation. The patient samples were mostly
small and, more importantly, poorly defined. With the possible exception of one study (Edelstein et al., 1981), the schizophrenic patients
involved were very chronic and treatment-resistant. The findings fell
into four categories.

(A) Where schizophrenia subtypes were recognized and considered,
there was a rather consistent observation of improvement in patients
with catatonic type of schizophrenia. During the short periods of
study, the therapeutic change was evident in the form of increased
verbal and emotional communication and improved alertness and awareness of the environment; the thought process and content, however,
remained psychotic. Studies reporting this effect all involved
cholinergic agonists.

(B) Chronic schizophrenics generally did not improve with one or
two parentral administrations of physostigmine, in doses ranging from
0.75 mg to 4 mg, but tended to become more dysphoric, lethargic and
withdrawn. In contrast, manic patients, especially those of euphoric
type, showed a decrease in many of these symptoms, while also tending
to become slower and dysphoric; irritable manics got more irritable.
Depressed patients also got worse and became agitated, while psychiatric patients with neither schizophrenia nor affective disorder mostly
became dysphoric with physostigmine. Unfortunately, unpleasant somatic symptoms such as nausea, vomiting and lethargy following intravenous physostigmine often complicated the clinical picture. It is

noteworthy, however, that a general pattern of psychomotor inhibition found in these studies with physostigmine contrasted with the alerting and activating effect of cholinergic agonists in catatonic schizophrenics.

(C) In the only study where physostigmine was given orally for a period of several weeks, all the five chronic, neuroleptic-resistant schizophrenics involved improved appreciably, especially in the area of thought disorder, although tolerance seemed to develop quickly. Neuroleptics were continued throughout, so that a neuroleptic-physostigmine interaction may have been involved in the observed therapeutic effect. Interestingly, despite the sizable dosages of physostigmine used (4 to 12 mg/day), few peripheral parasympathetic or toxic effects were noted.

(D) An acute exacerbation of psychosis induced by intravenous methylphenidate in chronic schizophrenics was reversed by subsequently administered physostigmine. Correspondingly, at least some of the acutely psychotic schizophrenics seemed to improve with a single intravenously administered dose of physostigmine; these patients seemed to recover on a subsequent two-week course of lithium.

3.   ACETYLCHOLINE PRECURSORS

3.1. Choline Feeding

A number of studies have suggested that choline chloride feeding can lead to increased brain acetylcholine concentrations and cholinergic activity (Haubrich et al., 1975; Cohen and Wurtman, 1975; Ulus and Wurtman, 1976). Based on this, Davis and Berger (1978) treated six drug-free chronic schizophrenic patients with up to 20 g per day of choline chloride. As compared to the baseline, three patients had lower psychopathology ratings after three to four weeks of this treatment; this improvement persisted during the subsequent one week on placebo. Neuroleptic treatment given thereafter to five patients seemed to produce a greater reduction in psychopathology than in the preceding choline treatment period. However, one patient who appeared to show the most dramatic response to choline treatment was not included in this part of the study. Also, the possibility of previous choline treatment acting to potentiate subsequent neuroleptic treatment was not considered.

3.2. Deanol

Deanol, or, 2-dimethylaminoethanol, is a tertiary amine analogue of choline which crosses the blood brain barrier and is believed to act as a precursor of acetylcholine in the brain, (Pfeiffer, 1959; Re, 1974). Murphree et al. (1959) first conducted a six-week double-blind trial in medical student volunteers who either received a placebo or deanol 10 to 30 mg/day. The results indicated that deanol produced an increase in muscle tone, increased ability for mental concentration, greater daytime energy, more affable mood and a change in sleep habits towards a lesser requirement of sleep. It is noteworthy that, unlike previously mentioned trials with cholinergic agents, deanol did not produce a dysphoric state.

An uncontrolled trial of deanol treatment was then conducted in 70 chronic schizophrenic patients who, after an initial two week period on 250 mg/day of deanol, received 50 mg/day of the drug for an average of nine months. A comparison group of 30 patients received a phenothiazine, Vesprin. Most patients slowly but definitely improved with deanol, and the improvement was thought to be equal to that with a phenothiazine neuroleptic. Thus moderate improvement to complete social remission was seen in 48 percent of deanol cases and 42 percent Vesprin cases. No clinical details concerning patient diagnosis or methods of assessment were provided.

3.3. Summary

The data on the effects of acetylcholine precursors in schizophrenia are quite limited and based on two, rather crude, nonblind studies. However, they are of interest in that they suggest some beneficial effect in at least some patients with this type of treatment. Deanol is particularly intriguing because, although slow in action, it seems to have therapeutic action equal to that of a phenothiazine. Also interesting is the fact that, unlike cholinergic agonists and anticholinesterases, deanol does not seem to produce a dysphoric state. If anything, it appears to produce a state of well-being, which should make it a preferable drug in the long-term treatment of schizophrenia, because neuroleptic treatment is sometimes attended with the emergence of a dysphoric state (Singh and Kay, 1979a). Also, the treatment may not have the most serious drawback of long-term neuroleptic treatment, that is, the development of tardive dyskinesia. Controlled studies of deanol, given alone or in combination with neuroleptics, in chronic schizophrenics may be quite worthwhile.

4.   IRREVERSIBLE ANTICHOLINESTERASES

A number of organophosphorous compounds developed as therapeutic agents (DFP, TEPP, OMPA), agricultural insecticides (Parathion, Mipafox, HETP, TEPP) or warfare agents (Sarin and Tabun or GA) produce an irreversible inhibition of cholinesterases, thus leading to an increase of central and peripheral cholinergic activity which persists until new cholinesterases have been synthesized. Their cholinergic effects, therefore, are long-lasting, and intentional, as well as accidental, experiments with them are of a chronic nature. As such, data from these may be expected to be different from those with acutely acting cholinergic drugs discussed in Section 2 (Bignami et al., 1975).

The effects of organophosphorous drugs in humans were extensively studied in the 1940's and 1950's both for civilian and military pur- poses. The symptoms produced by these agents represented both the muscarinic and nicotinic effects of acetylcholine, so that muscarinic blockers such as atropine only partially reversed their effects (Grob et al., 1947; Rowntree et al., 1950; Grob and Harvey, 1958).

4.1. Effects in Normal Humans

Normal persons receiving these drugs for short periods of two to four days generally developed a picture of dysphoria, restlessness, poor concentration, slowing of intellectual and motor functions, thought blocking, difficulty in expressing thoughts, insomnia, exces- sive dreaming and nightmares (Grob et al., 1947; Grob and Harvey, 1958; Bowers et al., 1964). The individuals appeared to have an altered state of awareness, but psychotic symptoms seldom appeared in acute studies involving small doses. With high doses and more chronic exposure, hallucinations and delusions began to develop. Psychologi- cal symptoms generally appeared when the whole blood cholinesterase activity fell below 40 percent of control (Bowers et al., 1964).

In a study involving 16 cases of 1.5 to 9 years long inadvertent exposure to organophosphorous insecticides, Gershon and Shaw (1961) found a clinical picture of a depressive state in seven persons, schizophrenic reactions in five persons, impaired memory and concen- tration in three persons, and a fugue state in one person. The schiz- ophrenic reactions were characterized by auditory hallucinations, per- secutory and religious delusions, ideas of reference, aggression, and apathy. Problems of memory and concentration were present in all 16 cases. Blood cholinesterase activity measured in two cases was 50 percent and 60 percent of normal. Similar but less severe abnormali- ties, lasting more than six months, were reported by Tabershaw and Cooper (1966) in 38 percent of 114 cases of acute organophosphate poisoning.

Metcalf and Holmes (1969) reported on the cognitive functioning in industrial workers acutely exposed to organophosphate pesticides in the early 1950's. Psychiatric interviews were conducted in 1952 in 56 cases with exposure and 22 unexposed controls. The exposed cases had significantly higher proportions of chronic complaints of forgetful- ness, difficulty in thinking, visual difficulty, aches and pains, drowsiness, fatigability and loss of interest in work. In 1965, i.e., 13 to 14 years after acute exposure, some of the same individuals, who in many instances had continued in the same employment, were adminis- tered a battery of tests of cognitive functions. The results revealed that, in comparison to controls, exposed persons had defective memory, difficulty in maintaining alertness and appropriate focus on attention,

a tendency towards fabrications on memory tests, perceptual distor-
tions on progressive geometric designs and a general impairment of
adaptiveness as shown in avoidance, delaying, inappropriate giving up
and slowing. In psychiatric interviews, exposed individuals especially those with high levels of exposure, complained of slowing, nervous-
ness and/or irritability, change in sleep and sexual habits and memory
difficulty. Thus, the suggestion was that organophosphate exposure
could produce long-lasting psychological impairment. However, precise
information on cholinesterase levels, work history and severity and
type of exposure was not known, so that it was not possible to judge
whether these impairments reflected chronic organophosphate exposure,
or long-term sequelae of acute exposures.

     In many of the studies noted above, electroencephalographic (EEG)
and other electrophysiological changes were looked for, and found, to
accompany central nervous system effects of organophosphates. With
doses producing mild to moderate behavioral symptoms, the EEG showed
desynchronization with increased frequency and reduced voltage, i.e.,
a cortical arousal pattern. However, with high doses and more intense
symptoms, bursts of high voltage slow waves appeared and the EEG rhythms and potentials became more irregular - a pattern similar to that
produced by cholinolytic psychotomimetics (Grob et al., 1947; Grob and
Harvey, 1958; Warburton, 1975; Burchfiel et al., 1976; Duffy and
Burchfiel, 1980). Muscarinic blockade with atropine reduced both the
psychological symptoms and electrophysiological changes. However,
this antagonistic effect was more complete and prolonged in terms of
the EEG abnormalities than in terms of the psychological disturbances
produced by the organophosphates (Grob et al., 1947). Indeed, in some
organophosphate-treated cases, pronounced psychological symptoms
developed after some time despite daily administration of atropine
and the concomitant absence of EEG changes. The withdrawal of atropine was followed within several days by the appearance of EEG abnormalities. Thus, it seemed that the EEG abnormalities represented
mainly the muscarinic aspects of cholinergic stimulation while the
psychological symptoms were relatd to both the muscarinic and nicotinic aspects of the cholinergic activity. The EEG changes also
tended to outlast the psychological symptoms after the organophosphate
treatment was stopped.

     In the Metcalf and Holmes (1969) study (see above), EEGs were
done in 1952 as well as in 1965. The outstanding finding in both sets
of recordings was the high incidence of low to medium voltage slow
activity in the theta, i.e., 4 to 6 Hz, frequency range. With high
levels of organophosphate exposure, the EEG became more irregular.
The presence of EEG abnormalities in the 1965 investigation suggested
the possibility that EEG changes due to organophosphates could persist
for long periods after exposure. All-night EEGs were also recorded in
12 cases; nine of them showed "narcoleptic records" and two "demonstrated disturbances of normal cycling of sleep stages." Interviews
with these cases indicated a high incidence of lethargy, drowsiness,

insomnia and narcolepsy-type symptoms. Auditory and visual evoked
responses studied in 1965 showed a tendency towards lower amplitudes
and longer peak latencies, suggesting impaired information processing
due to organophosphate exposure. Auditory evoked responses showed
more variability than the visual responses.

Duffy and Burchfiel (1980) provided the most systematic data on
the long-term effects of an organophosphate on EEGs. In a carefully
controlled study, they first demonstrated that a single large dose
($5\mu g/kg$) of Sarin, as well as 10 small doses ($1\mu g/kg$) given at weekly
intervals, produced EEG changes which were present on re-examination
one year later. The most prominent change that distinguished the experimental from the control animals consisted of an increase in beta
or fast activity. Later they compared the EEGs of 77 industrial
workers who had one to three exposures to Sarin within the previous
six years with the EEGs of 38 unexposed workers from the same plant.
Conventional EEGs as well as all-night sleep EEG recordings were obtained and then subjected to visual as well as computer analyses.
Both univariate and multivariate statistics showed highly significant
differences between the groups. The most prominent abnormality was
an increase in beta activity in the Sarin-exposed cases. In addition,
there was an excessive amount of slow activity (i.e., delta and theta
waves) in the exposed cases. Their sleep EEGs showed a significant
increase in REM sleep which occurred at the cost of stage 2 non-REM
sleep. All of these abnormalities tended to be more prominent in
cases with multiple exposures to Sarin. Thus, the data clearly established long-lasting EEG effects of short-term exposure to an organophosphate. In considering these data, the authors noted that
after an organophosphate exposure the cholinesterase recovery would
generally be complete within three to four months, while the behavioral recovery frequently would take only a few weeks (Grob and
Harvey, 1958; Milby, 1971). This meant that the tissue cholinesterase
levels were probably normal at the time the EEG abnormalities were
recorded, thus suggesting that organophosphate exposure had either
produced long-term changes in synaptic morphology or biochemistry,
which rendered postsynaptic receptors more sensitive to endogenous
acetylcholine, or the organophosphate Sarin had neurotoxic actions
unrelated to its anticholinesterase activity.

4.2.   Effects in Schizophrenic and Manic-Depressive Patients

Rowntree et al. (1950) studied the effects of difluorophosphate
(DFP) treatment in 17 chronic schizophrenics (five paranoid, nine
hebephrenic, two catatonic and one simple), nine manic depressives
(six hypomanic, one depressed, two in remission) and 10 normal subjects. DFP was dissolved in peanut oil and administered as intramuscular injection. Thirteen schizophrenics and all nine manic
depressives were given a total dose of 13 mg over a period of seven
days (1 mg on the first day, 2 mg on each succeeding day). The
remaining four schizophrenics continued to get the drug after the

seventh day and, over an average period of 37 days, received a mean total dosage of 43 mg; one patient received 63 mg in 35 days. An attempt to give DFP to normal controls in doses comparable to those administered to most of the patients, i.e., 13 mg, was unsuccessful, because six of them were unable to tolerate more than 7 mg due to severe toxic effects. Even with the co-administration of atropine, only two of the remaining four tolerated 13 mg doses, with the other two tolerating only 11 mg and 7 mg respectively. The inhibition of the cholinesterase activity in erythrocytes was 60 to 90 percent in schizophrenics, 58 to 84 percent in manic depressives, and 43 to 80 percent in controls.

Perhaps the most interesting observation was the great physical tolerance of the chronic schizophrenics to DFP effects. The physical muscarinic effects (anorexia, vomiting, diarrhoea, pallor, fainting) and EEG changes (see below) were quite similar in manic depressives and normals. However, in chronic schizophrenics, these effects were both less intense and less frequent, suggesting an unresponsivity of their muscarinic cholinergic mechanisms. This was most convincingly seen in one schizophrenic who received 63 mg of DFP without showing any characteristic effects of the drug. In some respects, the reactions of schizophrenics were paradoxical. Thus, while manic depressives showed a gradual fall in blood pressure, the schizophrenics had a tendency for the blood pressure to rise. This might indicate a preponderance of nicotinic over muscarinic activity in chronic schizophrenia. Only the paranoids among schizophrenics showed muscarinic effects comparable to those of the manic depressives and controls.

The EEG changes were essentially similar in all the cases. In the records taken within 24 hours of the last DFP injection, characteristically there was a lowering of amplitude along with a reduction in the amount and spread of alpha and, in some cases, an intermittent appearance of irregular low voltage theta in 4 to 7 Hz range. In the records obtained later, the amplitude had increased beyond the baseline along with an increase in the dominance and spread of alpha, and increased appearance of higher voltage 2 to 7 Hz theta and an increased instability on hyperpnoea. However, in general the EEG changes, especially the appearance of slow activity, were less marked in schizophrenic than in manic depressive patients.

The effects of atropine on EEG were also studied in four normal controls. The results indicated a gradual but intermittent lowering of amplitudes, an increase in irregular slow activity and an increase in alpha frequency. Apart from the increase in alpha frequency, these changes were similar to those produced by DFP. Not surprisingly, therefore, atropine given with DFP did not prevent the EEG changes characteristic of DFP. This suggested that DFP-induced EEG changes were in some respects similar to those produced by muscarinic blockade.

Mentally, dysphoric effects predominated in manic depressive patients and controls. One case of hypomania with schizophrenic

symptoms (schizo-affective disorder) improved considerably during two
separate courses of DFP treatment, developing a relapse each time the
drug was stopped. Two other hypomanics improved during DFP administration and remained well afterwards. One partially recovered recurrent hypomanic became maniacal two days after the DFP course was completed. In the only depressive studied, there was a marked deepening
of depression. Two remitted manic depressives and two of six hypomanics showed only slight dysphoria, insomnia, and increased dreaming
with DFP treatment.

Three out of five paranoid schizophrenics had a pronounced activation of psychosis with DFP, but of the nonparanoids, only two out of
nine hebephrenics and the lone simple schizophrenic worsened. The
activation was attended with the reappearance of symptoms that characterized the onset of illness and persisted for a number of months
after the withdrawal of DFP. One hebephrenic schizophrenic showed
marked improvement which was "associated with diminution of anxiety."

4.3.   Summary

The behavioral and electrophysiological effects of organophosphate anticholinesterases are complex and varied. Even after considering the fact that muscarinic and nicotinic aspects of cholinergic
stimulation are different, all of the consequences of organophosphate
exposure cannot be seen as being due to cholinergic stimulation. Considering the convincing evidence for the development of behavioral
tolerance to cholinergic stimulation (Bignami et al., 1975) and also
for the phenomenon of depolarization block and/or refractoriness of
cholinergic receptors resulting from local accumulation of acetylcholine (Burns and Paton, 1951; Katz and Thesleff, 1957), some of the
consequences of intense or prolonged cholinergic activity should probably be regarded as functionally similar to cholinergic blockade
rather than stimulation. At the same time, the findings reviewed here
suggest the possibility that organophosphates may change cholinergic
receptors through intense cholinergic stimulation or cause neurotoxic
effects unrelated to this action, so that behavioral and neurophysiological changes can last well beyond the period of cholinesterase inhibition, and certainly beyond the period when cholinergic tolerance
may be expected. Keeping these considerations in mind, the following
summary statements regarding the data in this section can be made:

(A) With acute, relatively low level exposure to organophosphates, the clinical picture was essentially that of generalized psychomotor inhibition with slowing of thinking, motor functions and
concentration, and a subjective state of dysphoria. In addition,
there was insomnia with excessive dreaming and nightmares. The behavioral symptoms usually occurred after a reduction of erythrocyte
cholinesterases to below 40 percent of control levels. The EEG effects consisting of increased low voltage fast activity along with
periods of increased theta range slow activity were suggestive of
cortical arousal, especially that seen in REM sleep.

(B) With relatively high doses and/or chronic exposures, the
clinical picture was suggestive of more profound disorders resembling
schizophrenia, toxic confusional state, or organic brain syndrome with
or without a significant depressive state. The EEG was more unstable
and showed greater amounts of high voltage slow activity. The sleep
EEG had excessive REM activity and a decrease in non-REM sleep. Auditory and visual evoked responses suggested impaired information processing. Many of the EEG features resembled those with atropine,
which, interestingly, failed to reverse the behavioral or electrophysiological consequences of severe or chronic organophosphate exposure.

(C) Persistent cognitive impairment, instability of mood, sleep
disturbance and EEG abnormalities could be detected months and years
after organophosphate exposure, suggesting long-lasting neurotoxic
effects or changes in cholinergic receptors leading, possibly, to
supersensitivity to endogenous acetylcholine.

(D) Treatment with an organophosphate (DFP) essentially produced
similar electrophysiological, physical and mental effects in affective
disorder patients and normal controls. As a consequence, the hypomania was reduced, psychomotor inhibition increased and subjective
dysphoria worsened.

(E) Chronic nonparanoid schizophrenic patients showed remarkable
resistance to muscarinic effects of DFP treatment. In comparison with
manic depressive patients and normal controls, they tolerated much
higher amounts of DFP and showed much milder physical muscarinic and
electrophysiological changes. Mentally also, these patients changed
infrequently. At the same time, in contrast to other groups, they
showed an increase in blood pressure. These data suggested an under-
reactivity of muscarinic mechanisms and a relative preponderance of
nicotinic mechanisms in chronic non-paranoid schizophrenia.

(F) Chronic paranoid schizophrenics resembled the manid depressive and normal individuals in terms of muscarinic response to DFP
treatment. Mentally, their condition tended to get worse. This suggested that paranoid schizophrenia might be different from nonparanoid
schizophrenia in having normally reactive muscarinic mechanisms.

5.   ANTICHOLINERGIC AGENTS

There are many types of anticholinergic agents known. Of these,
drugs such as atropine, scopolamine and belladonna are constituents of
the commonly occurring plants of the Solanaceae group. Priests, magicians and witches of many cultures used these plants ceremonially to
produce hallucinatory experiences, which varied in content and character according to the cultural beliefs and attitudes of the persons
involved (Lewin, 1964; Warburton, 1979). Accidental or intentional
cases of poisoning with these plants have also been frequently recorded. With the presenting picture of hallucinations and illusions

of various kinds as well as disturbances of attention and awareness, these cases are not infrequently given an initial diagnosis of acute schizophrenia (Warburton, 1979). Purified atropine, scopolamine and belladonna from the Solanaceae plants have also long been used as therapeutic agents and are commonly to be found in various over-the-counter sleep and asthma preparations. Psychotic reactions from the overuse of these preparations are well-known in emergency medicine (Hall et al., 1981).

A second group of anticholinergic agents are synthetic atropinics such as benztropine, trihexyphenidyl, biperidin, procyclidine and cycrimine, which are used in the treatment of Parkinsonism and neuro-leptic-induced pseudo-Parkinsonism. These drugs have relatively greater central than peripheral anticholinergic activity (Yahr and Duvoisin, 1972) and are, therefore, preferred over those in the first group for the treatment of Parkinsonism. However, to varying degrees, these anticholinergic agents also increase dopaminergic activity by blocking synaptosomal reuptake of dopamine (Snyder et al., 1970), so that, while their predominant effects are anticholinergic, their observable actions may also be in some degree due to dopaminergic effects. Then there is a class of synthetic anticholinergic drugs, the piperidyl glycolate esters such as Ditran, which are particularly psychotogenic (Abood and Biel, 1962). Their unusually strong psycho-tomimetic propensity may be due to the fact that, besides being exceedingly potent cholinolytics, these drugs also increase membrane permeability in the brain and elsewhere and have antiserotonic, anti-histaminic, and a variety of metabolic effects (Abood and Biel, 1962). Finally, one should mention cholinesterase, which reduces cholinergic activity by virtue of being a cholinolytic enzyme.

It is important to recognize that these anticholinergic drugs are all mainly antimuscarinic agents. Although both nicotinic and musca-rinic receptors are found in the brain, the muscarinic receptors are by far the most abundant, and the central nervous system effects of cholinergic stimulation are predominantly muscarinic in nature. For the understanding of the role of cholinergic mechanisms in behavior, therefore, antimuscarinics are of the greatest interest. Furthermore, most of the literature on the behavioral and psychophysiological con-sequences of cholinergic blockade is really based on muscarinic block-ade. However, in considering this literature, it is important to remember that the changes due to muscarinic blockade are in fact a mixture of the results of muscarinic blockade per se and the conse-quences of "released" nicotinic receptor activity.

5.1. Psychological Effects in Healthy Individuals

The clinical and experimental literature on this subject is ex-tensive (for bibliography see Warburton, 1975, pp. 125-127; Warburton, 1979). Many of the pertinent studies are reviewed in this monograph by Warburton and Wesnes and will be mentioned here only briefly to highlight certain issues.

It is well established that all anticholinergic drugs are capable
of producing a psychosis. This psychosis, especially at high doses,
resembles a toxic delirium or stupor because of marked disorientation,
confusion, illusions and dominant visual hallucinosis (Meduna and
Abood, 1959; Hoffer and Osmond, 1960) and is, therefore, often characterized as exogenous psychosis. However, in many ways the anticholinergic psychosis, especially in its less extreme form, resembles the
schizophrenic psychosis, and it is justifiable to consider it as a
"model psychosis" (Warburton and Wesnes, Chapter 8). Certain authors
have described it as "model psychosis" resembling that produced by
amphetamines (Abood and Meduna, 1958; Meduna and Abood, 1959; Shopsin
and Gershon, 1971) and similar to the paranoid forms of schizophrenia
(Stephens, 1967).

Two types of studies in healthy individuals have been reported;
those using piperidyl glycolates which were designed to produce a psychotic state in trained volunteers, and those using various anticholinergic therapeutic agents to test the effects of different levels
of cholinergic blockade on specific aspects of information processing.

Abood and Biel (1962) conducted studies on the effects of piperidyl glycolates in small groups of observers including psychiatrists,
psychologists, nurses and medical students. The effects depended on
the dose of the agent used and the psychological idiosyncracies of the
subject. In general, the piperidyl glycolates produced a state of
alienation, depersonalization, "lack of ego mastery," confusion and
disorganization, which in a comparative test resembled that produced
by LSD. Both drugs produced a similar profile on the Minnesota Multi-
phasic Personality Inventory and induced a pessimistic outlook which
affected self-evaluation, self-trust and psychological functioning.
LSD produced more irritability, hostility and brooding, while the
anticholinergic drug produced more anxiety and preoccupation with the
body.

The most dramatic characteristic of the anticholinergic psychosis
was hallucinations. Most often, the hallucinations were visual and
involved clearly defined objects, persons, animals or colors. However, frequently there were also auditory, tactile, olfactory and
gustatory hallucinations, thus contradicting the common belief that
the so-called exogenous psychosis produced by anticholinergic drugs
differs from schizophrenic psychosis in having visual rather than
auditory hallucinations. The auditory hallucinations involved musical
instruments and familiar voices. As the psychosis progressed, the
individuals began to respond to hallucinations and carried on extended
conversations with phantom voices.

At low doses on the drugs, the subjects were able to describe
their experiences coherently, but with increasing doses they began to
talk aimlessly and incoherently, losing their train of thought often,
and progressing sometimes to complete mutism. Emotionally, they were

labile, bewildered, apprehensive, panicky, and prone to angry out-
bursts. In addition, they showed negativism and paranoia. Some individuals were able to vividly recall their experiences after recovery
from the drug influence, while those who had become so confused as to
lose contact with the environment were partially or completely amnesic
afterwards.

Essentially similar findings have been reported by Wilson and
Shagass (1964) who compared the psychotomimetic effects of Ditran and
LSD.

It should be recalled at this point that, as was mentioned earlier (2.2), some workers have suggested that a relative or absolute
excess of central cholinergic activity may be the neurobiological
substrate of depression. One reason for this view has been reports
of euphoriant effects of anticholinergic drugs (Janowsky et al.,
Chapter 10). On this basis, cholinergic blockade should provide us
with a model of manic disorder. This seems not to be the case. The
studies with potent cholinergic blockers described above produced a
clinical picture resembling schizophrenia in many respects, but not
of mania. If anything, the mood changes with these drugs were the
opposite of those associated with mania. Similar conclusions were
suggested by the studies in which Ditran given to depressed patients
produced the characteristic psychotic state rather than a manic state,
or relief of depression (Meduna and Abood, 1959). After oral doses
of 10 to 20 mg of Ditran, 75 percent of the depressed patients studied
developed a dream-like state with hallucinations, disorientation, and
confusion, lasting for 12 to 48 hours. However, in the subsequent
days and weeks, i.e., corresponding to the period of recovery of cholinergic transmission, many of the patients who had become psychotic
with Ditran showed improved mood and, at times, developed a period of
elation and increased activity for a period of days!

Experimental studies with anticholinergic therapeutic agents have
produced a wealth of evidence which supports the possibility that
central cholinergic mechanisms may play a role in the pathophysiology
of at least some forms of schizophrenia. These studies concern attentional and cognitive dysfunctions which represent major if not fundamental aspects of schizophrenic pathology (Warburton and Wesnes,
Chapter 8).

Difficulty in sustaining attention or concentration is a well
recognized clinical feature of schizophrenia (McGhie and Chapman,
1961). Using a temporal measure of the ability to sustain attention,
Kay and Singh (1979) observed marked impairment in acute, particularly
non-paranoid, schizophrenics. Similar problems characterize the anticholinergic syndrome (White et al., 1956; Callaway and Band, 1958;
Michelson, 1961; Ostfeld et al., 1960; Crowell and Ketchum, 1967;
Ketchum et al., 1973). Experimental evidence has shown that even
relatively small amounts of an anticholinergic, such as scopolamine

1 mg, can produce a measurable impairment in sustaining attention
(Colquhoun, 1962; Mackworth, 1965). With the small doses of the drugs
used in these studies, there would be no impairment of sensorium nor
development of a confused state, yet difficulty in sustaining attention was evident.

With or without difficulty in sustaining attention, schizophren-
nics often seem to have problems in screening out redundant or irrelevant inputs (from within or without), so that they are more susceptible to distraction and show impaired rapid information processing of
the kind involved in dealing with language (McGhie and Chapman, 1961;
Weckowicz, 1960; Shakow, 1962; McGhie et al., 1964; Lawson et al.,
1967). Probably related to these dysfunctions, are problems in thinking, such as loosening of associations, disorganization and loss of
abstract reasoning, which characterize many schizophrenics and are
often regarded as one of the cardinal features of schizophrenia
(Kraepelin, 1919; Bleuler, 1950; Cameron, 1938, 1939; Payne, 1973;
Singh and Kay, 1978a; Kay and Singh, 1979). These abnormalities in
general are much more evident in nonparanoid than in paranoid forms
of schizophrenia. As examples may be mentioned studies which demonstrated (a) marked impairment in auditory or visual information processing by auditory or visual distracting stimuli in hebephrenic but
not in paranoid schizophrenics (McGhie et al., 1964; Lawson et al.,
1967); (b) much worse than normal performance by hebephrenic but not
by paranoid schizophrenics in a rapid information processing task
involving detection of consecutive odd or even numbers in a series of
random numbers spoken at a rate of 60 per minute (Claridge 1967); (c)
poor performance by unmedicated schizophrenics on the Continuous Performance Test designed to measure sustained attention, which improved
after neuroleptic treatment but worsened again during remission when
the task had to be performed in the presence of distracting or irrelevant stimuli (Orzack et al., 1967; Wohlberg and Kornetsky, 1973).

Healthy individuals receiving high doses of anticholinergic drugs
(e.g., atropine 15 mg/kg or scopolamine 24 mg/kg) show difficulty in
comprehending speech and following a train of thought in a fashion
similar to that seen in schizophrenics (Crowell and Ketchum, 1967).
They cannot adequately carry out instructions, follow complex conversations, explain proverbs or identify word similarities and differences (Ketchum et al., 1973; Ostfeld et al., 1960; White et al., 1956).

However, with anticholinergic doses much lower than those needed
for producing a psychosis, significant impairment in fast information
processing, distractibility, poor selective attention and thinking
disorder can still be demonstrated by using tests similar to those
which show abnormalities in these areas among schizophrenics, particularly those of the non-paranoid type, e.g., Embedded Figures Test,
Stroop Test and other tests for distractibility (Callaway and Band,
1958; Callaway and Dembo, 1958; Ostfeld and Aruguete, 1962); rapid
information processing of number sequences (Warburton and Wesnes, this

book); Luchins Jar test for problem solving using convergent and divergent modes of thinking (Warburton and Wesnes, this book).

These findings suggest that antimuscarinics in various amounts can reproduce important aspects of psychopathology seen in nonparanoid types of schizophrenia.

5.2. Psychological Effects in Psychotic Individuals

There are numerous reports indicating activation of true schizo-phrenic symptomatology by centrally active antimuscarinics of various kinds given in toxic as well as non-toxic doses to schizophrenic pa-tients (Tourlentes et al., 1960; Gershon and Olariu, 1960; Finkelstein, 1961; Davis et al., 1964; Itil et al., 1969; Shopsin and Gershon, 1971; El-Yousef et al., 1972, 1973; Singh and Smith, 1971, 1973a,b; Singh and Kay, 1975a,b,c, 1978a,b, 1979a,b). The studies of most heuristic value will be reviewed here.

One of the earliest systematic investigations was carried out by Tourlentes et al. (1960). They studied the effects of a piperazinoal-kylglycolate in 32 severely chronic schizophrenic patients, using a triple-blind, double-placebo research design. The results of a three-month long trial indicated a worsening in characteristic schizophrenic symptomatology such as withdrawal, autism, open masturbation, impul-sive acting out and regressed behavior.

Gershon and Olariu (1960) observed a similar worsening of psycho-pathology in chronic schizophrenic patients with Ditran, piperidylgly-colate, given in daily doses of 5 to 10 mg for a period of two to four weeks. Interestingly, these effects were most pronounced in paranoid schizophrenics. Fairly rapid tolerance developed for peripheral auto-nomic actions, but any adaptation to central actions developed slowly or not at all, thus suggesting differences in the central and periph-eral cholinergic mechanisms.

Abood and Biel (1962), citing work by their group on the effects of Ditran in chronic schizophrenic, neurotic and normal individuals, observed that anticholinergic or autonomic responsiveness to Ditran was generally reduced in the schizophrenic group as compared to both the neurotic and the normal groups. The schizophrenics who reacted to Ditran most like the controls as a rule showed a favorable response to psychotherapeutic agents and other treatment measures. This suggested that poor prognosis, chronic schizophrenics had deficient or under-responsive cholinergic mechanisms, and that intact responsivity of these mechanisms may be needed for recovery from psychosis.

Itil and Fink (1968) gave intravenous injections of various doses of Ditran or atropine to 65 patients diagnosed as schizophrenic states and 19 patients diagnosed as affective, emotional or personality dis-orders. For two months before the investigation, the patients had

received no psychotropic medication. The results, which did not take
into account any patient distinctions in terms of diagnostic types,
chronicity, etc., suggested that behavioral changes were quite different at different dose levels. With relatively small doses of Ditran
(0.005 to 0.05 mg/kg) or atropine (0.04 to 0.30 mg/kg), the patients
became restless, agitated and uncoordinated, and showed emotional
changes of anxiety, fear, depression or euphoria. There were periods
of drowsiness and occasional reports of perceptual disturbance. With
moderate doses (Ditran 0.04 to 0.25 mg/kg, atropine 0.20 to 0.40
mg/kg), there was increased delirious excitement with hallucinations
and disturbance of thought, association and memory. In contrast, at
the highest doses used (Ditran 0.04 to 0.30 mg/kg, atropine 0.25 to
0.50 mg/kg), psychomotor activity decreased and a state of deep sleep
or stupor developed in some cases. Thus, there seemed to be a dual or
biphasic action. Intravenous chlorpromazine, given in very small
doses (0.02 to 0.25 mg/kg) 30 to 40 minutes after Ditran or atropine
injections, suppressed the psychomotor activation and delirium produced by the anticholinergic medication but increased the stupor. Similarly used, d-amphetamine (0.15 to 0.30 mg/kg) increased the alertness
but decreased psychomotor activity.

Sherwood (1952, 1958) injected cholinolytic enzyme cholinesterase
or an anticholinergic agent, pentamethonium iodide, into the lateral
cerebral ventricles of stuporous chronic catatonic schizophrenics.
Fifteen patients received one or more injections of these drugs. According to the author, six returned to normal at one time or another;
in one case the improvement lasted four years, in another two years,
after the last injection. Thus, the results suggesting a therapeutic
action of cholinergic blockade in catatonic schizophrenia seemed to
contradict studies indicating worsening of schizophrenia by anticholinergic drugs. However, in many ways the recorded observations suggested an increase in parasympathetic, i.e., cholinergic, activity
rather than cholinergic blockade, e.g., pupillary constriction, brady-
cardia and decrease in blood pressure. This might mean that the clinical improvement was related less to cholinergic blockade but to a
possible cholinergic rebound or a mobilization of cholinergic circuits
following intense cholinergic blockade.

A similar conclusion is suggested by a series of studies in
which atropine or scopolamine-induced coma was used as a treatment
for schizophrenia and affective disorders (Forrer, 1956; Grissel and
Bynum, 1956; Miller, 1957; Schwartz, 1957; Forrer and Miller, 1958;
Goldner, 1967) and others in which Ditran-induced activation of
psychosis was used to improve the effectiveness of antipsychotic
medication (Itil et al., 1969).

The coma treatment involved intramuscular administration of massive doses of atropine sulphate (32 to 212 mg) or scopolamine (5 to
100 mg). Large numbers of patients with diagnoses of schizophrenia,
mania and depression were reportedly treated in the 1950's and 1960's

with atropine or scopolamine comas, administered three to six times a week in courses averaging 20 treatments. Concurrent psychotropic medications or other forms of treatment were frequently used. However, the treatment was found to be remarkably safe when conducted by trained personnel. The results were considered to be comparable to those with insulin coma, also in vogue at that time. For example, in the 500-patient series reported by Goldner (1967), the improvement rates for schizophrenic patients were as follows: acute undifferentiated schizophrenia under age 20 years, 77 percent; acute undifferentiated schizophrenia over age 20 years, 58 percent; chronic undifferentiated schizophrenia, zero percent; schizoaffective schizophrenia, 71 percent; paranoid schizophrenia, 63 percent. Improvement rates for affective disorder patients ranged from 84 to 96 percent for various groups. Unfortunately, no clinical criteria for diagnosis or assessment of improvement were given. In a somewhat more sophisticated study, using psychometric instruments, Grisell and Bynum (1956) confirmed the earlier clinical impression of Forrer (1956) that the schizophrenics to benefit most from the coma treatment were those with high manifest anxiety and affective symptoms in the clinical picture, i.e., the schizophreniform or schizoaffective patients. The results by Goldner (1967) were consistent with this view.

During the coma treatment, the observed changes were essentially biphasic (Forrer and Miller, 1958). Initially, the patients showed increased psychotic manifestations, restlessness, tachycardia, rise in blood pressure, tachypnea and dry mouth. Later, the patients became increasingly stuporous and showed reductions in heart rate, blood pressure and respiration and, sometimes, increased salivation. Improved accessibility was noted soon after recovery from each coma, and gradually there was a reduction in psychosis and improvement in "ego-strength." Since the improvement in mental functioning actually corresponded to recovery from intense cholinergic blockade, the mechanisms for this may be cholinergic rebound or mobilization of cholinergic circuits rather than cholinergic blockade per se.

Itil et al. (1969) used escalating doses of intravenously administered Ditran for symptom provocation in six chronic schizophrenics who had proven to be highly resistant to long courses of intensive psychopharmacological treatment. These patients were distinguished also by the presence of excessive amounts of high voltage slow waves and/or hypersynchronous alpha rhythms in their EEGs. One of the objectives of Ditran treatment was to desynchronize and accelerate the EEG pattern. After the occurrence of this change and symptom provocation (which was manifested as increased inappropriateness and instability of affect and mood, blocking, irrelevance and disorganization of thinking, and disturbance of orientation, consciousness and motor behavior), the patients were given the doctor's choice of antipsychotic medication. This resulted in marked clinical improvement so that, in general, patients were judged to be better than after intensive pharmacotherapy prior to symptom provocation. Four of the

six patients recovered sufficiently to be discharged from the hospital.
Prior to this treatment they had been continuously hospitalized for
an average of 5.5 years. In the same study, LSD was used in six other
intractable schizophrenics to produce symptom provocation and EEG
desynchronization. On subsequent psychopharmacological treatment,
again the therapeutic change was found to be greater than before the
provocation, and three patients could be discharged from the hospital.

Despite the small number of patients involved, this study is of
considerable theoretical interest because it suggests that antipsychotic treatment previously ineffective became effective in chronic
schizophrenia after some change produced by two psychotogenic agents.
The EEG changes, i.e., desynchronization and acceleration, produced by
these agents were quite similar to those produced by cholinergic stimulation (4.1, 4.2; Karczmar, 1978, 1979). Therefore, it may be justified to suggest that this study provided further evidence in support
of the view proposed above, i.e., strong but temporary cholinergic
blockade (and possibly other conditions producing a toxic psychosis)
mobilizes cholinergic circuits and that such a mobilization is con-
ducive to recovery from schizophrenic psychosis.

5.3. Electroencephalographic (EEG) Effects

There is extensive literature on the involvement of cholinergic
mechanisms in electrocortical aspects of arousal, attention and consciousness (e.g., Rinaldi and Himwich, 1955; Bradley and Elkes, 1957;.
De Feudis, 1974; Karczmar, 1979). The EEG changes produced by anticholinergic drugs are well-known, and consist mainly of the appearance, in all areas of the cortex, of high voltage, synchronized slow
waves and bursts of 12 to 15 Hz spindles of the type seen in states of
drowsiness and sleep (Bradley and Elkes, 1957; Longo, 1966). The
accompanying behavioral state, however, is usually not that of sleep
but of wakefulness and, at times, excitement. Another consequence of
anticholinergic treatment is that EEG desynchronization or arousal
normally produced by sensory input or electrical stimulation of the
brain stem reticular activating system is blocked (Rinaldi and
Himwich, 1955; Bradley and Elkes, 1957; Longo, 1966), thus suggesting
that interference with central cholinergic mechanisms may impair input
processing in the brain (De Feudis, 1974; Vanderwolf and Robinson,
1981).

Through the use of quantitative and computerized EEG analyses,
it has been found that, in addition to highly synchronized slow waves
and spindle bursts, the anticholinergic drugs, especially those with
psychotomimetic effects, produce an increase in fast beta (20 to 50
Hz) activity (Danielopolu et al., 1955; Fink, 1960; Lechner, 1956;
Itil and Fink, 1966). Corresponding to these changes is a decrease
or dissolution of alpha rhythms and the disappearance of alpha blocking in response to sensory stimulation. In studies with anticholinergic psychotogens, the EEG shift towards very fast beta (30 to 50 Hz)
along with 2 to 5 Hz slow activity was noted to correspond to delirium,

hallucinations, and other autistic experiences, which could be blocked by chlorpromazine, while a quieter, sleep-like or stuporous state was associated with a predominance of high voltage, slow-wave activity and 8 to 12 Hz spindle patterns, which were accentuated by chlorpromazine (Itil and Fink, 1968). These observations, unfortunately, came from studies with schizophrenics, and their generalizability may be suspect. In general, the EEG changes by both cholinergic and anticholinergic drugs are not accompanied by behaviors normally associated with similar changes in other circumstances. Indeed, the dissociation between behavioral and electrocortical arousal is a unique characteristic of drugs acting on the central cholinergic mechanisms (Karczmar, 1979).

The EEG changes produced by anticholinergic drugs are of considerable theoretical interest because they closely resemble the EEG abnormalities seen in certain types of schizophrenia.

In some early EEG studies, involving visual inspection of the records, abnormal amounts of slow waves with, at times, a paroxysmal character, were frequently found in schizophrenic patients, especially those with atypical or a good prognosis form of schizophrenia (Sawa, 1957; Yamada, 1960; Fukuda and Matsuda, 1969). Mitsuda (1967) noted a high incidence of epilepsy in the pedigrees of atypical schizophrenics and suggested that at least a subset of atypical schizophrenia may be related to temporal lobe epilepsy. Consistent with this position was a number of studies reviewed by Saletu (1980) which suggested the occurrence of abnormal EEG reminiscent of epilepsy in catatonic syndromes. More recent investigations reviewed by Itil (1977) and Saletu (1980), in which EEG records, taken under drug-free and then neuroleptic-treatment conditions, were subjected to quantitative digital computer analyses, show that the schizophrenic population as a whole has more delta, theta and fast beta activity, and less alpha and slow beta activity than normals, and that such a pattern successfully discriminates 78 percent of the patients from controls. Similar EEG patterns are said to differentiate between psychotic children and normal controls, as well as between children at high risk for schizophrenia and matched controls. Further, it has been observed that treatment responsive schizophrenics are distinguished by having a high amount of fast beta activity, i.e., a cortical hyperarousal pattern, in their pretreatment EEGs, while the treatment-resistant cases have a predominance of slow activities. However, the differences between the two groups were relative rather than absolute, and the general pattern of more than normal theta and delta and fast beta activity, but less than normal alpha and slow beta activity, was characteristic of both types of schizophrenic patients. At the same time, it should be noted that the patients involved in these studies were all chronic schizophrenics and probably did not include the good prognosis atypical schizophrenics or those with catatonic states in which previously mentioned workers had found a high incidence of paroxysmal type of slow wave activity.

It should be obvious that, in general, the EEG pattern in the schizophrenic population resembles that produced by cholinergic block-ade. This similarity extends to neuroleptic responsiveness, in that neuroleptics proved to be therapeutic in those patients with schizophrenia or anticholinergic drug-induced psychosis, in which the EEG showed excessive amounts of fast beta activity. On this basis, it may not only be suggested that a relative or absolute insufficiency of brain cholinergic mechanisms exists in schizophrenia (Saletu, 1976) but that the neuroleptic-responsive component of schizophrenia may be akin to the delirious state produced by drugs like Ditran. On the other hand, it may be noted that, in terms of EEG parameters, some of the cases with atypical schizophrenia, schizophreniform states or cat-atonic states have a psychophysiological disorder similar to that seen in Ditran-induced stupor. The beneficial effects of cholinergic agon-ists in cases of this type discussed earlier would support the idea of decreased cholinergic function in these patients.

5.4 Summary

At first glance, the observations on the effects of anticholin-ergic agents seem as contradictory as those on the effects of cholin-ergic agents. However, on careful analysis, the contradictions can be resolved, and it seems reasonable to make the following summary statements:

(A) Anticholinergic drugs in various doses can reproduce dis-turbances in attention and cognitive processing that seem to charac-terize nonparanoid forms of schizophrenia.

(B) Anticholinergic psychotogens exacerbate true symptoms of schizophrenia. Chronic paranoid schizophrenics may be more suscep-tible than chronic nonparanoid schizophrenics, suggesting relative unresponsivity of cholinergic mechanisms in nonparanoid schizophrenia.

(C) The apparent therapeutic effects of intense cholinergic blockade in schizophrenia may be due to subsequent mobilization of cholinergic circuits rather than to cholinergic blockade itself. Such a mobilization also seems to make intractable schizophrenics respon-sive to antipsychotic pharmacotherapy.

(D) The characteristic EEG changes produced by anticholinergic drugs are remarkably similar to those in schizophrenia, i.e., an in-crease in delta, theta, and fast beta and a decrease in alpha and slow beta activity.

(E) Considering both the behavioral and EEG changes produced by anticholinergic drugs, three schizophrenic syndromes may be recognized. The excited, disorganized, delirious state associated with excessive fast beta activity may be the pathophysiological counterpart of the neuroleptic-responsive component of schizophrenia. The inhibited, withdrawn, mute and stuporous state accompanied by predominantly high voltage, slow wave activity may be the pathophysiological analogue of atypical schizophrenia or catatonic states. In both these syndromes, the brain cholinergic mechanisms appear to be responsive but underactive. In the neuroleptic-resistant chronic schizophrenia, however, excessive slow wave activity seems to be accompanied by excessive but not intense fast beta activity, and cholinergic mechanisms may be relatively unresponsive.

6. ANTICHOLINERGIC-NEUROLEPTIC INTERACTION

As mentioned in the introduction, a major reason for discounting the role of cholinergic mechanisms in schizophrenia has been the observation that neuroleptic drugs such as chlorpromazine and thioridazine have antipsychotic activity despite having built-in anticholinergic activity, and also the general belief that, in clinical practice, combining anticholinergic antiParkinsonism (AP) agents with neuroleptics does not adversely affect the antipsychotic efficacy of these drugs. Indeed, so strong has been this view that one of the four criteria given by Matthysse and Haber (1974) for an animal model of schizophrenia was that the effects of antipsychotic drugs on this model should not be blocked by anticholinergic agents. On this basis, all the currently available animal paradigms of relevance to human schizophrenia, such as amphetamine-induced stereotypy, brain self-stimulation, conditional avoidance behaviors and arousal, were found wanting because anticholinergic drugs block neuroleptics in all these test models (Weiss et al., 1976). In this section, we will analyze the available research data on anticholinergic-neuroleptic interactions in terms of schizophrenic psychosis to see if this position is valid.

6.1. Clinical Effects of Adding Anticholinergic Drugs to Neuroleptic Treatment

There is surprisingly little systematic information on this issue because anticholinergic AP drugs have been studied mainly in terms of their effects on the undesirable extrapyramidal motor system changes produced by neuroleptics. In a series of multi-hospital studies, no significant relationship was found between the appearance of coarse extrapyramidal reactions such as Parkinsonism and the antipsychotic activity of neuroleptics (Cole and Clyde, 1961; Goldman, 1961; Ayd, 1961; NIMH Collaborative Study Group, 1964; Bishop et al., 1965). Since the extrapyramidal reactions involved increased cholinergic activity in the brain, and hence the beneficial effect of anticholinergic drugs, this lack of a relationship suggested that cholinergic mechanisms were not involved in psychosis and the antipsychotic activity of neuroleptics. In some studies of AP effects on extrapyramidal reactions, in fact, it was observed that the desired antipsychotic actions of neuroleptics may be lessened by the addition of AP drugs,

but the issue received only a passing comment. Thus, in a study by
Hanlon et al. (1966) which was designed to evaluate the prophylactic
value of benztropine against coarse extrapyramidal reactions produced
by a phenothiazine, perphenazine, in a group of acute psychotics and
nonpsychotics, it was noted but parenthetically that psychotic manifestations such as thought disorder and perceptual dysfunctions as
well as hostile behavior improved significantly better with perphenazine alone than with a perphenazine-benztropine combination. Similarly, Goldstein et al. (1968), noted in a study concerned with haloperidol perphenazine comparisons in acute schizophrenics that patients who
received neuroleptic alone did better overall than those who had benztropine added as a doctor's choice, but felt that its significance was
unclear.

     Haase (1954, 1965) was probably the first investigator to con-
sider seriously the possibility of a countertherapeutic interaction
between AP drugs and neuroleptics in schizophrenia. He distinguished
between the fine extrapyramidal hypokinesia and the coarse extrapyramidal symptoms produced by neuroleptics. Whereas the first, reflected
in mild to moderate handwriting changes (cramping, stiffening and
miniaturization), clearly seemed to be linked to the antipsychotic
effects of neuroleptics, the second, manifesting as rigidity, tremor,
akathisia, dyskinesia, akinesia, and severe handwriting changes, appeared to have no such relationship and, if anything, had the opposite
connotation. He regarded the appearance of fine extrapyramidal hypokinesia as a conditio sine qua non for the antipsychotic action of
neuroleptics, and believed that the inhibition of "psychokinetic conation," that is the process of translating drives, ideas and impulses
into motor action, through extrapyramidal hypokinesia, was the mechanism by which neuroleptics exercised their antipsychotic action. On
the other hand, the coarse extrapyramidal symptoms, he maintained,
were therapeutically disturbing and undesirable - a position which is
consistent with the reports of a negative correlation between severity of coarse extrapyramidal symptoms and improvement (Bishop et al.,
1965; Crane, 1967; May and Goldberg, 1978). Mattke (1968) found that
variability in fine motor inhibition accounted for 69 percent of the
variation in antipsychotic drug action, thus providing support for
Haase's hypothesis. This would suggest that "the therapeutic neuroleptic range lies between the occurrence of fine motor extrapyramidal
manifestations and the occurrence of subjectively disturbing coarse
motor extrapyramidal symptoms." (May and Goldberg, 1978, p1149).

     Within this framework, Haase interpreted the results of his clin-
ical studies of anticholinergic-neuroleptic interactions as follows:
the anticholinergic AP agents were beneficial to the extent that they
reduced coarse extrapyramidal symptoms, but when they reversed the
fine extrapyramidal hypokinesia, there was a reversal also of the
antipsychotic action of the neuroleptics. This would mean that the AP
drugs are likely to be countertherapeutic within the therapeutic neuroleptic range.

Haase's studies were usually nonblind and may be criticized for lacking proper controls. However, his insightful hypothesis is of considerable heuristic interest and has been supported in some respects by careful work carried out since then.

The most systematic investigations of the effects of anticholinergic AP agents on the course of therapeutic changes with neuroleptics in schizophrenia have so far been conducted by Singh and Smith (1971, 1973a,b,c) and Singh and Kay 1975a,b,c, 1978a,b, 1979a,b). These studies will be discussed in some detail because they provide data of practical and theoretical importance concerning not only the possible role of cholinergic mechanisms in schizophrenia but also the definition of psychobiological subtypes of this syndrome.

Three studies were carried out according to a double-blind, longitudinal, ABA' research design, in which neuroleptic alone was given during periods A and A' while an AP drug was added to constantly held neuroleptic treatment during the intervening B period. In two studies, more than one AP intervention was made along the course of the neuroleptic treatment, and in one study the AP effect during the baseline placebo period was examined. The lengths of the AP intervention periods varied from two to four weeks in different studies. Two prototypic neuroleptics were involved: haloperidol, which is a high-potency, low-dose neuroleptic with little built-in anticholinergic activity, and chlorpromzaine, which is a low-potency, high-dose neuroleptic with appreciable built-in anticholinergic activity. In two studies, these drugs could be compared in terms of therapeutic effects as well as interactions with AP agents. The neuroleptic dosages were individually titrated in the initial period so as to maximize therapeutic effects and minimize coarse extrapyramidal reactions. Therefore, AP medication was added to neuroleptics given within their optimal therapeutic range (haloperidol, 1.5 mg to 60 mg/day; chlorpromazine, 300 mg to 1800 mg/day). Two different AP drugs were employed in quite small doses: benztropine, 2 mg b.i.d., trihexyphenidyl, 2 mg t.i.d. A total of 47 carefully selected acute (0 to 2 years duration of illness) and subacute (3 to 5 years duration of illness) schizophrenic patients was involved in the three studies. Most of the patients were in the teens and early to mid twenties, and for 12 patients, it was their first psychotic breakdown. All the patients were actively psychotic and drug-free when included in the study, and none had been continuously hospitalized. A diagnostic as well as a prognostic classification was prospectively given to each patient. Measures of psychopathology, social functioning, sleeplessness and resting pulse rate were obtained at different points along the course of each study.

Besides the question of AP effects on antipsychotic efficacy of neuroleptics, the studies could address a number of other issues, namely: What is the relationship between the longitudinal characteristics of the pharmacotherapeutic process and the effects of AP intervention? Do the prototypic neuroleptics differ in terms of

therapeutic actions and interaction with AP drugs? Do the AP drugs
have any differential effects on various aspects of psychopathology
and pathophysiology? Do the AP effects differ in terms of nosological
and prognostic subtypes?

The statistical assessments were quite conservative and based on
the difference values obtained by subtracting period B (AP period)
ratings from a combined average of ratings in the period before (A)
and the period after (A'). By combining A and A' ratings, the order
effect was controlled. Parametric as well as nonparametric tests
indicated that in all three studies, the AP interventions had been
countertherapeutic (Singh and Kay, 1979b). Combined parametric analyses of 26 psychopathology dimensions plus sleeplessness and resting
pulse rate showed statistically significant AP effects in nine characteristics: thought disorganization ($p<0.05$), difficulty in abstract
thinking ($p<0.05$), bizarre and unusual thought content ($p<0.01$), delusions ($p<0.05$), suspiciousness and paranoid ideas ($p<0.05$), uncooperativeness ($p<0.10$), disorientation ($p<0.05$), sleeplessness ($p<0.001$)
and pulse rate ($p<0.05$). With the exception of pulse rate, which
paradoxically decreased during the AP period, all the affected features worsened with AP intervention. On nonparametric analyses (chi
square test), thirteen of the 28 parameters had statistically significant AP effects. Again, with the exception of pulse rate, the changes
indicated a countertherapeutic effect of anticholinergic medication.
The signs and symptoms involved were clearly those considered characteristic of schizophrenia and represented cognitive, social, as well
as physiological realms of pathology. It could be concluded, therefore, that anticholinergic AP drugs opposed the antipsychotic actions
of neuroleptic medication. This confirmed Haase's view that within
the therapeutic neuroleptic range, anticholinergic drugs reverse the
therapeutic activity of antipsychotic drugs.

Given in the baseline placebo period, benztropine seemed to further worsen the psychosis. In terms of longitudinal aspects of the
therapeutic process, a study-by-study analysis suggested that the
antagonistic anticholinergic effects were most likely to be apparent
in the aspects of the clinical picture which were undergoing the most
active therapeutic change at the time of the AP intervention. Thus
paralleling the observations (Singh and Smith, 1973a) that significant
therapeutic changes in social dysfunctions (e.g., uncooperativeness,
social withdrawal, hostility) antedate by many weeks those in cognitive disturbances (e.g., thought disorganization, difficulty in abstract thinking, bizarre and unusual thought content, delusions), the
countertherapeutic anticholinergic effects were most conspicuous in
social parameters when AP was introduced early in the therapeutic
course, whereas, later on it was increasingly evident in the cognitive
parameters (Singh and Kay, 1975c, 1979b).

The countertherapeutic effects with benztropine and trihexyphenidyl were essentially similar (Singh and Kay, 1979b). However, the

changes noted in the benztropine tests were more dramatic than those in the trihexyphenidyl tests. This may have been merely a reflection of the fact that the 6 mg dose of trihexyphenidyl used was only half as potent as the 4 mg dose of benztropine. Also trihexyphenidyl was often used against relatively larger amounts of antipsychotic medication and in patients (see below) who were less likely to show countertherapeutic AP effects.

Longitudinal as well as cross-sectional therapeutic comparisons between the two neuroleptics suggested that chlorpromazine, both at 50 mg to 1 mg and 100 mg to 1 mg ratios with respect to haloperidol, was somewhat inferior in its range and depth of therapeutic effects. At the same time, its therapeutic activity seemed to be much more susceptible to antagonism by the anticholinergic AP medication. This suggested that built-in anticholinergic activity may not only account for the lower potency of neuroleptics such as chlorpromazine, but also confer certain therapeutic inferiority on them and make them more vulnerable to the countertherapeutic effects of added AP drugs.

Perhaps the most interesting observations were those related to diagnostic and prognostic subtypes (Singh and Kay, 1978a). With respect to prognostic classification, the countertherapeutic AP effects were predominantly seen in the schizophreniform or good prognosis group (N = 19). With correlated t tests (two-tailed), the following ten measures showed significant AP effects in this group: social withdrawal ($p<0.05$), uncooperativeness ($p<0.02$), disorganized thinking ($p<0.10$), impoverishment and stereotypy of thought ($p<0.05$), poor judgment and insight ($p<0.10$), bizarre and unusual thought content ($p<0.02$), suspiciousness and paranoid ideas ($p<0.05$), disorientation ($p<0.05$), disturbance of volition ($p<0.02$), pulse rate ($p<0.05$). With the exception of pulse rate, all the parameters indicated an adverse effect of AP medication.

In the nuclear or poor prognosis schizophrenia group (N = 28), only the following parameters reached significance: disorganized thinking ($p<0.10$), delusions ($p<0.10$), sleeplessness ($p<0.002$). When the patients were grouped according to actual therapeutic outcome at the time of discharge from the research ward, both the predictive validity of the prognostic classification as well as the relationship between this classification and the AP effects were confirmed (Singh and Kay, 1978a).

When the patients were analyzed according to the three diagnostic subtypes (paranoid = 18; hebephrenic = 16; catatonic = 13), the significant AP effects appeared mostly in the nonparanoid, especially catatonic, schizophrenic patients. There was only one significant AP effect in the paranoid group (impoverishment and stereotypy of thought $p<0.05$), which could be regarded as a chance finding. Of the nonparanoid groups, the catatonics (excited and withdrawn types combined) had the following significant AP effects: social withdrawal ($p<0.02$),

hostility (p<0.05), uncooperativeness (p<0.05), disorganized thinking
(p<0.10), bizarre and unusual thought content (p<0.05), suspiciousness
and paranoid ideas (p<0.02), grandiosity (p<0.10), suicidal ideas and
actions (p<0.05), disorientation (p<0.10), anxiety (p<0.10), tension
(p<0.05), disturbance of volition (p<0.05). All the effects were
countertherapeutic. The hebephrenic group had the following significant AP effects: difficulty in abstract thinking (p<0.10), bizarre
and unusual thought content (p<0.02) anxiety (p<0.05) tension (p<0.05)
sleeplessness (p<0.05). Of these, anxiety and tension showed therapeutic augmentation with AP intervention, thus suggesting that the AP
drug decreased dysphoria in hebephrenics but increased it in
catatonics.

Considering these data along with those related to prognostic and
therapeutic outcome groupings, it seemed that the countertherapeutic
AP effects were most evident in the good prognosis, nonparanoid,
mostly catatonic, type of schizophrenia. The paranoid schizophrenia
seemed to be a condition apart, whereas nonparanoid schizophrenia
could be conceptualized as consisting of two disease factors: a psychotic factor responsive in opposite ways to neuroleptic and anticholinergic drugs, which was most prominent in the nonparanoid schizophreniform or catatonic patients, and a disease factor most evident in
the nonparanoid nuclear or hebephrenic schizophrenics, which was
resistant to both neuroleptics and AP drugs. These conclusions were
supported by a number of other studies by the same authors, which provided the following information: (a) Wheat gluten feeding worsened
schizophrenia despite ongoing neuroleptic treatment, but this worsening was most evident in poor outcome, nuclear types of cases (Singh
and Kay, 1976; Singh, 1978); (b) Data from the use of developmentally-
based tests of cognitive functions and measures of arousal and attention suggested the existence of a drug-responsive disorganizational
component associated with high psychomotor arousal, reflected in
sleeplessness and very poor ability to sustain concentration on a
simple motor task, and one or more drug-resistant components which
related to both early and late stages of cognitive development in
hebephrenic schizophrenics but to only the late stages of development
in paranoid schizophrenics (Kay and Singh, 1979); (c) In nonparanoid
schizophrenics, but not in paranoid schizophrenics, there emerged a
dysphoric state along with an increase in resting pulse rate following the introduction of neuroleptics, which presaged poor therapeutic
outcome (Singh and Kay, 1979a); (d) Data from the use of ethological-
ly-based measures of social bonding, territoriality and group organizational behavior suggested the existence of two abnormal patterns:
one pattern, most pronounced in catatonic schizophrenics, consisted of
a breakdown in territorial boundaries and maladaptive fight/flight
behavior, which were associated with global arousal (i.e., both pulse
rate and sleeplessness were high) and showed improvement with neuroleptic treatment; the second pattern, which was most evident in the
hebephrenic schizophrenics, was characterized by poor social bonding
and group integration, marked restrictive form of territoriality, high

autonomic arousal (pulse rate) but not psychomotor activation (sleep-lessness), and lack of response to neuroleptic treatment (Singh et al., 1981a,b). The paranoid schizophrenics did not show either of these patterns.

The studies of Singh and associates concerning anticholinergic neuroleptic interactions led to vigorous controversies of a technical nature, and their conclusions were questioned for that reason (Meltzer and Stahl, 1976; Ziemba et al., 1978; Singh and Kay, 1978b). Since then, however, there has been an independent corroboration of their work by Crow et al. (1981) and Johnstone et al. (1983) in England. These investigators studied 36 schizophrenics in a double-blind, AB design trial in which patients were first observed for ten days on flupenthixol alone (period A), given in individually adjusted amounts, and then on a combination of flupenthixol with an anticholinergic-AP drug, procyclidine (5 mg t.i.d.), or placebo. The flupenthixol dose was determined by increasing the number of tablets in the first five days of the trial until significant side effects appeared or total sleep time was in excess of ten hours per day. The assignment to the placebo or procyclidine in period B was done randomly. Patients were assessed every two weeks for psychopathology and extrapyramidal symptoms. Blood samples were also taken every week to determine serum neuroleptic and prolactin concentrations. The analyses showed that, as expected, the extrapyramidal symptoms were diminished by the addition of procyclidine, but that with this, the course of improvement in psychotic symptoms was also reversed. After the tenth day of the trial, the psychotic symptoms remained higher in the AP group than in the placebo group. The symptoms to be adversely affected by procyclidine included delusions, hallucinations and thought disorder. Sleep records revealed that procyclidine caused a significant decrease in total sleep time. The countertherapeutic procyclidine effect was seen mainly in patients who developed extrapyramidal reactions in period A and was found to be unrelated to any changes in serum neuroleptic concentrations. Thus, the study supported the observations of Singh et al. in terms of anticholinergic AP effects on both the symptoms of active schizophrenic psychosis as well as on sleeplessness. In addition, it demonstrated that the clinical changes were not due to a pharmacokinetic factor.

6.2. Pharmacokinetic Studies

Rivera-Calimlim et al. (1973) first raised the possibility that anticholinergic AP drugs may reduce the efficacy of neuroleptics by lowering their plasma concentrations through absorption interference or some other peripheral effect. In a study involving five schizo-phrenic patients, they found that plasma concentrations of chlorpromazine, measured 0 to 4 hours after drug administration, were lowered by the addition of trihexyphenidyl. In three patients, trihexyphenidyl (2 mg t.i.d. or q.i.d.) was added as a doctor's choice after three weeks of treatment with varying doses of chlorpromazine; the plasma

chlorpromazine concentrations seemed to decline thereafter. Two
patients received chlorpromazine-trihexyphenidyl combinations for two
weeks and then chlorpromazine alone; the withdrawal of trihexyphenidyl
seemed to be followed by an increase in plasma chlorpromazine concentrations. There was a suggestion that very low plasma chlorpromazine
concentrations (<30 ng/ml) were associated with lack of clinical
response. However, apparent reductions in plasma chlorpromazine concentrations by trihexyphenidyl were not consistently associated with
deterioration in clinical conditions. Patients often received other
conjunctive treatments. In a subsequent study involving a somewhat
larger group of patients, Rivera-Calimlim et al. (1976) reported an
average of 44 percent reduction in plasma chlorpromazine concentrations following trihexyphenidyl addition and an accompanying reduction
in clinical efficacy.

A number of other investigators have since reported confirmatory
as well as contradictory data on pharmacokinetic interactions between
anticholinergic AP drugs and neuroleptics. Cooper (1978) published a
critical review of the available data in 1978. He found that apart
from Rivera-Calimlim et al. (1973, 1976), an apparent reduction in
plasma levels of neuroleptics by AP medication had been reported by
Loga et al. (1975), Gautier et al. (1977) and Chouinard et al. (1977),
while El-Yousef and Manier (1974), Forsman and Ohman (1977), Lee et
al. (1978), and Simpson et al. (1980) had found the AP medication not
to have any effect on plasma neuroleptic concentrations. In one study
(Kolakowska et al., 1976), concomitant AP medication was found to
increase plasma chlorpromazine levels.

Cooper (1978) noted that apart from the studies by Lee et al. and
Simpson et al. the published investigations were seriously flawed in
their methodology. They did not meet the basic requirements for controls or split cross-over design and suffered from a variety of
defects including reliance on a single blood sample for comparisons,
small study samples, concomitant use of drugs other than those of
interest, and pooling of data for several neuroleptics and AP drugs.
In contrast, the studies by Lee et al. and Simpson et al. had a
placebo-controlled split cross-over design, a minimum number of 20
patients, a period of four weeks for stabilization on medication
before entering the patient into the study, multiple samples in each
study period to decrease the compounding effects of intra-individual
variations and strict prohibition against drugs other than those in
the protocol. Interactions between benztropine and butaperazine and
between trihexyphenidyl and chlorpromazine were investigated. No
significant alteration in the plasma levels of antipsychotic medication by the AP drugs was found.

Cooper (1978) concluded that it was doubtful that AP drugs could
lower plasma levels of antipsychotic medication to the point of possible interference with treatment. He further noted that after much
research over two decades, it remained uncertain that there was any

predictable relationship between the plasma concentrations of neuroleptics and the clinical response to these drugs. It would be very
difficult, therefore, to explain any changes in clinical response to
neuroleptics by AP drugs in terms of pharmacokinetic factors.

To the evidence reviewed by Cooper (1978), we must, of course,
now add the evidence by Crow et al. (1981) which shows that AP drugs
can reduce therapeutic efficacy of neuroleptics without significantly
affecting their pharmacokinetics.

6.3. Effects of Anticholinergic Drug Withdrawal on Neuroleptic
      Treatment

The acute studies of anticholinergic-neuroleptic interactions we
have reviewed so far cannot answer the question of whether the AP
drugs in any way influence the long-term efficacy of antipsychotic
medication. The clinicians could point to the fact that many schizophrenic patients receive AP drugs with neuroleptic medication for
extended periods without apparent detriment to their clinical condition. Unfortunately, no prospective, longitudinal studies, comparing
AP drugs with placebo in terms of chronic effects on the therapeutic
actions of neuroleptics, have been conducted to deal effectively with
this question. The only studies of some interest in this context are
those in which AP medications used chronically in conjunction with
neuroleptics were withdrawn.

Many of these studies focused solely on the effects of AP withdrawal on extrapyramidal symptoms of neuroleptic treatment (Cahan and
Parrish, 1960; Mandel and Oliver, 1961; Mandel et al., 1961; Stratas
et al., 1963; St. Jean et al., 1964; DiMascio and Demirgian, 1970;
Orlov et al., 1971; Klett and Caffey, 1972; McClelland et al., 1974;
Fleischhauer, 1975; Martini and Frassanito, 1975). In every instance,
the AP medication, given for unspecified reasons and for different
lengths of time, was abruptly withdrawn in a variety of neuroleptic-
treated patients. The patients were then observed, clinically, or by
the use of rating scales, for the resurgence of extrapyramidal disorders while the patients had a placebo or nothing added to their neuroleptic medication, which was usually held constant. Most of the
studies were double-blind, with the control group continuing on the
AP-neuroleptic combination it had been receiving. The results showed
a wide variation in the recurrence rates for drug-induced extrapyramidal symptoms: Cahan and Parrish (1960), 21 percent; Mandel et al.
(1961), 80 percent; Mandel and Oliver (1961), 41 percent; Stratas et
al. (1963), 27 percent; St. Jean et al. (1961), 0 percent with placebo substitution for AP and 67 percent with no substitution for AP;
DiMascio and Demirgian, (1970), 30 percent; Orlov et al. (1971), 9
percent; Klett and Caffey, (1972), 18 percent; McClelland et al.
(1974), 4 percent; Fleischhauer, (1975), 8 percent; Martini and
Frassanito, (1975), 27 percent. Thus, the recurrence probability may
be 0 to 80 percent. However, on the basis of most of the data,

especially those of Klett and Caffey (1972) whose study was by far the
largest with a sample of 500 patients, the typical probability would
seem to be less than 30 percent. Klett and Caffey (1972) observed
that patients who worsened tended to be older and those who had been
given AP medication in response to extrapyramidal disturbance rather
than for prophylaxis. The studies by DiMascio and Demirgian (1970)
and Orlov et al. (1971) together suggested that in patients who had
been on AP medication for three months or more, the recurrence rate
was only 9 percent while in cases who had been receiving AP drugs for
less than one month, AP withdrawal was attended with the return of
extrapyramidal symptoms in 67 percent of the cases (DiMascio, 1971).
On the other hand, St. Jean et al. (1964) observed that AP withdrawal
resulted in no symptom recurrence when placebo was substituted for the
AP drug but a 67 percent recurrence when no placebo substitution was
made, thus suggesting a strong placebo effect in the emergence of
withdrawal symptoms.

     In all the studies, the neuroleptic dosage was essentially an
uncontrolled factor, i.e., the neuroleptics had not been titrated to a
particular end point, so that there was apt to be much variation in
terms of dose-response equations. According to Haase's model discussed earlier in this section, patients who had a resurgence of coarse
extrapyramidal symptoms after AP withdrawal were probably getting more
neuroleptic medication than they needed for therapeutic control. This
was, to some extent, supported by the study of Stratas et al. (1963),
in which neuroleptic dosage adjustment or substitution with thioridazine obviated the need to reinstitute AP medication in all the 27 percent of their 88 cases who developed a relapse of drug-induced Parkinsonism after AP withdrawal. Another significant issue not addressed
by any of the studies is that the relapse of extrapyramidal symptoms
might have been due to cholinergic or other kind of neurochemical
rebound effect resulting from sudden withdrawal of anticholinergic
medication. The possibility of such a rebound is suggested by Luchins
et al. (1980); Schaffer et al. (1981) and Lieberman (1981). It seems
quite plausible that with a gradual withdrawal of AP medication, the
recurrence of drug-induced extrapyramidal symptoms might have been
less severe and less frequent.

     Only four published reports, to our knowledge, have concerned
themselves with both the extrapyramidal as well as the psychopathological consequences of AP withdrawal in neuroleptic-treated chronic
schizophrenics (Ananth et al., 1970; Jellinek et al., 1981; Manos and
Gkiouzepas, 1981; Manos et al., 1981). In these studies, the AP withdrawal was again abrupt.

     Ananth et al. (1970) studied 80 chronic hospitalized psychotic
patients, of whom 65 were schizophrenic. They had a mean age of 45.2
years and had been receiving neuroleptics with antiParkinsonism drugs
with no serious extrapyramidal symptoms. Using random assignment, AP
medication was stopped for half the patients but continued as before

for the other half. Fifty-two patients received the equivalent of
less than 800 mg/day of chlorpromazine, and only 28 patients received
neuroleptic dosages higher than this. Psychopathology ratings showed
no significant change after eight weeks of the trial, while extrapyramidal symptoms ratings showed worsening sufficient to require AP medication in 10 percent of the experimental group. These patients were
on medium to high doses of neuroleptic medication. The study, it
should be noted, was nonblind, since no placebo substitution was used
in the AP withdrawal group.

     Jellinek et al. (1981) took a sample of 32 schizophrenic out-
patients receiving various neuroleptic-AP combinations. Half the
patients were on fluphenazine decanoate injections while others
received high as well as low potency drugs by mouth. After baseline
evaluations, they were assigned double-blind for four weeks either to
continued AP medication (N = 8) or to placebo instead (N = 24) and
assessments were repeated every two weeks. Psychopathology was rated
using the 12-item Short Clinical Rating Scale (SCRS) and self rated
65-item Profile of Mood States (POMS), both of which are loaded with
features of mood disturbance rather than schizophrenia. Three scales
were used to assess extrapyramidal symptoms. The mean dose of antipsychotic medication, converted into chlorpromazine equivalent (formu-
la not given), was 345 mg/day for the test group and 640 mg/day for
the control group. The average age of test patients was 41.8 years
compared to 33.8 years for the control patients. They observed that
37.5 percent of the AP withdrawal patients had to leave the study pre-
maturely because of increased anxiety, restlessness or dystonia, and
that a total of 62 percent from this group showed adverse neurological
and psychopathological effects. At Week 2, they had significantly
higher ratings of dyskinesia of the lower extremities, POMS depression, and SCRS motor agitation, hallucinations, physical complaints
and total score, most of the difference being attributable to the
drop-outs. At Week 4, when the dropouts were not in the study, there
were no significant differences between the two groups on extrapyramidal symptoms scales. The POMS depression score was significantly
different but mainly due to a decrease in the control group scores
rather than to an increase in the test group scores. Total SCRS score
was the only other item to show significant difference. Thus, there
was a suggestion that dysphoric symptoms appeared in patients together
with the emergence of coarse extrapyrimidal symptoms, especially dyskinesia, following sudden AP discontinuation. This is consistent with
Haase's hypothesis and would suggest that some of the patients were
receiving excessive neuroleptic medication. The authors concluded
that a sizable proportion of chronic schizophrenics require antiParkinsonism drugs for controlling drug reactions as well as for clinical
stability. This does not seem justified on the basis of a small
sample study with a lopsided distribution of patients between various
groups and the appearance of a small number of significant differences
from among a very large number of measures.

The remaining two reports were by Manos and Gkiouzepas (1981) and Manos et al. (1981), which were based on one study. In 75 chronic schizophrenics, placebo replaced AP medication for six weeks, while 23 patients continued as before on AP-neuroleptic combinations and served as a control group. Nineteen patients received haloperidol (mean = 20.8 mg/day, range 10 to 70 mg), nine patients chlorpromazine (mean = 300 mg/day, range 100 to 600 mg), five patients trifluoperazine (mean = 30 mg/day, range 15 to 45 mg), five patients fluphenazine decanoate injections every two weeks (mean = 100 mg, range 37.5 - 150 mg), ten patients a combination of haloperidol (mean = 26.8 mg/day) and chlorpromazine (mean = 250 mg/day), six patients a combination of haloperidol (mean = 19 mg/day) and levomepromazine (mean = 37.5 mg/day), and thirteen patients a combination of three antipsychotic drugs. Forty-one patients (41.8 percent) were treated with haloperidol either alone or in combination with one or more antipsychotic drugs. Thus, in general, patients received rather large amounts of high potency neuroleptics. The extrapyramidal symptoms were formally rated but psychopathology was observed clinically. Of the experimental group, 68 percent showed sufficient worsening of extrapyramidal symptoms to necessitate early termination from the study, while another 28 percent showed less severe worsening. In the control group, the corresponding figures were 4.35 and 8.70 percent. In addition, it was noted that in 22.6 percent of the experimental group patients, mostly those with severe extrapyramidal reactions, a psychotic flare-up accompanied the extrapyramidal symptoms. This flare-up consisted of delusions and hallucinations related to rigidity, akathisia or akinesia, aggression or violence related to restlessness or akathisia, suicidal attempts related to akathisia, and social withdrawal related to akinesia. Other patients in the early termination group complained of a variety of dysphoric symptoms. The authors concluded that continued AP medication was the advisable course in neuroleptic-treated schizophrenics because its discontinuation was attended with severe extrapyramidal symptoms, psychotic flareups and subjective distress. They did not, however, consider the more likely possibility suggested by Haase's formulation, that is, the patients were simply getting too much potent neuroleptic medication which caused distressing coarse extrapyramidal symptoms after AP withdrawal. This would seem even more pertinent in this study than it was in the Jellinek et al. (1981) study. In addition, the possibility of "rebound" phenomena resulting from sudden AP withdrawal must be considered. Therefore, contrary to the authors' view, the more appropriate conclusions from this study might be that instead of using AP drugs, the neuroleptic dosages should be titrated downwards when there are coarse extrapyramidal symptoms, and that when AP drugs have to be stopped, this should be done gradually.

Thus, while these studies do not support the idea that long-term AP use in neuroleptic-treated schizophrenics is beneficial, they also do not help resolve the question of whether such AP use may be countertherapeutic. They do seem to provide some support for Haase's hypothesis concerning the relationship between the antipsychotic and extrapyramidal effects of neuroleptic medication. To answer the question of any long-term countertherapeutic effects of AP medication, one would either have to design prospective studies suggested before, or modify the AP withdrawal studies as follows: withdraw AP drug gradually, replace it with a placebo, down-titrate the neuroleptics to eliminate coarse extrapyramidal symptoms and then observe the therapeutic consequences in a double-blind controlled study for several months. It is quite possible that once active psychosis is brought under control by neuroleptics and the patient is in a stable state, the small therapeutic doses of AP drug used do not have any detrimental effect, but this has yet to be proved.

6.4.   Summary

The data on anticholinergic-neuroleptic interactions in schizophrenia are neither extensive nor conclusive. However, they clearly bring home the point that the heterogeneity of schizophrenia must be a major consideration in assessing the role of cholinergic mechanisms in this group of conditions. With this in mind, the case for the direct or indirect involvement of cholinergic processes in schizophrenias is certainly strengthened by these data, which may be summarized as follows:

(A)   In relatively acute experiments, the anticholinergic AP agents seem to reverse the antipsychotic actions of neuroleptics. This is evident both in terms of psychopathology of active schizophrenic psychosis and also in signs of psychomotor activation such as sleeplessness.

(B)   This interaction appears to be unrelated to pharmacokinetic factors and is probably central. There is no convincing evidence for clinically significant pharmacokinetic interactions between AP drugs and neuroleptics.

(C)   The countertherapeutic AP effects seem to be confined to the nonparanoid forms of schizophrenia and are most evident in the catatonic or nonparanoid schizophreniform types, in which psychosis is characterized by high levels of arousal, psychomotor symptoms and disorganization. Paranoid schizophrenia may be a condition apart.

(D)   It is not clear at this point whether chronic use of AP drugs with neuroleptics in the therapeutic range has any countertherapeutic effects.

(E)   The AP withdrawal studies seem to support Haase's concept that the appearance of coarse extrapyramidal symptoms with neuroleptic treatment is subjectively distressing and possibly countertherapeutic, and that it suggests the neuroleptic dose to be beyond the therapeutic range. The AP medication may be useful to correct this neuroleptic excess, but a better course would be to reduce the neuroleptic dose.

7.   CHOLINERGIC ASPECTS OF CHEMICAL NEUROPATHOLOGY OF SCHIZOPHRENIA

Pharmacological studies can at best provide indirect evidence for
any neurobiological hypothesis of mental dysfunction. Search for direct evidence in the brain of afflicted individuals has to be a part
of the process of discovering the causes and mechanisms of the illness.
With regard to cholinergic functions of schizophrenia, such direct
information is exceedingly limited. However, what little is available
is briefly reviewed here to round off the consideration of cholinergic
involvement in schizophrenic disorders.

7.1. Intracranial Stimulation

Almost two decades ago, Heath (1966) observed that direct injection of atropine, but not of several other drugs including putative
neurotransmitters, into the septum of schizophrenics rapidly produced
a psychotic episode. This is of considerable interest because a
strong cholinergic input from the septum to the hippocampus is a major
component of the cholinergic limbic circuit (see Robinson, Chapter 2).
Heath (1966), further observed that the stimulation of the hippocampus
of schizophrenic patients produced spiking in the septum, and the
occurrence of psychotic symptoms. A return circuit from the hippocampus to the septum and nucleus accumbens via the fimbria is known
(De France and Yoshihara, 1975; Siegel et al., 1974).

7.2. Postmortem Studies

Abnormalities of cholinergic parameters, particularly the synthesizing enzyme choline acetyltransferase (CAT) and metabolizing enzyme
acetylcholinesterase (AChE), have been reported in the septal-hippocampal system and other limbic areas of postmortem brains from schizophrenics.

Domino et al. (1973a,b) examined various enzymes involved with
putative neurotransmitters in several areas of the brain. As compared
to controls, they found significant alterations in cholinergic system
enzymes in the amygdala, septum, and visual system in schizophrenic
brains. Both AChE and CAT were over twice the control levels in the
amygdala but less than half the control levels in the septum. Considering a major projection via the stria terminalis from the amygdala to
the septum (Brodal, 1969), Lloyd (1978) raised the question of whether
the cholinergic path in the stria terminalis was "malfunctioning in a
manner that would prevent the normal axoplasmic flow of cholinergic
enzymes from cell bodies to terminalis?" In portions of the visual
system, Domino et al. (1973b) found significant decreases of CAT and
increases of AChE in schizophrenic brains.

Essentially consistent with the findings of Domino et al. (1973a)

are observations by Wise et al. (1974) as well as by Bird et al. (1977), who have reported a significant decrease in CAT activity in the hippocampus, which receives cholinergic input from the septum. Bird et al. (1977) also found a CAT reduction in the nucleus accumbens. A recent report of disarray and disorientation of hippocampal pyramidal cells and their dendritic systems, which are major recipients of cholinergic input from the septum, in the postmortem brains of schizophrenic patients (Kovelman and Scheibel, 1983) would seem to lend further support to the idea that cholinergic functions in the limbic circuit may be deranged in schizophrenia.

In disagreement with these findings is a report by McGeer and McGeer (1977) of increased CAT activity in the caudate, putamen, nucleus accumbens and hippocampus of 11 schizoprenic brains compared to 18 control brains. They did not think that this was due to postmortem changes or prior drug treatment and suggested that CAT increase might be compensatory to defective cholinergic receptor sites in schizophrenia.

In considering this disagreement, one must first look at factors such as differences in drug treatment, measurement techniques and postmortem handling of materials. If such factors do not apply and both types of abnormalities seem to be "real," then one should consider the possibility of two or more biological subtypes of schizophrenia. It is quite conceivable that the brain cholinergic parameters, like the pharmacological responses reviewed earlier, are different in various schizophrenic subpopulations.

One other abnormality of brain cholinergic parameters has been reported. Pope et al. (1952), found that the cholinolytic enzyme AChE was 50 percent higher in biopsy samples of the frontal lobes of psychotic as compared to nonpsychotic patients, a difference which they believed was related to electroshock treatment. No corroboration of this has been reported. If confirmed by others and found to be unrelated to treatment, this may be of considerable interest because of recent findings indicating that in very chronic, nonparanoid schizophrenics, frontal cerebral blood flow is relatively reduced, and also unresponsive to tasks which produce circulation increases in normal persons (Ingvar and Franzen, 1974; Franzen and Ingvar, 1975). Branches of cholinergic neurons have been demonstrated in the pial and other cerebral blood vessels, where they seem to be associated with processes of vasoactive intestinal peptide neurons (Owman et al., 1974; Larsson et al., 1976). In vitro as well as in vivo studies have shown that acetylcholine increases cerebral blood flow and that vasoactive intestinal peptide acts as a facilitatory modulator (Larsson et al., 1976; Heistad et al., 1980; Krieger and Martin, 1981a,b). It is quite conceivable, therefore, that cerebral blood flow problems and frontal lobe hypofunctioning in chronic nonparanoid schizophrenia are related to impaired cholinergic functions and possibly to the associated peptidergic functions.

7.3. Cholinergic Regulation of Neuromuscular Functions

     Finally, a mention should be made of one other type of evidence
which suggests cholinergic impairment in schizophrenia. Cantor et al.
(1980) have reported that in schizophrenic children with thought disorder there are muscle hypotonia, abnormal muscle fiber morphology and
other peripheral features indicative of a decrease in cholinergic
function.

7.4. Summary

     There is some evidence suggesting impairment of the limbic cho-
linergic circuit. In addition, in some cases there may be impaired.
cholinergic regulation of neuromuscular function and brain circulation.

8.   CONCLUSIONS AND PERSPECTIVES

     The literature we have reviewed is of highly uneven quality. The
studies, especially those involving psychiatric patients, were often
uncontrolled, involved small, poorly characterized samples, and lacked
consideration of factors such as dose-response relations, the narrow
physiological range of cholinergic activity, tolerance, noncholinergic
actions of drugs, and heterogeneity of populations. The situation was
further complicated by the fact that in many circumstances the effects
of cholinergic manipulations are not unitary and tend to be biphasic
(see Section1). Still another type of problem was the failure to
distinguish between nonspecific effects, such as the generalized inhibitory state due to cholinergic stimulation, and specific actions
on behaviors under study. Yet, when we pieced the different fragments
of evidence together, certain regularities were apparent. The following statements reflect on those regularities and the future directions
suggested by them.

8.1. Is a Cholinergic Hypothesis of Schizophrenia Justified?

     There is nothing we have reviewed which conclusively proves the
involvement of cholinergic functions in schizophrenia. However, the
possibility that cholinergic mechanisms may be relevant for understanding the pathophysiology and treatment of some components or
types of schizophrenia is supported by several lines of evidence.

(i) Anticholinergic AP drugs significantly reverse the therapeutic
actions of neuroleptics in terms of characteristic symptoms of schizophrenic psychosis and sleeplessness (6.1).

(ii) Anticholinergic drugs in themselves tend to accentuate pre-
existing symptoms of schizophrenia (5.2).

(iii) Anticholinergic drugs, given in various doses to normal individuals, can reproduce the attentional and cognitive processing dysfunctions characteristic of some forms of schizophrenia (5.1).

(iv)   Anticholinergic drugs can reproduce the EEG characteristics of the schizophrenic population (5.3).

(v)   Methylphenidate exacerbation of schizophrenic psychosis is reversed by parenteral physostigmine (2.2). Similarly, in acutely psychotic schizophrenics, improvement is evident with a single intravenous dose of physostigmine (2.2). In chronic schizophrenics, no improvement is seen with acute, parenteral physostigmine treatment, but chronic, oral physostigmine treatment does seem to be beneficial in some cases (2.2).

(vi)   Deanol, which is believed to be a precursor of acetylcholine in the brain, may have slow but progressive therapeutic effects in chronic schizophrenia (3.2).

(vii)   In postmortem brain material from schizophrenics, abnormalities on cholinergic parameters have been found in the septum, hippocampus and amygdala (7.2). These structures, especially the septum and hippocampus, are important parts of the cholinergic limbic circuit (Robinson, Chapter 2) and also of the circuits involved in emotional regulation and expression (Papez, 1973; Stevens, 1973). Most of the data suggest reduced cholinergic function in the septal-hippocampal system. Consistent with this are observations of worsening in schizophrenic psychosis by atropine injection in the septum, and of disarray and disorientation in the hippocampal cells which receive cholinergic input from the septum (7.1, 7.2). Evidence of generalized decrease in peripheral cholinergic activity in childhood schizophrenics (7.3) and also of reduced frontal brain activity and vascular reactivity (7.2) may be further indications of seriously impaired cholinergic function in some schizophrenics.

A number of observations seem at first to serve against the hypothesis; however, on close scrutiny many of them can be reconciled. The following are examples of this type:

(a)   Relatively high level or chronic exposure to organophosphate irreversible cholinesterase inhibitors can produce a state resembling schizophrenia or an organic brain syndrome with depressive features in normal individuals, and can worsen pre-existing symptoms in schizophrenics (4.1, 4.2). This would seem to contradict the idea that cholinergic impairment contributes to schizophrenia. However, poor effectiveness of atropine against the consequences of severe or chronic organophosphate exposure, the atropinic rather than cholinergic type EEG changes, and long-term persistence of the effects of organophosphate exposure would suggest that the functional consequences may be more akin to cholinergic blockade than to cholinergic stimulation and result from factors such as "depolarization block," receptor desensitization, receptor damage or general neurotoxicity.

(b) Psychotogenic or coma-producing amounts of anticholinergic drugs
can be therapeutic in schizophrenia (5.2), which would appear to be
inconsistent with the cholinergic deficiency hypothesis of schizophrenia. However, when it is recognized that features of parasympathetic activity appeared during atropine coma and that improvement in
psychosis occurred after the anticholinergic activation or coma, when
cholinergic activity would be recovering, this contradiction too disappears.

(c) There is no evidence to suggest that long-term use of anticholinergic drugs is harmful to neuroleptic-treated schizophrenics. It is
not possible to confirm or deny this because studies needed to resolve
the question have not been carried out. The experiments involving
withdrawal of anticholinergic drugs after chronic use have not been
helpful in providing a resolution (6.3).

(d) The countertherapeutic AP effects may be due to pharmacokinetic
factors rather than to central interactions (6.2). The best available
data do not support the possibility of a clinically significant AP
drug effect on the pharmacokinetics of neuroleptic medication.

(e) The countertherapeutic AP effects may be due to the demonstrable
ability of these drugs, especially benztropine, to block synaptosomal
uptake of dopamine (Snyder et al., 1970; Lloyd, 1978). Such an action
would make more dopamine available at the synaptic site where neuroleptics act. To explain countertherapeutic AP effects on this basis
would require the implausible assumption that weak dopamine-enhancing
effects of AP drugs can overcome receptor blockade by neuroleptics
which is powerful enough to overcome dopaminergic effects of amphetamines and dopamine agonists like apomorphine (Singh and Lal, 1982).
The only experiment concerning this leaves the question unresolved.
As described by Wauquier and Clincke in this book, the brain self-
stimulation inhibition by a dopamine blocker, pimozide, was reversed
almost completely by dexetimide (anticholinergic and dopamine-uptake
blocker) as well as by cocaine and nomifensine (dopamine and norepi-
nephreine uptake blockers), while amphetamine, which releases catecholamines at the receptor, was only partially antagonistic. However,
the inhibition of self-stimulation by chlorpromazine, which blocks
both norepinephrine and dopamine receptors, was not significantly
affected by dexetimide but was reversed to various degrees by amphetamine, nomifensine and cocaine. These data might be interpreted to
mean that dopamine-uptake blocking effects of AP drugs play a significant part in their antagonism of neuroleptic activity related to dopamine receptor blocking effects. Two facts speak against this being
the explanation for AP reversal of antipsychotic activity of neuroleptics. Firstly, in contrast to the experiment just described, the
anticholinergic AP drugs seemed to reverse therapeutic actions of
chlorpromazine much more completely than those of haloperidol (6.1).

Secondly, and even more importantly, it is not possible on the basis of this thesis to explain the observation that therapeutic actions of neuroleptics were reversed by AP drugs in the catatonic schizophrenics but not in the paranoid schizophrenics (6.1).

8.2.   Cholinergic Functions and Affective Disorders

Acute parenteral administration of physostigmine produces a state of psychomotor inhibition and dysphoria which worsens the clinical condition of depressed patients but is therapeutic, to some degree, in euphoric manic patients (2.2). Acute treatment with organophosphate anticholinesterases has similar effects in manic depressive patients, while chronic exposure to these toxic agents can sometimes produce a clinical picture of depression, lethargy and organic brain dysfunctions (4.1, 4.2).

These observations suggest the possibility that a relative cholinergic excess may be involved in depression and a relative cholinergic deficit in mania (Janowsky et al., Chapter 10). They may also be considered as evidence against the cholinergic hypothesis of schizophrenia, particularly since in some of the same studies, the anticholinesterases were not found to show obvious antischizophrenic activity (2.2, 4.2).

To accept these positions, one would need to show that the mood effects of cholinergic agents were specific and not reflections of nonspecific generalized inhibition which these drugs are known to produce (Karczmar and Richardson, Chapter 7), nor the result of toxic apathetic state caused by them. Also, for the data in question to serve as an argument against cholinergic involvement in schizophrenia, one would need to show that within the framework of the experiments, the cholinergic effects were different from those produced by antipsychotic drugs in affective disorders and chronic schizophrenia.

Weiss et al. (1976) pointed out that a major behavioral effect in these experiments was "the induction of a nonspecific state of generalized retardation suggestive of delirioid incapacitation qualitatively distinct from psychological sadness and pessimism." We should like to point out that many of the changes produced by cholinergic stimulation are similar to those with neuroleptics. The powerful inhibitory effects of these drugs are well documented and can be demonstrated in a variety of behavioral pharmacological tests (Singh and Lal, 1982). They are also often depressiogenic, and this effect can be seen after a single injection (Van Putten and May, 1978; Singh and Kay, 1979a). They have nonspecific antimanic effects, while their well-recognized specific antipsychotic effects may take days or weeks to become evident (Singh and Smith, 1973a; Singh and Lal, 1982).

The studies with the acetylcholine precursor, deanol, are also of interest in this context (3.2). In contrast to physostigmine and

organophosphates, this drug produced a state of well-being in normal
individuals, thus raising the possibility that some of the depressiogenic effects of anticholinesterases may be toxic in nature. Also,
deanol seemed to have some antischizophrenic properties.

Besides these arguments, the findings from studies with antimuscarinics provide probably the most serious objection to the cholinergic hypothesis of affective disorders (5.1, 5.2). If mania represented cholinergic deficit, then anticholinergic drugs should be able
to produce a manic state. They do not and, instead, produce many
aspects of the psychopathology and psychophysiology of schizophrenia
(5.1, 5.2, 5.3).

8.3. Schizophrenia Subtypes and Cholinergic Functions

Perhaps the most significant conclusions to be drawn from this
review is that schizophrenia is heterogenous in terms of cholinergic
functions and that not one but three cholinergic hypotheses of schizophrenia may be recognized. Indeed, our analysis suggested that,
besides the variable and often biphasic character of cholinergic
system responses, the heterogeneity of schizophrenia was probably the
most significant source of variability of effects seen in the psychotic population. Unfortunately, clinical subclassification of schizophrenics was not always considered in these studies, but sufficient
information could be gleaned to formulate the following three biological subgroups of schizophrenia in terms of the cholinergic system
functions:

(i) The first group might be characterized as suffering from reversible inhibition or insufficiency of cholinergic mechanisms, which
remain responsive and, when stimulated within a physiological range,
can produce clinical improvement. The patients in this class would
tend to belong to clinical types designated as catatonic, acute
schizophreniform or good prognosis schizophrenia (Singh and Kay,
1978a, 1982, 1984). They would show global over-arousal evidenced by
marked sleeplessness and high pulse rate (Singh and Kay, 1982) and an
excess of fast beta activity in EEG (5.3). Their EEG would be most
like that produced by atropinics, and they would be highly responsive
to neuroleptic treatment (5.2, 5.3). Moderate cholinergic stimulation
would improve their condition (2.1, 2.2) while cholinergic blockade
would worsen their condition and seriously antagonize the therapeutic
actions of neuroleptics (6.1). In other words, they would be reactive
to cholinergic manipulations. Consistent with this, the mobilization
of cholinergic circuits by treatments such as atropine coma would be
therapeutic in such cases (5.2).

(ii) The second group might be characterized as suffering from an
under-activity as well as from an under-reactivity of cholinergic
mechanisms. Patients of this type would tend to fall into the poor
prognosis, or nuclear, nonparanoid categories such as hebephrenia and

chronic undifferentiated schizophrenia. They would lack clinical evidence of global over-arousal (Singh and Kay, 1978a, 1982, 1984) and their EEG would have an excess of slow wave activity but much less of fast beta (5.3, also Singh and Kay, 1984). They would be most likely to show relatively decreased frontal cerebral circulation and reactivity (7.2). Their response to neuroleptic treatment would be poor, so that AP intervention would have little to undo (6.1). However, a decrease in dysphoria might be seen with AP medication in these cases. At the same time, these patients would be distinguished by showing a paradoxical increase in pulse rate with neuroleptic treatment (6.1). They would tend to be highly resistant to both muscarinic stimulation (4.2) and muscarinic blockade (5.2), and on intense exposure to organophosphate anticholinesterases, they might show some paradoxical effects indicating perhaps an excessive activity of nicotinic receptors (4.2). Extended treatment with oral physostigmine or the acetylcholine precursor, deanol, may be of some therapeutic benefit in such cases (2.2, 3.2). Also, the presumed mobilization of cholinergic circuits through intense, psychotogenic, muscarinic blockade may sometimes make these patients treatment-responsive (5.2).

(iii) Patients with paranoid schizophrenia would typify the third class. AP reversal of neuroleptic action would not be seen in these cases even when response to antipsychotic medication is good. They would react to cholinergic stimulation (4.2) and cholinergic blockade (5.2) much like normals or manic depressives. However, in contrast to the schizophrenics of the second type, these patients might be particularly sensitive to the psychotogenic effects of both cholinergic (4.2) and anticholinergic (5.2) toxins. This could suggest overly sensitive cholinergic receptors, an abnormality which some workers have also found to be present in affective disorder patients (Janowsky et al., Chapter 10). Could supersensitive cholinergic mechanisms be an abnormality common to, and characteristic of, both paranoid schizophrenia and manic depressive illness? A relationship between these conditions has been suggested by a phenomenological, family, and treatment-response study (Taylor and Abrams, 1974).

8.4. Implications for the Treatment of Schizophrenia

The data we have reviewed do not suggest any breakthrough in the treatment of schizophrenia. Most of the drugs which increase cholinergic activity tend to be susceptible to the development of tolerance and are too toxic to be useful as therapeutic agents. It is possible that with careful individualized dosage titration, these disadvantages may be less apparent. Still, evidence for any long-term therapeutic efficacy of cholinergic agents has yet to be obtained. Furthermore, if our analysis is correct, an important conclusion is that the cholinergic mechanisms may be more or less unresponsive in chronic non-paranoid schizophrenics, who represent a major segment of the therapy-resistant schizophrenic population. If this were the case, suggesting refractoriness of some or all cholinergic receptors, then giving cholinergic drugs would seem to be an illogical treatment. Rather, the search would have to be for the means of understanding and undoing this presumed receptor refractoriness.

There does seem to be some treatment possibilities for future research. One of these concerns the cholinergic precursor, deanol, which in one open clinical trial was found to be non-toxic and therapeutic in schizophrenia (3.2). Furthermore, unlike other cholinergic drugs, deanol appeared not to be a dysphoric agent. This might mean that some of the toxicity and dysphoria produced by cholinominetics may be unrelated to their cholinergic activity per se. This is an important issue for further research, as is the apparent antischizophrenia activity of deanol. There is evidence to suggest that certain types of schizophrenics, especially those categorized as nonparanoid nuclear or hebephrenic, develop a dysphoric state accompanied by an increase in autonomic arousal during neuroleptic treatment, which is associated with poor prognosis (Singh and Kay, 1979a). In such cases, deanol may well prove to be of particular use.

Another area of promise is the use of anticholinergic drugs to activate psychosis in therapy-resistant schizophrenics. If further study confirms the observation (5.2) that such an activation changes intractable chronic schizophrenia into treatment-responsive schizophrenia, then the treatment and study of schizophrenia would be clearly advanced.

Still another, but at present only a theoretical, possibility concerns the refractoriness of cholinergic mechanisms. We noted earlier the coexistence of, and interaction between cholinergic and vasoactive intestinal peptide mechanisms in cerebral blood vessels and possibly in other areas of the brain (7.2). In a situation like this, the peptide mechanism might act as a facilitory or inhibitory receptor modulator, and a defect in the modulatory mechanism rather than the primary neuronal mechanism might lead to abnormal functioning. With such a possibility in mind, it might be of interest to determine if a combined treatment with a cholinergic drug and vasoactive intestinal peptide can change the brain circulation and reactivity defects in chronic nonparanoid schizophrenics and whether this or another type of a change can produce a therapeutic benefit (Singh and Kay, 1983).

With these sort of possibilities for the future, the only treatment-related statement that could be made unequivocally at present is that anticholinergic AP drugs should not be combined with neuroleptics, because they appear to reduce the clinical efficacy of the latter. Even here, one will have to say that more work is needed with respect to a number of issues such as generalizability of findings to various types of neuroleptics and AP drugs, the pharmacokinetic factors and relations between AP effects and schizophrenia subtypes. Further, the available data relate only to the acute stages of treatment, and it is not possible to judge whether long-term AP use is good or bad for neuroleptic-treated schizophrenics.

9.   SUMMARY

We have systematically reviewed the literature on the pharmacological effects of cholinergic agonists, reversible and irreversible
anticholinesterases, acetylcholine precursors, and various types of
anticholinergic agents on normal mental and neurophysiological functions, affective disorders, and schizophrenic disorders. While no
study leads to an unequivocal conclusion, piecemeal evidence from many
sources of variable quality suggests that cholinergic mechanisms
should be seriously considered in understanding the pathophysiology of
schizophrenia and in searching for new treatment approaches to this
syndrome. An important conclusion from the review is that, in terms
of cholinergic functions, there might be three quite different biological subtypes of schizophrenia, each with a different set of cholinergic parameters and problems. Any unitary cholinergic hypothesis of
schizophrenia would, therefore, seem simplistic, if not ill-advised.

ACKNOWLEDGEMENT

We wish to thank Barbara Mason for her help in preparing the
manuscript.

REFERENCES

Abood, L. G., and Biel, J. H., 1962, Anticholinergic psychotomimetic
    agents, Int. Rev. Neurobiol. 6:218-273.
Abood, L. G., and Meduna, L. J., 1958, Some effects of a new psychoto-
    gen in depressive states, J. Nerv. Ment. Dis. 127:546-550.
Ananth, J. V., Horodesky, S., Lehmann, H. E., and Ban, T. A., 1970,
    Effect of withdrawal of antiparkinsonian medication of chronical-
    ly hospitalized psychiatric patients, Laval Medical 41:934-938.
Ayd, F. J., 1961, Neuroleptic and extrapyramidal reactions in psych-
    iatric patients, in "Extrapyramidal System," J. M. Bordeleau, ed.,
    pp. 355-365 Editions Psychiatrique, Montreal.
Bignami, C., Rosic, N., Michalek, H., Milosevic, M., and Gatti, G. L.
    1975, Behavioral toxicity of anticholinesterase agents: Methodo-
    logical, neurochemical and neuropsychological aspects, in "Behav-
    ioral Toxicity," B. Weiss and V. G. Laties, eds., pp. 155-215,
    Plenum Press, New York.
Bird, E. D., Barnes, J., Iversen, L. L., Spokes, E. G., Mackay, A. V.
    P., and Shepherd, M., 1977, Increased brain dopamine and reduced
    glutamic acid decarboxylase and choline acetyl transferase activ-
    ity in schizophrenia and related psychoses. Lancet ii:1157-1159.
Bishop, M., Gallant, D., and Syke, T., 1965, Extrapyramidal side ef-
    fects and therapeutic response, Arch. Gen. Psychiatry. 13:155-162.
Bleuler, E., 1950, "Dementia Praecox, Or The Group of Schizophrenias,"
    trans. J. Zinkin, International Universities Press, New York.

Bowers, M. B., Jr., Goodman, E., and Sim, V. M., 1964, Some behavioral changes in man following anticholinesterase administration, J. Nerve. Ment. Dis. 138:383-389.

Bowery, N. G., Collins, J. F., and Hill, R. G., 1976, Bicyclic phosphorus esters that are potent convulsants and GABA antagonists, Nature 261:601-602.

Bradley, P. B., and Elkes, J., 1957, The effects of some drugs on the electrical activity of the brain, Brain 80:77-117.

Brodal, A., 1969, "Neurological Anatomy," Oxford University Press, Toronto.

Burchfiel, J. L., Duffy, F. H., and Sim, V. M., 1976, Persistent effects of sarin and dieldrin upon the primate electroencephalogram, Toxicol. Appl. Pharmacol. 35:365-379.

Burns, B. D., and Paton, W. D. M., 1951, Depolarization of the motor end-plate by decamethonium and acetylcholine, J. Physiol. (Lond.) 115:41.

Cahan, R. B., and Parrish, D. D., 1960, Reversibility of drug-induced parkinsonism, Am. J. Psychiatry 116:1022-1023.

Callaway, E., and Band, R. K., 1958, Some psychopharmacological effects of atropine, Arch. Neurol. 79:91-102.

Callaway, E., and Dembo, D., 1958, Narrowed attention: A psychological phenomenon that accompanies a certain physiological change, J. Neurol. Psychiatry 79:74-90.

Cameron, N., 1939, Deterioration and regression in schizophrenic thinking, J. Abnorm. Soc. Psychol. 34:265-270.

Cameron, N., 1938, Reasoning, regression and communication in schizophrenics, Psychol. Mono. 50:(221) 1-34.

Cantor, S., Trevenen, C., Postuma, R., Dueck, R., and Fjeldsted, B., 1980, Is childhood schizophrenia a cholinergic disease? Arch. Gen. Psychiatry 37:658-667.

Chouinard, G., Annable, L., and Cooper, S., 1977, Antiparkinsonism drug administration and plasma levels of penfluridol, a new long-acting neuroleptic, Comm. Psychopharmacol. 1:325-331.

Claridge, G. S., 1967, "Personality and Arousal: A Psychophysiological Study of Psychiatric Disorder," Pergamon Press, London.

Cohen, E. L., and Wurtman, R. J., 1975, Brain acetylcholine: Increase after systematic choline administration, Life Sci. 16:1075-1102.

Cohen, L. H., Thale, T. and Tissenbaum, M. J., 1944, Acetylcholine treatment of schizophrenia, Arch. Neurol. Psychiatry 51:171-175.

Cole, J. O., and Clyde, D. J., 1961, Extrapyramidal side effects and clinical response to the phenothiazines, in "Extrapyramidal Systems," J. M. Bordeleau, ed., pp. 469-478, Editions Psychiatrique, Montreal.

Collard, J., Lecoq, R., and Demaret, A., 1965, Un essai de therapeutique pathogenique de al schizophrenie par un acetocholinique: L'oxotremorine, Acta Neurol. Belg. 65:122-126.

Colquhoun, W. P., 1962, Effects of hyoscine and meclozine on vigilance and short-term memory, Br. J. Ind. Med. 19:287-298.

Cooper, T. B., 1978, Plasma level monitoring of antipsychotic drugs Clin. Pharmacokinet. 3:14-38.

Crane, G. E., 1967, A review of the clinical literature on haloperidol
     Int. J. Neuropsychiatry 3: Suppl. 1, 110-123.
Crow, T. J., Frith, C. D., Johnstone, E. C., and Owens, D. G. C., 1981
     The influence of anticholinergic medication on the extrapyramidal
     and antipsychotic effects of neuroleptic drugs in the treatment of
     acute schizophrenia, "Proc. IIIrd World Cong. Biol. Psychiatry,"
     Elsevier/North-Holland Press, Amsterdam.
Crowell, E. B., and Ketchum, J. S., 1967, The treatment of scopolamine
     induced delirium with physostigmine, Clin. Pharmacol. Ther.
     8:409-414.
Danielopolu, D., Giurgea, C., and Drocon, G., 1955, Electroencephalo-
     graphic study of the non-specific pharmacodynamics of the stimula-
     tory effects of atropine on the cerebral cortex, Fiziol. Zh.
     41:601-611.
Davis, C. S., and Richardson, R. J., 1980, Organophosphorous compounds
     in "Experimental and Clinical Neurotoxicology," R. S. Spencer and
     H. H. Schaumburg, eds., pp. 527-544, Williams and Wilkins,
     Baltimore.
Davis, H. K., Ford, H. F., Tupin, J. P., and Calvin, A., 1964, Clini-
     cal evaluation of JB-329 (Ditran), Dis. Nerv. Syst. 25:179-183.
Davis, K. L., and Berger, P. A., 1978, Pharmacological investigations
     of the cholinergic imbalance hypotheses of movement disorders and
     psychosis, Biol. Psychiatry 13:23-49.
Davis, K. L., Berger, P. A., Hollister, L. E., and Barchas, J. D.,
     1978, Cholinergic involvement in mental disorders, Life Sci.
     22:1865-1872.
De Feudis, F. V., 1974, "Central Cholinergic Systems and Behavior,"
     Academic Press, London.
De France, J. F., and Yoshihara, H., 1975, Fimbria input to the
     nucleus accumbens septi, Brain Res. 90:159-163.
DiMascio, A., 1971, Toward a more rational use of antiparkinson drugs
     in psychiatry, Drug Therapy 1:23-29.
DiMascio, A., and Demirgian, E., 1970, Antiparkinson drug overuse,
     Psychosomatics 11:596-601.
Domino, E. F., Krause, R. R., and Bowers, J., 1973a, Regional distri-
     bution of some enzymes involved with putative neurotransmitters
     in the human visual system, Brain Res. 58:179-189.
Domino, E. F., Krause, R. R., and Bowers, J., 1973b, Various enzymes
     involved with putative neurotransmitters, Arch. Gen. Psychiatry
     29:195-201.
Douglas, R. J., 1972, Pavlovian conditioning and the brain, in
     "Inhibition and Learning," R. A. Boakes and M. S. Halliday, eds.,
     pp. 529-553, Academic Press, London.
Douglas, R. J., 1975, The development of the hippocampal function:
     Implications for theory and for therapy, "The Hippocampus, Vol.
     2," R. L. Isaacson nd K. H. Pribram, eds., pp. 327-361, Plenum
     Press, New York.
Duffy, F. H., and Burchfiel, J. L., 1980, Long-term effects of the
     organophosphate Sarin on EEG in monkeys and humans, Neurotoxicol.
     1:667-689.

Edelstein, P., Schultz, J., Hirschowitz, J., Kanter, D. R., and
    Garver, D. L., 1981, Physostigmine and lithium response in the
    schizophrenias, Am. J. Psychiatry 138:1078-1081.
El-Yousef, M. K., Janowsky, D. S., Davis, J. M., and Sekerke, H. J.,
    1972, Reversal by physostigmine of cogentin toxicity, "Abstracts
    125th Meeting of the American Psychiatric Association."
El-Yousef, M. K., Janowsky, D. S., Davis, J. M., and Sekerke, H. J.,
    1973, Reversal of antiparkinsonian drug toxicity by physostigmine:
    A controlled study, Am. J. Psychiatry 130:141-145.
El-Yousef, M. K., and Manier, D. H., 1974, The effect of benztropine-
    mesylate on plasma levels of butaperazine maleate, Am. J.
    Psychiatry 131:471-472.
Feldberg, W., 1964, Discussion on extrapolation from animals to man:
    Catatonia, in "Animal Behavior and Drug Action," H. Steinberg,
    ed., pp. 429-439, Churchill, London.
Fiamberti, A., 1946, L'acetocolina nelle sindromi schizofreniche,
    Riv. Patol. Nerv. Ment. 66:1.
Fink, M., 1960, Effect of anticholinergic compounds on post-convulsive
    EEG and behavior of psychiatric patients, Electroencephalogr.
    Clin. Neurophysiol. 12:359-369.
Finkelstein, B. A., 1961, Ditran, a psychotherapeutic advance: A
    review of one hundred and three cases, J. Neuropsychiatry
    2:144-148.
Fleischhauer, J., 1975, Open withdrawal of antiparkinson drugs in the
    neuroleptic-induced Parkinson syndrome, Int. Pharmacopsychiatry
    10:222-229.
Forrer, G. R., 1956, Symposium on atropine toxicity therapy, J. Nerv.
    Ment. Dis. 124:257-283.
Forrer, G. R., and Miller J. J., 1958, Atropine coma: A somatic
    therapy in psychiatry, Am. J. Psychiatry 115:455-458.
Forsman, A., and Ohman, R., 1977, Applied pharmacokinetics of haloper-
    idol in man, Curr. Ther. Res. 21:396-408.
Frankenhaeuser, M., Myrsten, A. L., Johansson, G., and Post, B., 1971,
    Behavioral and physiological effects of cigarette smoking in a
    monotonous situation, Psychopharmacologia 22:1-7.
Franzen, G., and Ingvar, D. J., 1975, Absence of activation in frontal
    structures during psychological testing of chronic schizophrenics,
    J. Neurol. Neurosurg. Psychiatry 38:1027-1032.
Fukuda, T., and Matsuda, Y., 1969, Comparative characteristics of slow
    wave EEG, autonomic function and clinical picture in typical and
    atypical schizophrenia during and following electroconvulsive
    shock treatment, Int. Pharmacopsychiatry 3:13-14.
Fulcher, J. H., Gallagher, W. J., and Pfeiffer, C. C., 1957, Compara-
    tive lucid intervals after amobarbital, CO_2 and arecoline in
    the chronic schizophrenic, Arch. Neurol. Psychiatry 78:392-395.
Gautier, J., Jus, A., Villeneuve, A., Jus, K., Peires, P., and
    Villeneuve, R., 1977, Influence of the antiparkinsonian drugs on
    the plasma levels of neuroleptics, Biol. Psychiatry 12:389-399.
Gershon, S., and Olariu, J., 1960, J.B. 329°:   A new psychotomi-
    metic, its antagonism by tetrahydroaminocrin and its comparison
    with LSD, mescaline and sernyl, J. Neuropsychiatry 1:283-292.

Gershon, S., and Shaw, F. H., 1961, Psychiatric sequelae of chronic exposure to organophosphorous insecticides, Lancet, i:1371-1374.

Goldman, D., 1961, Parkinsonism and related phenomena from the administration of drugs, their production and control under clinical conditions and possible relation to therapeutic effect, in "Extrapyramidal System," J. M. Bordeleau, ed., p. 453-464, Editions Psychiatrique, Montreal.

Goldner, R. D., 1967, Scopolamine sleep treatment in private practice, Int. J. Neuropsychiatry 3:234-247.

Goldstein, B. J., Clyde, D. J., and Caldwell, J. M., 1968, Clinical efficacy of the butyrophenones as antipsychotic drugs, in "Psychopharmacology: A Review of Progress 1957-1967," D. H. Efron, J. O. Cole, J. Levine and J. R. Wittenborn, eds., pp. 1085-1091, U.S. Government Printing Office, Washington, D.C.

Greengard, P., 1978, Cyclid nucleotides, phosphorylated proteins, and neuronal function, "Disting. Lect. Ser. Soc. Gen. Physiol. Vol. 1," Raven Press, New York.

Grisell, J. L., and Bynum, H. J., 1956, Symposium on atropine toxicity therapy: A study of the relationship between anxiety level, ego strength and response to atropine toxicity therapy, J. Nerv. Ment. Dis. 124:265-268.

Grob, D., and Harvey, A. M., 1958, Effects on man of anticholinesterase compound sarin (isopropyl methyl phosphorafluoridate), J. Clin. Invest. 37:350-358.

Grob, D., Harvey, A. M., Langworthy, O. R., and Lilienthal, J. L., Jr. 1947, The administration of di-isopropylfluorophosphate (DFP) to man: III - The effect on the central nervous system, with special reference to the electrical activity of the brain, Bull. Johns Hopkins Hosp. 81:257-266.

Haase, H.-J., 1965, Clinical observations on the actions of neuroleptics, in "Actions of Neuroleptics: A Psychiatric, Neurologic and Pharmacological Investigation," H.-J. Haase and P. A. J. Janssen, eds., pp. 1-118, North Holland Publishing Company, Amsterdam.

Haase, H.-J., 1954, Über vorkommen and deutung des psychomotorischen Parkinson syndroms bei megaphen-bzw. Largactil-daurbehandlung, Nervenarzt. 25:486-492.

Hall, R. W., Feinsilver, D. L., and Holt, R. E., 1981, Anticholinergic psychosis: Differential diagnosis and management, Psychosomatics 22:581-587.

Hanlon, T. E., Schoenrich, C., Freiner, W., Turek, I., and Kurland, A. A., 1966, Perphenazine-benztropine mesylate treatment of newly admitted psychiatric patients, Psychopharmacologia 9:328-339.

Haubrich, D. R., Wang, P. F. L., Clody, D. E., and Wedeking, P. W., 1975, Increase in rat brain acetylcholine induced by choline or deanol, Life Sci. 17:975-980.

Heath, R. G., 1966, Schizophrenia: Biochemical and physiologic alterations, Int. J. Neuropsychiatry 2:597-610.

Heistad, D. D., Marcus, M. L., Said, S. I., and Gross, P. M., 1980, Effect of acetylcholine and vasoactive intestinal peptide on cerebral blood flow, Am. J. Physiol. 239:473-80.

Hery, F., Giorguieff, M. F., Hamon, M., Besson, M. J., and Glowinski, J., 1978, Role of cholinergic receptors in the release of newly synthesized amines from the serotonergic and dopaminergic terminals, in "Interactions Between Putative Neurotransmitters in the Brain," S. Garattini, J. F. Pujol and R. Samanin, eds., pp. 39-51, Raven Press, New York.

Hoffer, A., and Osmond, H., 1960, in "The Chemical Basis of Psychiatry," Charles C. Thomas, Springfield, Illinois.

Ingvar, D. H., and Franzen, G., 1974, Abnormalities of cerebral blood flow distribution in patients with chronic schizophrenia, Acta Psychiatr. Scand. 50:425-462.

Itil, T., 1977, Qualitative and quantitative EEG findings in schizophrenia, Schizophr. Bull. 3:610-679.

Itil, T., and Fink, M., 1966, Anticholinergic drug-induced delirium: Experimental modification, quantitative EEG and behavioral correlations, J. Nerv. Ment. Dis. 143:492-507.

Itil, T., and Fink, M., 1968, EEG and behavioral aspects of the interaction of anticholinergic hallucinogens with centrally active compounds, Prog. Brain Res. 28:158-168.

Itil, T. M., Keskiner, A., and Holden, J. M. C., 1969, The use of LSD and ditran in the treatment of therapy-resistant schizophrenics, Dis.Nerv. Syst. 30:93-103.

Janowsky, D. S., El-Yousef, M. K., Davis, J. M., and Sekerke, H. J., 1973, Antagonistic effects of physostigmine and methylphenidate in man, Am. J. Psychiatry 130:1370-1376.

Jellinek, T., Gardos, G., and Cole, J. O., 1981, Adverse effects of antiparkinson drug withdrawal, Am. J. Psychiatry 138:1567-1571.

Johnstone, E. C., Crow, T. M., Frith, C. D., and Owens, D. G. C., 1983, Adverse effects of anticholinergic medication in positive schizophrenic symptoms; theoretical and practical implications, Psychol. Med. 13:513-527.

Karczmar, A. G., 1979, Brain acetylcholine and animal electrophysiology, in "Brain Acetylcholine and Neuropsychiatric Disease," K. L. Davis and P. A. Berger, eds., pp. 265-310, Plenum Press, New York.

Karczmar, A. G., 1978, Exploitable aspects of central cholinergic functions, particularly with respect to the EEG, motor, analgesic and mental functions in "Cholinergic Mechanisms and Psychopharmacology," D. J. Jenden, ed., pp. 679-708, Plenum Press, New York.

Karczmar, A. G., 1967, Pharmacologic, toxicologic and therapeutic properties of anticholinesterase agents, in "Physiological Pharmacology, Vol. 3," W. S. Root and F. G. Hofman, eds., pp. 163-322, Academic Press, New York.

Karczmar, A. G., and Ohta, Y., 1981, Neuropsychopharmacology as related to anticholinesterase action, Fund. Appl. Toxicol. 1:135-142.

Karczmar, A. G., and Van Meter, W. G., 1963, Reports, Subcontract No. SU-630505-63, Melpar, Inc.

Katz, B., and Thesleff, S., 1957, A study of the "desensitization" produced by acetylcholine at the motor end-plate, J. Physiol. (Lond.) 138:63.

Kay, S. R., and Singh, M. M., 1979, Cognitive abnormality in schizo-
    phrenia: A dual-process model, Biol. Psychiatry 14:155-176.
Ketchum, J. S., Sidell, F. R., Crowell, E. B., Aghajanian, G. K., and
    Hayes, A. H., 1973, Atropine, scopolamine and ditran: Comparative
    pharmacology and antagonists in man, Psychopharmacologia
    28:121-133.
Klett, C. J., and Caffey, E., 1972, Evaluating the long-term need for
    antiparkinson drugs by chronic schizophrenics, Arch. Gen. Psy-
    chiatry 26:374-379.
Kolakowska, T., Wiles, D. H., Gilder, M. G., and McNeilly, A. S., 1976
    Clinical significance of plasma chlorpromazine levels, Psycho-
    pharmacology 49:101-379.
Kovelman, J. A., and Scheibel, A. B., 1983, A neurohistological corre-
    late of schizophrenia. Paper presented at the 38th Annual Conven-
    tion of the Society of Biological Psychiatry, New York.
Kraepelin, E., 1919, "Dementia Praecox and Paraphenia," (Trans. R. M.
    Barclay), Livingstone, Edinburgh.
Krieger, D. T., and Martin, J. B., 1981a, Brain peptides, N. Engl. J.
    Med. 304:876-885.
Krieger, D. T., and Martin, J. B., 1981b, Brain peptides, N. Engl. J.
    Med. 304:944-951.
Ladinsky, H., Consolo, S., Bianchi, S., Ghezzi, D., and Samanin, R.,
    1978, Link between dopaminergic and cholinergic neurons in the
    striatum as evidenced by pharmacological, biochemical and lesion
    studies, in "Interactions Between Putative Neurotransmitters in
    the Brain," S. Garattini, J. F. Pujol and R. Samanin, eds.,
    pp. 3-21, Raven Press, New York.
Larsson, L-I., Edvinsson, L., Fahrenkrug, J., Hakanson, R., Owman,
    Ch., Schaffalitzky de Muckadell, O., and Sundler, F., 1976,
    Immunohistochemical localization of a vasodilatory polypeptide
    (VIP) in cerebrovascular nerves, Brain Res. 113:400-404.
Lawson, J. S., McGhie, A., and Chapman, J., 1967, Distractibility in
    schizophrenic and organic cerebral disease, Br. J. Psychiatry
    113:527-535.
Lechner, H., 1956, On the influence of anticholinergic drugs on the
    EEG of recent closed cranio-cerebral injuries, Electroencephalogr.
    Clin. Neurophysiol. 8:714-715.
Lee, J. H., Cooper, T. B., Srivastava, R. K., and Simpson, G. M.,
    1978, A study of butaperazine plasma levels with or without anti-
    parkinsonism agents. Cited in Cooper, T. B., Plasma level
    monitoring of antipsychotic drugs, Clin. Pharmacokinet. 3:14-38.
Lewin, L., 1964, "Phantastica, Narcotic and Stimulating Drugs,"
    Routledge, Kegan Paul, London.
Lewis, J. J., 1964, "An Introduction to Pharmacology," Williams and
    Wilkins, Baltimore.
Lieberman, J., 1981, Cholinergic rebound in neuroleptic withdrawal
    syndromes, Psychosomatics 22:253-254.
Lloyd, K. G., 1978, Observations concerning neurotransmitter interac-
    tion in schizophrenia, in "Cholinergic-Monoaminergic Interactions
    in the Brain," L. L. Butcher, ed., pp. 363-392, Academic Press,
    New York.

Loga, S., Curry, S., and Lader, M., 1975, Interaction of orphenadrine and phenobarbitone with chlorpromazine plasma concentrations and effects in man, Br. J. Clin. Pharmacol. 2:197-208.

Longo, V. G., 1966, Mechanisms of the behavioral and electroencephalographic effects of atropine and related compounds, Pharmacol. Rev. 18:965-996.

Luchins, D. J., Freed, W. J., and Wyatt, R. J., 1980, The role of cholinergic supersensitivity in the medical symptoms associated with withdrawal of antipsychotic drugs, Am. J. Psychiatry 137:1395-1398.

Mackworth, J. F., 1965, The effect of amphetamine on the detectability of signals in vigilance tasks, Can. J. Psychol. 19:104-109.

Mandel, W., Claffey, B., and Margolis, L. H., 1961, Recurrent thioperazine-induced extrapyramidal reaction following placebo substitution for maintenance antiparkinson drug, Am. J. Psychiatry 118:351-352.

Mandel, W., and Oliver, W. A., 1961, Withdrawal of maintenance antiparkinson drug in the phenothiazine-induced extrapyramidal reaction, Am. J. Psychiatry 118:350-351.

Manos, N., and Gkiouzepas, J., 1981, Discontinuing antiparkinson medication in chronic schizophrenics: At what cost to the patient? Acta Psychiatr. Scand. 63:28-32.

Manos, N., Gkiouzepas, J., and Logothetis, J., 1981, The need for continuous use of antiparkinsonian medication with chronic schizophrenic patients receiving long-term neuroleptic therapy, Am. J. Psychiatry 138:184-188.

Martini, M., and Frassanito, L. S., 1975, Contributo clinico sugli effetti della sospensions di farmaci contro i disturbi extrapiramidali nei trattamenti prolungati con neurolettici, Rassegna Studi Psychiat. 64:641-671.

Matthysse, S., and Haber, S., 1974, Animal models of schizophrenia, in "Model Systems in Biological Psychiatry," D. I. Ingle and H. M. Shein, eds., M.I.T. Press, Cambridge.

Mattke, D. J., 1968, A pilot investigation in neuroleptic therapy, Dis. Nerv. Syst. 29:516-524.

May, P. R., and Goldberg, S. C., 1978, Prediction of schizophrenic patients' response to pharmacotherapy, in "Psychopharmacology: A Generation of Progress," M. A. Lipton, A. DiMascio and K. F. Killam, eds., pp. 1139-1153, Raven Press, New York.

McClelland, H. A., Blessed, G., Bhate, S., Ali, N., and Clarke, P. A., 1974, The abrupt withdrawal of antiparkinsonian drugs in schizophrennic patients, Br. J. Psychiatry 124:151-159.

McGeer, P. L., and McGeer, E. G., 1977, Possible changes in striatal and limbic cholinergic systems in schizophrenia, Arch. Gen. Psychiatry 34:1319-1323.

McGhie, A., and Chapman, J., 1961, Disorders of attention and perception in early schizophrenia, Br. J. Med. Psychol. 34:103-116.

McGhie, A., Chapman, J., and Lawson, J. S., 1964, Disturbances in selective attention in schizophrenia, Proc. R. Soc. Med. 57:419-422.

Meduna, L. J., and Abood, L. G., 1959, Studies of a new drug (Ditran) in depressive states, J. Neuropsychiatry 1:20-22.

Meltzer, H. Y., and Stahl, S. M., 1976, The dopamine hypothesis of schizophrenia: A review, Schizophr. Bull. 2:19-76.

Metcalf, D. R., and Holmes, J. H., 1969, EEG, psychological and neurological alterations in humans with or without organophosphate exposure, Ann. N.Y. Acad. Sci. 160:357-365.

Michelson, M. J., 1961, Pharmacological evidences of the role of acetylcholine in the higher nervous activity of man and animals, Act. Nerv. Super (Praha) 3:140-147.

Milby, T., 1971, Prevention and management of organophosphate poisoning, J.A.M.A. 216:2131-2133.

Miller, R. E., Murphy, J. V., and Mirsky, I. A., 1957, The effect of chlorpromazine on fear-motivated behavior in rats, J. Pharmacol. Exp. Ther. 120:379-387.

Mitsuda, H., 1967, Clinico-genetic study of schizophrenia, Bull. Osaka Medical School Suppl. 12:49-90.

Modestin, J., Hunger, J., and Schwartz, R. B., 1973a, Uber die depresogene wirkung von physostigmin, Arch. Psychiatr. Nervenkr. 218:67-77.

Modestin, J., Schwartz, R. B., and Hunger, J., 1973b, Zur frage der beeinflussung schizophrener symptome durch physostigmin, Pharmakopsychiatr. Neuropsychopharmakol. 9:300-304.

Murphree, H. B., Jenney, E. H., and Pfeiffer, C. C., 1959, 2-dimethylaminoethanol as a central nervous system stimulant: One aspect of the pharmacology of reserpine, Res. Publ. Assoc. Res. Nerv. Ment. Dis. 37:204-207.

NIMH Collaborative Study Group, 1964, Phenothiazine treatment in acute schizophrenia, Arch. Gen. Psychiatry 10:246-261.

O'Neill, J. J., 1981, Non-cholinesterase effects of anticholinesterases, Fund. Appl. Toxicol. 1:154-160.

Orlov, P., Kasparian, G., DiMascio, A., and Cole, J. O., 1971, Withdrawal of antiparkinson drugs, Arch. Gen. Psychiatry 25:410-412.

Orzack, M. H., Kornetsky, C., and Freeman, H., 1967, The effects of daily administration of carphenazine on attention in the schizophrenic patient, Psychopharmacologia 11:31-38.

Ostfeld, A. M., and Aruguete, A., 1962, Central nervous system effects of hyoscine in man, J. Pharmacol. 137:133-139.

Ostfeld, A. M., Machne, X. and Uhna, K. R., 1960, The effects of atropine on the electroencephalogram and behavior in man, J. Pharmacol 128:265-272.

Owman, C., Edvinsson, L, and Nielsen, K. C., 1974, Autonomic neuroreceptor mechanisms in brain vessels, Blood Vessels 11:2-31.

Papez, J. W., 1973, A proposed mechanism of emotion, Arch. Neurol. Psychiat. 38:725-743.

Payne, R. W., 1973, Cognitive abnormalities, in "Handbook of Abnormal Psychology," H. J. Eysenck, ed., pp. 420-483, Pitman Medical Press, London.

Petras, J. M., 1981, Human neurotoxicity, Fund. Appl. Toxicol. 1:242.

Pfeiffer, C. C., 1959, Parasympathetic neohumors: Possible precursors and effect on behavior, Int. Rev. Neurobiol. 1:195-244.

Pfeiffer, C. C., and Jenney, E. H., 1957, The inhibition of condition-
    al response and counter-action of schizophrenia by muscarinic
    stimulation of the brain, Ann. N.Y. Acad. Sci. 66:753-764.
Pope, A., Caveness, W., and Livingstone, K. E., 1952, Architectonic
    distribution of acetylcholinesterase in the frontal isocortex of
    psychotic and nonpsychotic patients, Arch. Neurol. Psychiat.
    68:425-443.
Pradhan, S. N., 1976, Balance of central neurotransmitter actions in
    self-stimulation behavior, in "Brain-Stimulation Reward," A.
    Wauquier and E. T. Rolls, eds., pp. 171-185, North-Holland
    Publishing Company, Amsterdam.
Randrup, A., and Munkvad, I., 1972, Evidence indicating an association
    between schizophrenia and dopaminergic hyperactivity in the brain,
    Orthomolec. Psychiatry 1:2-7.
Ré O., 1974, 2-dimethylaminoethanol (deanol): A brief review of its
    clinical efficacy and postulated mechanisms of action, Curr.
    Ther. Res. 16:1238-1242.
Rinaldi, R., and Himwich, H. E., 1955, A cholinergic mechanism invol-
    ed in the function of mesodiencephalic activating system, Arch.
    Neurol. Psychiat. 173:396-402.
Rivera-Calimlim, L., Castaneda, L., and Lasagna, L., 1973, Effects of
    mode of management on plasma chlorpromazine in psychiatric
    patients, Clin. Pharmacol. Thera. 14:978-986.
Rivera-Calimlim, L., Nasrallah, H., Strauss, J., and Lasagna, L.,
    1976, Clinical response and plasma levels: Effect of dose,
    dosage schedules and drug interactions of plasma chlorpromazine
    levels, Am. J. Psychiatry 133:646-652.
Rosenthal, R., and Bigelow, L. B., 1973, The effects of physostigmine
    in phenothiazine resistant chronic schizophrenic patients: Pre-
    liminary observations, Compr. Psychiatry 14:489-494.
Rowntree, D. W., Nevin, S., and Wilson, A., 1950, The effects of
    diisopropylfluorophosphonate in schizophrenia and manic depressive
    psychosis, J. Neurol. Neurosurg. Psychiatry 13:47-62.
Russell, R. W., 1969, Behavioral aspects of cholinergic transmission,
    Fed. Proc. 28:121-131.
Russell, R. W., 1966, Biochemical substrates of behavior, in
    "Frontiers in Physiological Psychology," R. W. Russel, ed.,
    pp. 185-246, Academic Press, New York.
Saletu, B., 1976, "Psychopharmaka, Gehrintatigkeit und Schlaf: Neuro-
    physiologische Aspekte der Psychopharmakologie und Pharmakopsy-
    chiatrie. Biblthca Psychiat. Nr. 155," Karger, Basel.
Saletu, B., 1980, Central measures in schizophrenia, in "Handbook of
    Biological Psychiatry II: Brain Mechanisms and Abnormal Behavior-
    Psychophysiology," H. M. Van Praag, M. H. Lader, O. J. Rafaelsen
    and E. J. Sachar, eds., pp. 97-144, Marcel Dekker, Inc., New York.
Sawa, M., 1957, Epileptogenic factors in atypical endogenous psychoses
    Psychiat. Neurol. Japan 5:73-111.
Schaffer, C. B., Shahid, A., Javaid, J. I., and Davis, J. M., 1981, A
    case report of vomiting related to the interactions of antipsycho-
    tics and benztropine, Am. J. Psychiatry 138:833-835.

Schwartz, H. 1957, Symposium on atropine toxicity therapy: Statisti-
    cal evaluation, J. Nerv. Ment. Dis. 124:281-286.
Shakow, D., 1977, Schizophrenia: Selected Papers Psychology Issues
    10, No. 2, Monograph No. 38," Raven Press, New York.
Shakow, D., 1962, Segmental set: A theory of the formal psychological
    deficit in schizophrenia, Arch. Gen. Psychiatry 6:17-33.
Sherwood, S. L., 1958, Consciousness, adaptive behavior and schizo-
    phrenia, in "Schizophrenia: Somatic Aspects," D. Richter, ed.,
    pp. 131-146, Pergamon, London.
Sherwood, S. L., 1952, Intraventricular medication in catatonic
    stupor, Brain 75:68-75.
Shopsin, B., and Gershon, S., 1971, Chemotherapy of manic-depressive
    disorder, in "Brain Chemistry and Mental Disease," B. T. Ho and
    W. M. McIsaac, eds., pp. 319-377, Plenum Press, New York.
Siegel, A., Edinger, H., and Ohgami, S., 1974, The topographical
    organization of the hippocampal projection to the septal region:
    A comparative neuroanatomical analysis in the gerbil, rat, rabbit
    and cat, J. Comp. Neurol. 157:359-378.
Simpson, G. M., Cooper, T. B., Bark, N., Sud, I., and Lee, J. H.,
    1980, Effect of antiparkinsonian medication on plasma levels of
    chlorpormazine, Arch. Gen. Psychiatry 37:205-208.
Singh, M. M., 1981, Cholinergic mechanisms and the psychobiology of
    schizophrenia in "Biological Psychiatry 1981." C. Perris, G.
    Strüwe and B. Jansson, eds., pp. 793-800, Elsevier/North-Holland
    Biomedical Press, Amsterdam.
Singh, M. M., 1978, Some insights into the pathogenesis of schizo-
    phrenia, in "The Biological Basis of Schizophrenia," G. Hemmings
    and W. A. Hemmings, eds., pp. 179-195, University Park Press,
    Baltimore.
Singh, M. M., and Kay, S. R., 1975a, A comparative study of haloperi
    dol and chlorpromazine in terms of clinical effects and thera-
    peutic reversal with benztropine in schizophrenia. Theoretical
    implications for potency differences among neuroleptics, Psycho-
    pharmacologia 43:103-113.
Singh, M. M., and Kay, S. R., 1975b, A longitudinal therapeutic com-
    parison between two prototypic neuroleptics (haloperidol and
    chlorpromazine) in matched groups of schizophrenics. Nonthera-
    peutic interactions with trihexyphenidyl. Theoretical implica-
    tions for potency differences, Psychopharmacologia 43:115-123.
Singh, M. M., and Kay, S. R., 1979a, Dysphoric response to neuroleptic
    treatment in schizophrenia, its relationship to autonomic arousal
    and prognosis, Biol. Psychiatry 14:275-292.
Singh, M. M., and Kay, S. R., 1983, Exogenous peptides and schizo-
    phrenia, in "Psychoneuroendocrine Dysfunction in Psychiatric and
    Neurological Illnesses: Influence of Psychopharmacological
    Agents," N. S. Shah and A. G. Donald, eds., Plenum Press, New
    York.
Singh, M. M., and Kay, S. R., 1978a, Nosological and prognostic dis-
    tinctions in schizophrenia: Pharmacological validation in terms
    of therapeutic antagonism between anticholinergic anti-Parkinson-
    ism drugs and neuroleptics, Neuropsychobiology 4:288-304.

Singh, M. M., and Kay, S. R., 1978b, Therapeutic antagonism between
    anticholinergics and neuroleptics: Possible involvement of anti-
    cholinergic mechanisms in schizophrenia, Schizophr. Bull. 4:3-6.
Singh, M. M., and Kay, S. R., 1979b, Therapeutic antagonism between
    anticholinergic anti-Parkinsonism agents and neuroleptics in
    schizophrenia: Implications for a neuropharmacological model,
    Neuropsychobiology 5:74-86.
Singh, M. M., and Kay, S. R., 1975c, Therapeutic reversal with benz-
    tropine in schizophrenia, J. Nerv. Ment. Dis. 160:258-266.
Singh, M. M., and Kay, S. R., 1982, Towards a psychobiological model
    of schizophrenia: A neuroscientist's view, in "Psychobiology of
    Schizophrenia," M. Namba and H. Kaiya, eds., pp. 93-107, Pergamon
    Press, Oxford.
Singh, M. M., and Kay, S. R., 1984, Typical (nuclear) vs. atypical
    (schizophreniform) schizophrenias: A multidimensional examination
    in search of external validation, in "Clinical Biology of Atypical
    Psychoses," Proc. 3rd Annual Meeting Japanese Soc. Biol. Psychiat.
    Oct. 23-24, 1981, Kyoto, Japan. In press.
Singh, M. M., and Kay, S. R., 1976, Wheat gluten as a pathogenic
    factor in schizophrenia, Science 191:401-402.
Singh, M. M., Kay, S. R., and Pitman, R. K., 1981a, Aggression control
    and structuring of social relations among recently admitted schiz-
    ophrenics, Psychiatry Res. 5:157-169.
Singh, M. M., Kay, S. R., and Pitman, R. K., 1981b, Territorial
    behavior of schizophrenics: A phylogenetic approach, J. Nerv.
    Ment. Dis. 169:503-512.
Singh, M. M., and Lal, H., 1982, Central cholinergic mechanisms,
    neuroleptic action and schizophrenia, in "Clinical Applications
    of Neuropharmacology," W. B. Essman and L. Valzelli, eds.,
    pp. 337-389, Spectrum Publications, New York.
Singh, M. M., and Smith, J. M., 1973a, Kinetics and dynamics of
    response to haloperidol in acute schizophrenics: A longitudinal
    study of the therapeutic process, Compr. Psychiatry 14:393-414.
Singh, M. M., and Smith, J. M., 1973b, Reversal of some therapeutic
    effects of an antipsychotic agent by an anti-Parkinsonism drug,
    J. Nerv. Ment. Dis. 157:50-58.
Singh, M. M., and Smith, J. M., 1971, Reversal of some therapeutic
    effects of haloperidol in schizophrenia by anti-Parkinsonism
    drugs, Pharmacologist 13:207.
Singh, M. M., and Smith, J. M., 1973c, Sleeplessness in acute and
    chronic schizophrenia in response to haloperidol and anti-
    Parkinsonism agents, Psychopharmacologia 29:21-32.
Snyder, S., Greenberg, D., and Yamamura, H. E., 1974, Antischizo-
    phrenic drugs and brain cholinergic receptors: Affinity for
    muscarinic sites predicts extrapyramidal effects, Arch. Gen.
    Psychiatry 31:58-61.
Snyder, S. H., Taylor, K. M., Coyle, J. T., and Meyerhoff, J. L.,
    1970, The role of brain dopamine in behavioral regulation and
    action of antipsychotic drugs, Am. J. Psychiatry 127:117-125.
Stephens, D. A., 1967, Psychotoxic effects of benzhexol hydrochloride
    (Artane), Br. J. Psychiatry 133:213-218.

Stevens, J. R., 1973, An anatomy of schizophrenia? Arch. Gen. Psychiatry 29:177-189.

St. Jean, A., Donald, M. W., and Ban, T. A., 1964, Uses and abuses antiparkinsonian medication, Am. J. Psychiatry 120:801-803.

Stratas, N. E., Philips, R. D., Walker, P. A., and Sandifer, M. G., 1963, A study of drug-induced parkinsonism, Dis. Nerv. Syst. 24:180.

Tabershaw, I. R., and Cooper, W. C., 1966, Sequelae of acute organic-phosphate poisoning, J. Occupat. Med. 8:5-20.

Taylor, M., and Abrams, R., 1974, Manic-depressive illness and paranoid schizophrenia: A phenomenological family and treatment-response study, Arch. Gen. Psychiatry 31:640-642.

Tourlentes, T., Axiotis, A., Hunsicker, A., Hurd, D., Vassilon, G., and Abood, L. C., 1960, Effects of new piperazinoglycolate on chronic schizophrenics, J. Neuropsychiatry 2:49-53.

Ulus, I. H., and Wurtman, R. J., 1976, Choline administration: Activation of tyrosine hydroxylase in dopaminergic neurons of rat brain, Science 194:1060-1061.

Van Andel, H., 1959, Neuropharmacological studies in catatonic phenomena, in "Neuropharmacology," P. B. Bradley, P. Deniker, G. Raduoco-Thomas, eds., pp. 701-703, Elsevier, Amsterdam.

Vanderwolf, C. H., and Robinson, T. E., 1981, Reticulo-cortical activity and behavior: A critique of the arousal theory and a new synthesis, Behav. Brain Sciences 4:459-514.

Van Meter, W. G., Karczmar, A. G., and Fiscus, R. R., 1978, CNS effects of anticholinesterases in the presence of inhibited cholinesterases, Arch. Int. Pharmacodyn. Ther. 231:249-260.

Van Putten, T., and May, P. R. A., 1978, Subjective response as a predictor of outcome in pharmacotherapy: The consumer has a point, Arch. Gen. Psychiatry 35:477-480.

Van Rossum, J. M., 1967, The significance of dopamine-receptor blockage for the action of neuroleptic drugs, in "Neuropsychopharmacology," H. Brill, ed., pp. 321-329, Exerpta Medica Foundation, The Hague. Warburton, D. M., 1972, The cholinergic control of internal inhibition in "Inhibition and Learning," R. Boakes and M. S. Halliday, eds., pp. 431-460, Academic Press, London.

Warburton, D. M., 1975, "Brain, Behavior and Drugs: Introduction to the Neurochemistry of Behavior," Chapters 1,3,4 and 7, John Wiley, London.

Warburton, D. M., 1979, Neurochemical basis of consciousness, in "Chemical Influences on Behavior," K. Brown, S. Cooper, eds., pp. 421-462, Academic Press, London.

Weckowicz, T. E., 1960, Perception of hidden figures by schizophrenic patients, Arch. Gen. Psychiatry 2:521-527.

Weiss, B. L., Gordon Foster, F., and Kupfer, D. J., 1976, Cholinergic involvement in neuropsychiatric syndromes, in "Biology of Cholinergic Functions," A. M. Goldberg and I. Hanin, eds., pp. 603-617, Raven Press, New York.

White, R. P., Rinaldi, F., and Himwich, H. E., 1956, Central and
    peripheral nervous effects of atropine sulfate and mepiperphenidal
    bromide ("Darstine") on human subjects, J. Appl. Physiol.
    8:635-642.
Wilson, R. E., and Shagass, C., 1964, Comparison of two drugs with
    psychotomimetic effects (LSD and Ditran), J. Nerv. Ment. Dis.
    138:277-286.
Wise, C. D., Baden, W. M., and Stein, L., 1974, Post-mortem measure-
    ment of enzymes in human brain: Evidence of a central noradren-
    ergic deficit in schizophrenia, J. Psychiat. Res. 11:185-198.
Wohlberg, G. W., and Kornetsky, C., 1973, Sustained attention in
    remitted schizophrenics, Arch. Gen. Psychiatry 28:533-537.
Yahr, M. D., and Duvoisin, R. C., 1972, Drug therapy of Parkinsonism,
    New Engl. J. Med. 287:20-24.
Yamada, T., 1960, Heterogeneity of schizophrenia as demonstrable in
    EEG, Bull. Osaka Medical School, 6:107-146.
Ziemba, T., Meltzer, H. Y., and Davis, J. M., 1978, Do anticholin-
    ergics antagonize antipsychotic drug action? Schizophr. Bull.
    4:7-12.

Chapter 10

BRAIN CHOLINERGIC SYSTEMS AND THE PATHOGENESIS OF AFFECTIVE DISORDERS

David S. Janowsky[1,2], Samuel Craig Risch[1,2],
Lewis L. Judd[2], Leighton Y. Huey[1,2] and
Donal C. Parker[3]

[1]Psychiatry Service
San Diego Veterans Administration Medical Center
San Diego, California 12161, U.S.A.

[2]Department of Psychiatry
University of California, San Diego
La Jolla, California 92093, U.S.A.

[3]Department of Medicine
San Diego Veterans Administration Medical Center and
University of California, San Diego
La Jolla, California 92093, U.S.A.

---

1.   INTRODUCTION

Extreme and debilitating fluctuations in mood have long been
thought to involve chemical imbalances in the central nervous system.
The role of catecholamines in the affective disorders has been emphasized since the pioneering work by Schildkraut and Kety (1967) and
others, who noted that drugs which elevate mood and which are effective in the treatment of depression facilitate catecholaminergic
transmission in the brain, and conversely, that drugs which may produce depression and that are used in the treatment of manic behavior
tend to antagonize the synaptic actions of dopamine and norepinephrine. Measurements of catecholamine metabolites in the urine and
cerebrospinal fluid of manic and depressed patients have also produced
some evidence consistent with the view that depression is associated
with reduced catecholaminergic synaptic transmission (Schildkraut,
1973; Schildkraut and Kety, 1967).

More recently, a variety of disturbances of other single neurotransmitters in the brain have been suggested as etiologic in affective disease, including a deficiency (Chase and Murphy, 1973) or an
excess of serotonergic activity (Tissot, 1975) and disturbances of the
GABA and the opioid systems (Gerner et al., 1981; Janowsky et al.,
(1979a).

During the past decade, theorists have explored the possibility
that, as with physiologic functions, mood states may reflect disturbances in the interaction of multiple neurotransmitters. Tissot (1975)
for example, has hypothesized that depression reflects a relative
increase in serotonergic activity, occurring in conjunction with a
decrease in catecholaminergic activity, while mania is presumed to
reflect the opposite imbalance. Similarly, in 1972, Janowsky and co-
workers (1972a) proposed their cholinergic-adrenergic balance hypothesis of affective disorders. This hypothesis suggests that affect may
represent a balance between cholinergic and adrenergic neurotransmitter activity in those areas of the brain that regulate mood, with depression being a disease of cholinergic predominance and mania being
the converse (Janowsky et al., 1972a).

In the following paragraphs we will discuss information supportive of a role for adrenergic-cholinergic interactions in the regulation of affect and affective disorders. We will discuss data from
animal-behavioral experiments and observations of the relationship of
mood change to adrenergic-cholinergic imbalances caused by medically
and psychiatrically prescribed drugs as supportive of the above hypothesis. We will also cite information regarding the effects of cholinomimetics on depressive and manic symptoms, and offer information
demonstrating that physiologic, neuroendocrine, and behavioral hyper-
responsiveness to cholinergic agents occurs in patients with affect
disorders. Lastly, we will discuss the antagonistic effects of cholinergic agonists and psychostimulants, and the euphorigenic properties of anticholinergic drugs, as supportive of an adrenergic-cholinergic balance hypothesis.

2.   BEHAVIORAL EFFECTS OF MANIPULATIONS OF CENTRAL CHOLINERGIC
      ACTIVITY IN ANIMALS

The possibility that adrenergic and cholinergic systems produce
divergent effects which influence behavior is supported by a variety
of animal studies. For example, centrally active cholinomimetics usually produce depressant and inhibitory behavioral effects, including
lethargy, decreased locomotion and decreased self-stimulation (Carlton,
1963; Pradhan and Kavat, 1972; Olds, 1958; Domino and Olds, 1968),
while centrally active sympathomimetics and anticholinergic agents
produce behavioral arousal, hyperactivity and increased self-stimulation and stereotyped behaviors (Janowsky et al., 1972b). Furthermore
there is evidence that adrenergic and cholinergic behavioral influences may antagonize each other with respect to locomotion, self-
stimulation and stereotyped behaviors (Janowsky et al., 1972b; Domino
and Olds, 1968). The fact that the above behaviors are increased and
decreased by adrenergic and cholinergic agents respectively is consistent with the hypothesis that mood is likewise regulated by a balance
between adrenergic and cholinergic factors. However, it is important
to note that the above animal behavioral models are not necessarily
accepted parallels of affective disorder and, indeed, that at least
stereotyped behavior is actually a better model of schizophrenia than
of affective disorder.

There is also indirect evidence that increases in central cholinergic activity may cause compensatory increases in central adrenergic
neurotransmitter associated behaviors such as locomotion (Fibiger et
al., 1971). A number of neurochemical studies also support the existence of induction of these acute and subsequent compensatory behavioral changes, with catecholamines initially decreasing and ultimately
increasing acetylcholine activity and vice versa (Mandell and Knapp,
1971).

3.   CHOLINERGIC-ANTICHOLINERGIC EFFECTS OF MEDICALLY PRESCRIBED DRUGS

3.1.   General Medical Drugs

Supporting a role for adrenergic-cholinergic balance in the regulation of affect are observations that many medications, such as propranolol, alphamethyldopa and reserpine which can cause depression,
have apparent cholinomimetic, as well as anti-adrenergic properties
(Janowsky et al., 1972a).

In animals, reserpine can cause parasympathetic somatic effects
such as miosis, lacrimation, salivation, diarrhea and tremor, and such
behavioral effects as sedation, decreased locomotor activity, decreased self-stimulation (Goodman and Gilman, 1975), decreased conditioned
responses, and antagonism of methylphenidate-induced stereotyped gnawing behavior. These are all effects which parallel those of the cholinomimetic drugs (Scheel-Krüger, 1971).

In man, the psychologic side effects of reserpine are remarkably
similar to those of centrally acting parasympathetic agents, and include depression of mood, nightmares, lethargy, anergy, and sleepiness
(Goodman and Gilman, 1975). Antipsychotic drugs, which block central
dopamine activity and increase acetylcholine activity can, in selected
patients, also cause at least some of the components of clinical depression, such as dysphoria and motor retardation. Thus, Van Putten
and May (1978) reported that a subgroup of antipsychotic drug treated
schizophrenics developed an 'akinetic depression,' which was reversible following administration of anticholinergic agents. However, in
contrast, Singh (1976) has noted some instances of neuroleptic-induced
euphoria, and furthermore, Singh (1976) and Singh and Kay (1979) did
not find the association between dysphoria, depression and extrapyramidal symptoms that Van Putten and May did. Rather, they found this
phenomenon to be related to an increase in resting pulse from a high
baseline, a phenomenon consistent with the central hypertensive and
tachycardiac effects of cholinomimetics (Risch et al., 1981a).

3.2.   Cholinergic Effects of Lithium Carbonate

Although the effects of lithium have often been conceptualized
as antiadrenergic, and consistent with a catecholamine hypothesis of
affective disorders, some findings from basic neurophysiology and behavioral neuropharmacology suggest that lithium may also affect central cholinergic processes (Pestronk and Drachman, 1980; Janowsky
et al., 1979b).

On the one hand, there is evidence that lithium decreases acetylcholine activity. In neurochemical and electrophysiologic studies,
lithium usually decreases acetylcholine efflux and acetylcholine turnover and increases intraneuronal acetylcholine in the brain. Also
following lithium administration, a decrease in postsynaptic peripher-

al cholinergic receptors has been reported (Pestronk and Drachman, 1980; Neil et al., 1976). Consistent with the possibility that lithium can antagonize central acetylcholine activity is the report that physostigmine's ability to antagonize methylphenidate-induced gnawing in rats was found to be partially reversed by sustained lithium pretreatment (Janowsky et al., 1979b).

Conversely, there is also evidence that treatment with lithium facilitates acetylcholine activity. Thus, for example, lithium treatment increased the lethality of physostigmine (Samples et al., 1977). Similarly, Jope et al. (1980) and Hanin (1982) have noted that red blood cell choline levels in man and brain acetylcholine turnover in rats increased dramatically with lithium pretreatment, a phenomenon which took about two weeks to reach a plateau and which paralleled in time lithium's antimanic effects (Domino et al., 1980). Thus, it appears that lithium ion profoundly affects acetylcholine, although the direction of the effect is uncertain and may depend on the length of lithium administration and the model used to test the interaction.

The implications of the above described research are uncertain with respect to an adrenergic-cholinergic balance hypothesis of affective disorders. If lithium indeed increases central acetylcholine activity, a rationale for its antimanic properties would be obvious within the context of an adrenergic-cholinergic balance hypothesis (Samples et al., 1977). However, such an effect would not explain lithium's ability to antagonize and prevent depression. Were lithium able to decrease acetylcholine activity and to also decrease norepinephrine activity, as postulated elsewhere (Janowsky et al., 1979b), its effects on mania and depression could be rationally explained.

4.   GENERAL EFFECTS OF CHOLINOMIMETICS IN MAN

4.1. Previous Studies

Some of the most convincing evidence that central cholinergic influences may play a role in the regulation of affect comes from descriptions of the psychologic effects of centrally acting cholinesterase inhibitors in man. Between 1950 and 1970, Rowntree et al., (1950), studying normals, depressives, and manics; Gershon and Shaw (1961), observing insecticide-poisoned normals; and Bowers et al. (1964), observing normals, reported that cholinesterase inhibitors exert anergic-inhibitory effects, as well as intensifying and inducing depressive symptoms and antagonizing manic symptoms.

4.2. Recent Studies

More recently, Janowsky et al. (1973a) gave intravenous physostigmine (a centrally acting cholinesterase inhibitor) and neostigmine (a similar cholinesterase inhibitor which does not cross the

blood brain barrier) to patients to study the behavioral sequelae to
central cholinergic stimulation. Physostigmine, in contrast to neostigmine or placebo, was found to rapidly exert behavioral effects in
virtually all patients who received it. These inhibitory effects
consisted of lethargy, anergy, feelings of tiredness, psychomotor
retardation, feelings of being drained, the perception of having no
thoughts or decreased thoughts, and social withdrawal, as well as
occasional late onset nausea or vomiting. Behavioral changes occurred
within 5 to 15 minutes of physostigmine administration, lasted between
20 and 90 minutes (corresponding to physostigmine's pharmacokinetic
profile), and were rapidly antagonized by small doses of the centrally
active antimuscarinic drug, atropine. The fact that atropine reversed
physostigmine's obvious behavioral effects suggests that these occur
via a muscarinic mechanism.

However, physostigmine-released acetylcholine also activates central nicotinic receptors, which generally are thought to cause euphoria or antianxiety effects. It is thus possible that physostigmine
causes opposite effects via muscarinic and nicotinic receptors, but
that the muscarinic receptor stimulation overbalances the nicotinic
effects.

5.   EFFECTS OF PHYSOSTIGMINE ON MANIC SYMPTOMS

Consistent with an adrenergic-cholinergic hypothesis of affective
disorders, and with the work of Rowntree et al. (1950), Janowsky et
al. (1973a) also found that physostigmine caused a dramatic but brief
reduction in hypomanic and manic symptoms in bipolar patients, whereas
placebo and neostigmine produced no such changes. Physostigmine rapidly converted mania to a syndrome consistent with a psychomotor retarded depression. After physostigmine, manics became significantly
less talkative, euphoric, active, cheerful, happy, friendly, or grand-
iose, and showed a decrease in flight of ideas. Patients also reported inhibitory symptoms, such as feeling drained, being without energy,
becoming apathetic, and having 'no thoughts,' and their responses frequently included depression, including crying and sadness. This observation was subsequently confirmed by others, with Modestin et al.
(1973a,b) showing a lessening of mania following physostigmine administration, Davis et al. (1978) reporting that physostigmine had significant and dramatic effects on a subgroup of manic patients who
showed low anger and irritability levels, and Carroll et al. (1973)
and Shopsin et al. (1975) showing a decrease in the mood and motor
components of mania after physostigmine, although not in manic thought
content as such.

In addition to alleviating manic symptoms, Shopsin, Janowsky and
colleagues (Shopsin et al., 1975) studied the late effects of relatively high doses of physostigmine in three manic patients. All initially developed the 'physostigmine inhibitory syndrome,' in addition

to a decrease in certain manic symptoms such as hyperactivity, cheerfulness, flight of ideas, tangentiality, pressure of speech and
talkativeness. In addition, in two subjects, a late rebound into a
'hypermanic state' occurred, with a marked exacerbation of mania
beyond baseline levels. This observation paralleled Fibiger's et al.
(1971) study in rats showing that although physostigmine initially
caused behavioral inhibition, a rebound increase in locomotor activity
occurred later, which was postulated due to compensatory increases in
adrenergic activity.

6.   EFFECTS OF PHYSOSTIGMINE AND ARECOLINE ON DEPRESSIVE SYMPTOMS

Physostigmine has also been found to cause a depressed mood,
possibly by shifting adrenergic-cholinergic balance to a cholinergic
predominance. Thus, consistent with work using other cholinesterase
inhibitors (Rowntree et al., 1950; Gershon and Shaw, 1961), Janowsky,
Davis and colleagues (1972a, 1973a) and later Davis et al. (1978) and
Modestin et al. (1973a) found induction of depressive symptoms in a
subgroup of actively ill manics given physostigmine, as well as in a
larger group of psychiatric patients including depressives and schizo-
affectives who had an affective component to their illness (Janowsky
et al., 1973b). Similar effects have been found in depressives given
the directly acting cholinergic agonist arecoline (Risch et al., unpublished data, 1982; Janowsky et al., 1982). Furthermore, physostigmine caused depression in the majority of a group of euthymic bipolar
patients maintained on lithium (Oppenheimer et al., 1979). Also,
Risch, Janowsky and colleagues (Risch et al., 1981b) have more recently discovered that some normals given physostigmine, as well as those
given arecoline, also become depressed, as will be described subsequently (Risch et al., unpublished data, 1982; Janowsky et al., 1982),
and that normals receiving marijuana pretreatment become profoundly
depressed after receiving physostigmine (El-Yousef et al., 1973).

7.   MOOD EFFECTS OF ACETYLCHOLINE PRECURSORS

Depressive moods have also been observed in subjects receiving
acetylcholine precursors such as deanol, choline, and lecithin. Davis
et al. (1979) and Tamminga et al. (1976) found an increase in depressive symptoms in schizophrenics with tardive dyskinesia treated with
choline, and others have noted, in a minority of cases, that depression is a side effect of choline and lecithin treatments used in
attempt to reverse the memory deficits of Alzheimer's disease. Furthermore, Casey (1979) has observed induction of depressed mood and,
in some cases, a paradoxical hypomania, in a minority of tardive dyskinesia patients treated with deanol. Thus, acetylcholine precursors
generally induce depressive symptoms, a finding consistent with an
adrenergic-cholinergic balance hypothesis, although the induction of
hypomanic symptoms is not consistent with such a simple explanation

of mood regulation. Conversely, Cohen et al. (1980) have independently reported preliminary data suggesting that administration of
the choline precursor lecithin may have antimanic effects in manic
subjects.

8.   SPECIFIC VS NON-SPECIFIC EFFECTS OF CHOLINOMIMETICS

      Physostigmine could cause its anergic, dysphoric and neuroendoc-
trine effects by inducing nausea or a syndrome akin to motion sickness.
We have doubted this possibility because the behavioral effects of
physostigmine usually precede the nauseating effects. Recently, however, we have made two observations which also help to refute a nausea
etiology for physostigmine's mode of action. First, in a subgroup of
inpatients recently studied at the University of California, San
Diego, physostigmine infusion caused increased negative affect and
anergia, increased cortisol and prolactin levels, and increased pulse
and blood pressure, without causing any nausea or emesis whatsoever,
although lightheadedness, and dizziness did occur. Second, Dr. Samuel
Craig Risch, giving arecoline to normals and affective disorder patients, observed induction of affective changes, as well as increases
in ACTH, cortisol, and beta-endorphin, without his subjects developing
nausea, and indeed, without the subjects being able to distinguish
arecoline from placebo (Risch et al., unpublished observations, 1982).
Nevertheless, it is possible that the subjective experience of physostigmine intoxication may be a stress as such, especially in patients
who are depressed or dysphoric to start with. Furthermore, it is
possible that increasing acetylcholine actually sets in motion the
neurochemistry and endocrinology of stress, with stress actually being
regulated by cholinergic mechanisms.

9.   DIFFERENTIAL BEHAVIORAL SENSITIVITY OF AFFECTIVE DISORDER
      PATIENTS TO CHOLINOMIMETIC DRUGS

9.1. Previous Studies of Behavioral Hypersensitivity

      The above paragraphs have indicated that manipulations of cholin-
ergic-adrenergic balance can cause depressive symptoms and antagonize
mania in man, and exert parallel effects in animals. However, such
manipulations could merely be a pharmacologic model of affective
states. They do not necessarily support the existence of a specific
defect of neurotransmitter function in affective disorder patients.
It is important, therefore, to determine if altered cholinergic function or adrenergic-cholinergic balance differentiates affective disorder patients from individuals without affective disease.

      Much literature suggests that the mood depressant effects of
various drugs may be specific to patients with affective disorder.
For example, individuals with a history of depression and/or a family

history of depression more often develop depressive responses to
reserpine, while anergy and lethargy, but not usually depression, are
noted in non-affective disorder patients. Similarly, there is growing evidence that affective disorder patients may be more sensitive
or vulnerable to the mood depressing and other effects of cholinomimetics than are other psychiatric patients or normals. Janowsky
et al. (1973b) noted that while almost all psychiatric inpatients
studied developed an inhibitory or anergic syndrome after receiving
physostigmine, a group of patients with depression, mania or a schizoaffective diagnosis, when compared to schizophrenics without a significant mood component to their illness, became significantly more sad
and depressed.

9.2.   Behavioral Hypersensitivity Studies in Affective Disorder
Patients

At the University of California at San Diego (U.C.S.D.), we have
recently studied the possibility that there is a selective exaggerated
responsiveness in affective disorder patients to the mood depressant
effects of intravenous physostigmine infusion (Risch et al., 1981a).
To date, 65 psychiatric inpatients have been studied after being classified by Research Diagnostic Criteria (RDC) following a Schedule of
Affective Disorder and Schizophrenia (SADS) diagnostic interview. The
primary psychiatric diagnoses were as follows: 32 patients had affective disorders (major affective disorder = 17; bipolar, manic type =
6; bipolar, depressed type = 9) and 36 additional psychiatric patients
were without affective disorder (schizoaffective disorder = 7; schizophrenia = 4; alcoholism = 8; drug use disorder = 3, other psychiatric
disorder = 14).

All subjects were kept medication-free for at least one week.
Using a double-blind counterbalanced order design, all were pretreated with IM methscopolamine (0.75 mg) or oral probanthene (45 mg),
administered prior to physostigmine (0.022 mg/kg) and placebo infusion.
Repeated blood samples were obtained at -30, -15, and -1 minutes before, and at +0, +10, +20, +30, +45 and +60 minutes after physostigmine and placebo infusions. At -15 minutes before and +10 and +60
minutes after experimental drug infusion, subjects rated themselves
and were rated using observer (BPRS, observer Activation Inhibition,
Beigel-Murphy Mania Scale) and self-rating scales (Subject Activation-
Inhibition, POMS).

Physostigmine caused a number of statistically significant
(p<0.01 to p<0.001) main effects including decreases on the Beigel-
Murphy Arousal and Activation subscales, the Euphoria-Grandiosity sub-
scale, and the Total Mania Scale, as well as significant increases on
the NIMH Anergia and Depression subscales, and the NIMH Total Scale.
On the Janowsky-Davis Activation-Inhibition Scale, rater-evaluated
and self-rated inhibition and dysphoria increased, and activation
decreased. Self-rated POMS Vigor, Elation and Friendliness subscales

significantly decreased and Tension-Anxiety, Depression-Dejection, Anger-Hostility, Fatigue and Confusion-Bewilderment subscales significantly increased.

Physostigmine differentiated the affective disorder patients on a number of behavioral variables. Behavioral hyper-responsiveness was generally noted in the patients with affective disorders, compared with a group of patients with non-affective psychiatric diagnoses. Thus, rater evaluated inhibition, patient-rated activation, and POMS anxiety, depression, hostility, confusion, and elation subscales statistically significantly differentiated ($p < 0.05$) the patient groups with one or another of the affective disorder diagnoses from other psychiatric patient groups, with the affective patients showing greater increases in negative affect and behavioral inhibition. With respect to differential behavioral effects of physostigmine within affective disorder diagnostic subgroups, the number of patients in each subgroup is too small to make definitive statements. However, it appears that a trend exists for patients with bipolar disease to show less physostigmine-induced negative affect than do patients with unipolar affective disorder.

Thus, our recent results show that, as a group, patients with affective disorder diagnoses are significantly more reactive to physostigmine's dysphoric and behavioral inhibition inducing effects than are other psychiatric patients. Consistent with this possibility, Oppenheimer et al. (1979) noted that a significant proportion of a small group of euthymic bipolar patients receiving lithium became depressed after receiving physostigmine, while normal controls receiving physostigmine did not. Also, Casey (1979) noted that those patients with a strong history of affective disorder selectively showed affective symptoms while receiving deanol for tardive dyskinesia, in contrast to patients without a history of affective disorder.

With respect to normals, Davis et al. (1976) and Greden (personal communication) noted no significant increases in depression in a group of normals receiving physostigmine, thus suggesting a relative lack of responsiveness to physostigmine in normals. However, during the past two years we have studied nine normals exactly as we had the methscopolamine pretreated psychiatric patients studied at U.C.S.D. and described above, except that 0.033 mg/kg intravenous physostigmine was given. Overall, the nine normal subjects showed statistically significant increases in self and observer-rated negative affect on the BPRS, POMS, and Activation-Inhibition rating scales (Risch et al., 1981b). Although there was a statistically significant negative affect inducing effect of physostigmine, this could be accounted for by only three of the nine normal subjects who obviously became dysphoric and depressed, while the other subjects became only mildly depressed, or merely experienced the non-specific, general inhibitory syndrome associated with physostigmine administration.

     More recently, we have been studying the effects of physostigmine
(0.022 mg/kg) in normals, screened using a SADS interview so as to
have no history of mood disorder. We have to date evaluated 20 normal
males. As with the nine NIMH normals given the 0.033 mg/kg dose of
physostigmine, overall statistically significant increases in self and
observer-rated negative affect and anergia have been found. Preliminary analysis of these results, compared with those occurring in the
similarly treated affective disorder patients described above, suggest
that the affective disorder patients are somewhat more reactive to
physostigmine than are the normals, but not nearly as dramatically so
as compared to non-affective disorder patients.

     The possibility that physostigmine may behaviorally differentiate
patients with an affective disorder diagnosis receives parallel support from the work of Edelstein et al. (1981). These investigators
used physostigmine in an attempt to differentiate schizophrenic patients who were responsive to lithium carbonate therapy from those for
whom lithium was not helpful. Presumably, lithium-responsive patients
represent an affective disorder variant. These investigators found
that patients who responded to physostigmine with a clearing of psychotic symptoms were significantly more likely to respond to a trial
of lithium than those who did not so respond.

9.3.   Physiologic and Neuroendocrine Hypersensitivity to
           Cholinomimetics in Patients with Affective Disorder

9.3.1.   Physiologic Studies

     With respect to physiologic hyper-responsiveness to cholinomi-
metics in affective disorder patients, Sitaram et al. (1980, 1982)
found that REM latency, an acetylcholine-sensitive sleep parameter
which is decreased by acetylcholine and increased by adrenergic
agents, and which is decreased in depression, shortened significantly
more following arecoline infusion in patients with an affective disorder diagnosis and in patients who had anorexia nervosa associated
with a history of having had an affective disorder episode, than in
normals and in 'pure' anorexia nervosa patients. They found that this
vulnerability to the effects of cholinomimetic drug occurred whether
or not their patients with an affective disorder diagnosis had remitted clinically, and whether or not they had been drug-free for a
period of months. Similarly, Sitaram (1982) has recently noted an
increased degree of pupillary constriction following instillation of
pilocarpine into the eyes of patients with affective disorder diagnoses, as compared to normals. Likewise, Janowsky et al. (1982),
using the patients described above, have reported that affective disorder patients are more prone to suffer nausea after a physostigmine
infusion than are normals or non-affective disorder patients: and M.
Berger et al. (unpublished observations, 1982) have found that
physostigmine induces awakening during the early phases of sleep more

frequently in affective disorder patients than in normals.

Finally, a growing body of information suggests that red blood cell choline utilization may reflect central acetylcholine dynamics. Hanin (1982) has observed that a subpopulation of patients with depression appeared to have high red blood cell choline levels, and Jope et al. (1980) noted that a subpopulation of manics with little likelihood of having been pretreated with lithium also had increased red blood cell choline levels, a finding not replicated in another study.

9.3.2. Neuroendocrine Studies

In addition to physiologic and behavioral parameters, evidence is accumulating that a neuroendocrine strategy may be useful in delineating the differential sensitivity to cholinergic drugs in patients with affective disorders. Here, as with similar strategies exploring the role of dopamine, norepinephrine and other neurotransmitter systems in affective and schizophrenic disorders, the differential effects between diagnostic groups of an acetylcholine altering drug on neuroendocrine function may lead to clues as to the role of acetylcholine in the affective disorders, and provide diagnostic markers of these disorders.

For example, there is animal evidence that cholinergic mechanisms may regulate prolactin secretion. Atropine inhibits the nocturnal surge and the proestrus prolactin surge in cycling rats (Blake and Sawyer, 1972; Grandison and Meites, 1976a,b; Blake et al., 1973, Subramanian and Gala, 1976; Libertun and McCann, 1973; 1974), and Gibbs et al. (1979) have shown that intraventricular injection of acetylcholine in rats resulted in a marked increase of prolactin secretion. On the other hand, cholinergic agonists have been reported to inhibit ovarian hormone-linked prolactin release (Grandison and Meites, 1976a; Blake et al., 1973).

Growth hormone is also affected by cholinergic drugs. Some studies show that cholinomimetics increase growth hormone levels in rats, an effect reversed by atropine (Bruni and Meites, 1978; Mendelson et al., 1981). Other evidence exists that cholinomimetics either have no effect, or a blunting effect on growth hormone (Kato et al., 1974; Burnett et al., 1978).

With respect to the hypothalamic-pituitary-adrenal axis, a number of in vitro studies support a role for acetylcholine in the regulation of ACTH secretion. In vitro preparations of rat hypothalamus show that cortocotropin releasing factor (CRF) is released in a dose dependent manner by acetylcholine (Bradbury et al., 1974; Edwardson and Bennett, 1974; Hillhouse et al., 1975), and acetylcholine-induced release of hypothalamic CRF was found to be inhibited by norepinephrine (Jones et al., 1969). Carbachol, implanted in the hypothalamus of a variety of animal species induces the release of corticosteroids from the adrenal, presumably via ACTH release (Naumenko, 1968; Endroczi et al., 1963; Krieger and Krieger, 1970), and conversely, hypothalamic implantation of atropine prevents stress-induced ACTH release (Hedge and Smelik, 1968; Kaplanski and Smelik, 1973; Hedge and De Weid, 1971). Also, the intravenous administration of cholinergic agonists in rats and dogs results in adrenocortical activation and the increased release of 17-OH-corticosteroids (Otsuka, 1966; Suzuki et al., 1975), an effect blocked by hypophysectomy or radiation-induced lesions of the anterior median eminence (Suzuki et al., 1975, 1964). Carbachol, injected into the lateral ventricles of rats, also results in activation of the hypothalamic-pituitary-adrenal axis. In man, inhalation of nicotine produces a dose dependent increase in serum cortisol (Hill and Wynder, 1974), and galanthamine, a centrally active acetylcholinesterase inhibitor, also increases serum cortisol concentrations (Cozanitis, 1974).

Central cholinergic mechanisms have also been implicated in the circadian variation of cortisol secretion. In both the cat (Krieger and Krieger, 1967; Krieger et al., 1968) and man (Ferrari et al., 1977), atropine given during a critical evening period blocks the subsequent diurnal rise in serum cortisol, while atropine, administered at other times, has no effect on the circadian periodicity of adrenal cortisol secretion.

Several studies (Janowsky et al., 1980; Risch et al., 1981a; Davis and Davis, 1979) have explored the effects of cholinomimetic drugs on neuroendocrine activity. We have recently studied the effects of physostigmine (0.022 mg/kg) on serum neurohormones in subgroups of the same patients described above, in whom we evaluated behavioral and physiological measures.

Serum samples were obtained sequentially, as described above, before and after placebo and physostigmine infusion and analyzed for serum prolactin, growth hormone and cortisol using radioimmunoassays (Risch et al., 1981a). Overall physostigmine caused significant increases in serum prolactin, cortisol, and growth hormone, and in the small number of cases in which it was assayed, serum luteinizing hormone did not change. These results are similar to the findings of Davis and Davis (1979), who found increased growth hormone, prolactin, and cortisol following physostigmine infusion.

In addition, decreases in positive mood and increases in self-rated negative affect caused by physostigmine were found to be correlated negatively and positively, respectively, with serum prolactin changes; and affective disorder patients showed significantly greater increases in prolactin after physostigmine than did non-affective disorder patients and normal controls. Furthermore, serum cortisol levels increased significantly more in affective disorder patients than in normal controls (Janowsky et al., 1982).

Similarly, we also found significant neuroendocrine effects in
the nine normal volunteers studied at NIMH who received the higher
(0.033 mg/kg) physostigmine dose. Physostigmine here again caused a
dramatic rise in serum prolactin, cortisol and growth hormone levels,
similar to our results in affective disorder patients. Associated
with the physostigmine-induced alterations in mood and behavioral in-
hibitions in the NIMH normals and in the subjects studied at U.C.S.D.
have been significant increases in plasma beta-endorphin and plasma
ACTH (Risch et al., 1980, 1982a).

In the NIMH normals, physostigmine associated increases in negative affect were highly correlated with increases in plasma beta-
endorphin and ACTH immunoreactivity. Plasma ACTH changes were also
highly correlated with plasma beta-endorphin changes, thus making ACTH
and beta-endorphin likely candidates as potential markers for physostigmine's differential cholinergic effects. Plasma beta-endorphin
and prolactin were likewise highly correlated, and we have suggested
that cholinergically stimulated increases in beta-endorphin are responsible for the stimulation of prolactin release (Risch et al.,
1982b).

More recently, we have demonstrated in a subset of the patients
studied at U.C.S.D. and receiving a 0.022 mg/kg dose of physostigmine,
that affective disorder patients show greater increases in beta-endorphin and serum ACTH immunoreactivity than do normals or nonaffective
disorder patients after the infusion of physostigmine (Risch et al.,
1982c; Janowsky et al., 1982).

Thus, it appears that physostigmine-induced increases in hypothalamic-pituitary-adrenal function parallel other phenomena noted in
endogenous depression, such as increased afternoon cortisol secretion
and cortisol resistance to suppression by dexamethasone (Carroll et
al. 1978). Possibly, the physostigmine-induced changes in ACTH, cortisol, and beta-endorphin ultimately will have diagnostic implications
similar to the observations in hypothalamic-pituitary-adrenal function
noted by others in affective disorder patients, and may suggest that
the hypothalamic-pituitary-adrenal alterations seen in depression have
a cholinergic component.

In spite of considerable converging evidence suggesting that cholinergic hypersensitivity occurs in affective disorder patients, some
caution is indicated in interpreting these findings. The major behavioral study described above by the authors did not show dramatic differences between normals and actively ill affective disorder patients,
and it is possible that the relatively dramatic differences between
affective disorder patients and other psychiatric patients lies in a
resistance to muscarinic agents in non-affective disorder psychiatric
inpatients, as has been noted in chronic non-paranoid schizophrenics
(Singh and Lal, 1982). Significantly, Nurnberger et al. (1982a) have
found no blood pressure, cortisol, prolactin, growth hormone, and

behavioral differences between the effects of arecoline in normals and euthymic affective disorder patients. Similarly, Berger et al. (1982) did not find an increased ability of physostigmine to reverse dexamethasone suppression in depressives. Furthermore, even when cholinergic hypersensitivity appears a feature of the affective disorder patient, the finding may reflect a tendency for norepinephrine or epinephrine to be turned off or to be antagonized, rather than a cholinergic hypersensitivity. To this end, Janowsky et al. (1982), reporting work by G. Groom, have noted that rat brain beta-adrenergic receptors are decreased in number and increased in their affinity for beta-adrenergic ligands 40 minutes after administration of physostigmine 0.8 mg/kg to Sprague Dawley rats.

Similarly, caution is necessary in interpreting the above described neuroendocrine and physiological results beyond their significance as markers of affective disorder. Whether relatively greater increases in serum cortisol, ACTH, prolactin, beta-endorphin; and nausea and the greater decreases in REM latency and pupillary contraction reflect true cholinergic supersensitivity in affective disorder patients, or whether balancing neurotransmitters such as norepinephrine, or systems mediating punishment and stress, are hyper-responsive in affective disorder patients cannot be ascertained from the above studies. Furthermore, with respect to the theoretical aspects of these findings, we have not noted prolactin, ACTH, and beta-endorphin blunting in acute manics after physostigmine infusion, as would be theoretically expected. Further studies will help clarify such issues.

10. MONOAMINE-ACETYLCHOLINE INTERACTIONS

Although our data suggest that affective disorder patients may have relatively exaggerated neuroendocrine and behavioral responses to a physostigmine infusion, it is also true that considerable heterogeneity of response exists within diagnostic subgroups, and that much overlap of patient values exists between the individuals in each group. This variability could derive in part from the relationship of acetylcholine to other neurotransmitter systems. Indeed, evidence exists which is consistent with this view.

10.1 Catecholaminergic-Cholinergic Interactions

A pharmacologic-behavioral model for naturally occurring adrenergic-cholinergic nervous system regulation of behavior may be found in the interactions and reciprocal effects of psychostimulants and cholinomimetics. Janowsky et al. (1972b) and others have noted that a model of schizophrenia, methylphenidate-induced stereotyped behavior and increased locomotion in rats (thought to represent a hyperdopaminergic phenomenon) is effectively antagonized by physostigmine, but not by neostigmine.

Likewise, methylphenidate-induced psychomotor stimulation in manic and schizophrenic patients (i.e., increased talkativeness, elevated mood, interpersonal interactions in manics, as well as activation of psychosis in schizophrenics) can be rapidly antagonized by physostigmine administration. Conversely, physostigmine's inhibitory-depressant effects can be reversed by methylphenidate administration (Janowsky et al., 1973c).

Possibly related to the ability of physostigmine to antagonize methylphenidate-induced psychomotor stimulation is the observation of Ostrow et al. (1980) that physostigmine infusion caused a rapid and dramatic drop in serum MHPG, presumed to reflect high central noradrenergic activity, in one of their extremely ill manic patients, associated with induction of a tearful depressed state and improvement in manic thinking.

Furthermore, there is evidence that a reciprocal relationship exists between a patient's response to a psychomotor stimulant and his separate response to a cholinomimetic agent. In one study by Nurnberger et al. (1982b), a negative correlation was noted between amphetamine-induced excitation in a given subject and the ability of arecoline given on another occasion to decrease REM latency. We have noted that in 26 psychiatric patients having a variety of psychiatric diagnoses, administration of 0.5 mg/kg dose of oral methylphenidate correlates with physostigmine (0.022 mg/kg) effects in the following way. Patients who have an intense inhibitory and negative affective response to physostigmine tend to show lower elevations of systolic blood pressure and self-rated positive mood ratings, and increased depression and anxiety after methylphenidate ingestion (Janowsky et al., 1982). Similarly, Siever et al. (1981) showed that in a mixed group of eight affective disorder patients and normals, those who had the most dramatic cholinomimetic induced anergy and negative affect showed a blunted growth hormone response to clonidine.

Thus, the interaction and reciprocal relationship between cholinomimetics and psychostimulants, as they affect or relate to each other in man, could suggest an adrenergic-cholinergic continuum model of behavior, in which behavior ranges from adrenergic activation (increased thoughts, cheerfulness, talkativeness, emotionality, mania, etc.) to cholinergic inhibition (decreased thoughts, dysphoria, lethargy, anergy, and depression). Clinically such a continuum could determine a normal individual's relative aggressiveness, talkativeness, and activation, and in the manic-depressive, such a balance could determine whether a psychiatric patient was activated and manic, or motor retarded and depressed.

10.2. Serotonergic-Cholinergic Interactions

In addition to adrenergic-cholinergic interactions, recent findings of decreased platelet serotonin uptake in depression prompted us

to examine platelet serotonin uptake after administration of physostigmine, since it is possible that serotonergic-cholinergic balance
may also regulate affect. To investigate the effect of physostigmine
on platelet serotonin uptake, ten subjects were administered intravenous physostigmine (0.022 mg/kg) using a double-blind, placebo controlled crossover design, using a platelet serotonin uptake analysis
described previously (Rausch et al., 1982). Analysis of variance
revealed a significant drug by time interaction, such that platelet
serotonin uptake was lower after physostigmine in comparison to placebo. Thus, physostigmine lowers platelet serotonin uptake in the
direction that occurs naturally in patients with depression. In addition, several significant correlations between physostigmine-induced
inhibition of platelet serotonin uptake and physostigmine-induced behavioral changes were found.

11. MOOD EFFECTS OF CENTRALLY ACTIVE ANTICHOLINERGIC AGENTS

In addition to the mood lowering and antimanic effects of cholinomimetic drugs, there is some evidence, albeit not from well-control-
led studies, that centrally active anticholinergic drugs have mood
elevating properties. Anticholinergic antiParkinsonian agents, given
to treat drug-induced Parkinsonian symptoms, may cause a feeling of
euphoria, associated with a sense of well-being, increased sociabil-
ity, and even a reversal of depressed feelings (Jellenek et al., 1981;
Smith, 1980). Furthermore, these euphoric effects can occur in patients who have not previously taken neuroleptics. In addition, several old reports suggest that high doses of atropine and other anticholinergics may cause alleviation of depression, and more recent reports have been published indicating that a tricyclic antidepressant-
induced central anticholinergic syndrome may alleviate depression
(Hoch and Maas, 1932; Abood and Medina, 1958; Finkelstein, 1961;
English, 1962; Safer and Allen, 1971). Furthermore, in the last year,
two reports have suggested that the anti-Parkinsonian agents biperiden
and trihexylphenidyl may be useful in alleviating depression. Conversely, neuroleptic treated patients may develop some aspects of depression including a depressed mood and hypoactivity several weeks
after discontinuing anticholinergic medications (Jellenek et al.,
1981), which is preventable with continued anticholinergic treatment.

12. DISCUSSION

As reviewed above, considerable evidence exists suggesting that
the cholinergic nervous system, alone and/or interacting with serotonin, catecholaminergic or other neurotransmitters, may have an
important role in the regulation of affect. Nevertheless, as with
all currently proposed biological hypotheses as to the etiology of
affective disorders, alternative explanations of the above data, and
data inconsistent with the above adrenergic-cholinergic balance
hypothesis do exist.

For example, antidepressant drugs do not consistently have equal degrees of anticholinergic activity, and indeed trazodone, a proven effective antidepressant, has virtually no anticholinergic properties. Furthermore, although atropine easily reverses the mood depressing effects of cholinomimetics, atropine is not known to be an immediately effective antidepressant, as is, for example, amphetamine. Furthermore, the most frequent effects of high doses of centrally acting anticholinergic drugs are hallucinations and agitation, rather than mood effects and euphoria. Conversely, although the antimanic and mood depressant effects of centrally acting cholinomimetic drugs are profound and obvious, it is possible that these drugs may cause their effects either by increasing acetylcholine's effects on other neurotransmitters such as norepinephrine, GABA or serotonin, or by affecting other aspects of neuronal function, such as membranes, nucleotides, or other neurotransmitters than those directly moderated by acetylcholine.

Thus, it is certainly possible that pharmacologically-induced changes in acetylcholine may be the cause of perturbations in other systems which are etiologic of affective disorders, and that acetylcholine alterations, secondary to cholinomemetics, may indirectly cause 'model depression' and excessively perturb the governing neurotransmitters of depression in affective disorder patients, but may not directly cause endogenous depression. Consistent with this possibility, it is worth noting that the EEG effects of anticholinergic and cholinomimetics most closely parallel the naturally occurring EEG's of schizophrenics, rather than affective disorder patients; and anticholinergics have not been noted to date to intensify mania, as do these agents intensify schizophrenic symptoms (Singh and Kay, Chapter 9).

However, even if cholinomimetics can only cause a 'model depression,' understanding this phenomena may ultimately offer important clues, and a window into the pathophysiology of affective disorders. If acetylcholine is not causally involved in the etiology of affective disorders, understanding the 'downstream' implications of cholinomimetics may give clues to the actual neurobiology of affective disorders. Alternatively, it is not beyond possibility that acetylcholine, or monoaminergic-cholinergic balance, actually is partially or fundamentally involved in the etiology, and/or the expression of the affective disorders.

REFERENCES

Abood, L. C., and Meduna, L. L., 1958, Some effects of a new psychotogen in depressive states, J. Nerv. Ment. Dis. 127:546-550.
Berger, M., Doerr, P., Lund, R., Bronisch, T., and Zerssen, D. von, 1982, Neuroendokrinologische befund und polygraphische schlafuntersuchungen bei patienten mit depressiven syndromen, in "Fortschritte Psychiatrischer Forschung," H. Beckman, ed., Huber-Verlag, Bern.

Blake, C. A., Norman, R. L., Scaramuzzi, R. J., and Sawyer, C. H., 1973, Inhibition of the proestrous surge of prolactin in the rat by nicotine, Endocrinology 92(5):1334-1342.

Blake, C. A., and Sawyer, C. H., 1972, Nicotine blocks the suckling induced rise in circulating prolactin in lactating rats, Science 177:619-621.

Bloom, F. E., Segal, D., Ling, N., and Guillemin, R., 1976, Endorphins: profound behavioral effects in rats suggest new etiological factors in mental illness, Science 194:630-633.

Bowers, M. B., Goodman, E., and Sim, V. M., 1964, Some behavioral changes in man following anticholinesterase administration, J. Nerv. Ment. Dis. 138:383.

Bradbury, M. W. B., Burden, J., Hillhouse, E. W., and Jones, M. T., 1974, Stimulation electrically and by acetylcholine of the rat hypothalamus in vitro, J. Physiol. (Lond.) 239:269-283.

Bruni, J. F., and Meites, J., 1978, Effects of cholinergic drugs on growth hormone release, Life Sci., 23:1315-1358.

Burnett, G. R., Prange, A. J., Wilson, E. C., and Snyder, S. H., 1978, Neuroendocrine-drug relations in tardive dyskinesia. Presented at the Annual Meeting of the American Psychiatric Association, Atlanta, Georgia.

Carlton, P. L., 1963, Cholinergic mechanisms in the control of behavior by the brain, Psychol. Rev., 70:19-39.

Carroll, B. J., Frazer, A., Schless, A., and Mendels, J., 1973, Cholinergic reversal of manic symptoms, Lancet i:427.

Carroll, B. J., Greden, J. F., Rubin, R. T., Haskett, R., Feinberg, M., and Schteingart, D., 1978, Neurotransmitter mechanism of neuroendocrine disturbances in depression, Acta Endocrinol Suppl. 220:14.

Casey, D. E., 1979, Mood alterations during deanol therapy, Psychopharmacology 62:187-191.

Chase, T. N., and Murphy, D. L., 1973, Serotonin and central nervous system function, Ann. Rev. Pharmacology 13:181-197.

Cohen, B. M., Miller, A. L., Lipinsky, J. F., and Pope, H. G., 1980, Lecithin in mania: a preliminary report, Am. J. Psychiatry 137:242-243.

Cozanitis, D. A., 1974, Galenthamine hydrobromide versus neostigmine, Anaesthesia 29:163-168.

Davis, K. L., Berger, P. A., Hollister, L. E., and Defraites, E., 1978 Physostigmine in man, Arch. Gen. Psychiatry 35:119-122.

Davis, K. L., and Davis, B. M., 1979, Acetylcholine and anterior pituitary hormone secretion, in "Brain Acetylcholine and Neuropsychiatric Disease," K. L. Davis and P. A. Berger, eds., Plenum Press, New York.

Davis K., Hollister, L. E., and Berger, P. A., 1979, Choline chloride in schizophrenia, Am. J. Psychiatry 136:1581-1584.

Davis, K. L., Hollister, L. E., and Overall, J., 1976, Physostigmine effects on cognition and affect normal subjects, Psychopharmacology 51:23-27.

Domino, E. F., and Olds, M. E., 1968, Cholinergic inhibition of self-stimulation behavior, J. Pharm. Exp. Ther. 164:202-211.

Domino, E. F., Riaz, A., Rodin, E., Dementriou, S., Mathews, B., and Tait, S., 1980, Effect of duration of lithium therapy on various psychiatric patients on red blood cell/plasma choline ratio. Presented at the 1980 American College of Neuropsychopharmacology Meeting.

Edelstein, P., Schultz, J. R., Hirschowitz, J., Kanter, D. R., and Garver, D. L., 1981, Physostigmine and lithium response in the schizophrenias, Am. J. Psychiatry 138:1078-1081.

Edwardson, J. A., and Bennett, G. W., 1974, Modulation of corticotropine-releasing factor release from hypothalamic synaptosomes, Nature 251:425-427.

El-Yousef, M., Janowsky, D. S., Davis, J. M., and Rosenblatt, J. E., 1973, Induction of severe depression by physostigmine in marijuana intoxicated individuals, Br. J. Addict. 68:321-325.

Endroczi, E., Schreiberg, G., and Lissak, K., 1963, The role of central nervous activating and inhibitory structures in the control of pituitary-adrenocortical function. Effects of intracerebral cholinergic and adrenergic stimulation, Acta Physiol. Acad. Sci. Hung. 23:211-221.

English, D. C., 1962, Reintegration of affect and psychic emergence with ditran, J. Neuropsychiat. 3:304-310.

Ferrari, E., Bossolo, P. A., Vailati, A., Martinelli, I., Rea., A., and Nosari, I., 1977, Variations ciracadiennes des effets d'une substance vagolytique sur le system ACTH - secretant chez l'homme, Ann. Endocrinol. (Paris) 38:203-213.

Fibiger, H. C., Lynch, G. S., and Cooper, H. P., 1971, A biphasic action of central cholinergic stimulation on behavioral arousal in rat, Psychopharmacologia 20:366-382.

Finkelstein, B., 1961, Ditran, a psychotherapeutic advance: a review of one hundred and three cases., J. Neuropsychiat. 2:144-148.

Gerner, R. H., Catlin, D. H., and Gorlick, D. A., 1981, Beta-endorphin, Arch. Gen. Psychiatry 37:642-647.

Gershon, S., and Shaw, F. H., 1961, Psychiatric sequelae of chronic exposure to organophosphorous insecticides, Lancet i:1371-1374.

Gibbs, D. N., Plotsky, P. M., deGreef, W. J., and Neill, J. D., 1979, Effect of histamine and acetylcholine on hypophyseal stalk plasma dopamine and peripheral prolactin levels, Life Sci. 24:2063-2070.

Goodman, L. S., and Gilman, A., 1975, "The Pharmacological Basis of Therapeutics," 5th Edition, Macmillan, New York.

Grandison, L., and Meites, J., 1976a, Evidence for adrenergic medication of cholinergic inhibition of prolactin release, Endocrinology 99:775-779.

Grandison, L., and Meites, J., 1976b, Inhibition of pseudopregnancy and stress-induced prolactin release in rats by pilocarpine, Fed. Proc. 35:306.

Hanin, I., 1982, RBC choline as a potential marker in psychiatric and neurologic disease, in "Proceedings of the Conference on Biologic Markers in Psychiatry and Neurology," E. Usdin and I. Hanin, eds., Pergamon Press, Oxford.

Hedge, G. A., and DeWeid, D., 1971, Corticotropin and vasopressin se-
    cretion after hypothalamic implantation of atropine, _Endocrinology_
    88:1257-1259.
Hedge, G. A., and Smelik, P. G., 1968, Corticotropin release: inhibi-
    tion by hypothalamic implantation of atropine, _Science_
    159:891-892.
Hernández-Peón, K., 1965, Central neuro-humoral transmission in sleep
    and wakefulness, _Prog. Brain Res._ 18:96-117.
Hill, P., and Wynder, E. L., 1974, Smoking and cardiovascular disease,
    Am. Heart J. 87(4):491-496.
Hillhouse, E. W., Burden, J., and Jones, M. T., 1975, The effect of
    various putative neurotransmitters on the release of corticotropin
    releasing hormone from the hypothalamus of the rat in vitro. I.
    The effect of acetylcholine and noradrenaline, _Neuroendocrinology_
    17(1):1-11.
Hoch, P. H., and Mauss, W., 1932, Atropin behandlung bei geisteckvank-
    heiten (Atropine treatment of depression), _Arch. Psychiatry_
    97:546-552.
Janowsky, D. S., Abrams, A. A., Groom, G. P., Judd, L. L., and
    Clopton, P., 1979b, Lithium administration antagonizes cholinergic
    behavioral effects in rodents, _Psychopharmacology_ 63:147-150.
Janowsky, D. S., Davis, J. M., El-Yousef, M. K., and Sekerke, H. J.,
    1973b, Acetylcholine and depression, _Psychosom. Med._ 35(5):459.
Janowsky, D. S., El-Yousef, M. K., Davis, J. M., and Sekerke, H. J.,
    1972a, A cholinergic-adrenergic hypothesis of mania and depression
    Lancet ii:6732-6735.
Janowsky, D. S., El-Yousef, M. K., Davis, J. M., and Sekerke, H. J.,
    1973c, Antagonistic effects of physostigmine and methylphenidate
    in man, _Am. J. Psychiatry_ 130:1370-1376.
Janowsky, D. S., El-Yousef, M., Davis, J. M., and Sekerke, H. J.,
    1972b, Cholinergic antagonism of methylphenidate-induced stereo-
    typed behavior, _Psychopharmacologia_ 27:295-303.
Janowsky, D. S., El-Yousef, M. K., Davis, J. M., and Sekerke, H. J.,
    1973a, Parasympathetic suppression of manic symptoms by physostig-
    mine, _Arch. Gen. Psychiatry_ 28:542-547.
Janowsky, D. S., Judd, L. L., and Groom, G., 1982, The influence of
    lithium on cholinergic function, in "Proceedings of the 13th
    Collegium Internationale Neuro-Psychopharmacologicum Congress,"
    Jerusalem, Israel.
Janowsky, D. S., Judd, L. L., Huey, L., and Segal, D.S., 1979a,
    Effects of naloxone on normals, manics and schizophrenics, in
    "Endorphins in Mental Health Research," E. Usdin, W. Bunney and
    N. Kline, eds., pp. 435-447, Macmillan, London.
Janowsky, D.S., Risch, S.C., Parker, D., Huey, L., and Judd, L.L.,
    1980, Increased vulnerability to cholinertgic stimulation in
    affect disorder patients, _Psychopharm. Bull._ 16(4):29-31.
Jellinek, T., Gardos, G., and Cole, J., 1981, Adverse effects of anti-
    Parkinsonian drug withdrawal, _Am. J. Psychiatry_ 138:1567-1571.

Jimerson, D. C., Nurnberger, J. I., Jr., Simmons, S., and Gershon,
    E. S., 1982, Anticholinergic treatment for depression, Presented
    at the 1982 American Psychiatric Association Meeting, Toronto,
    Canada, May 15-21.
Jones, M., Hillhouse, E., and Burden, J., 1969, The secretion of
    corticotropin-releasing hormone in vitro, in "Frontiers of
    Neuroendocrinology, Vol. 4," L. Martini and W. Granong, eds.,
    Raven Press, New York.
Jope, R. S., Jenden, D. J., Ehrlich, B. E., Diamond, J. M., and
    Gosenfeld, L. F., 1980, Erythrocyte choline concentrations are
    elevated in manic patients, Proceedings of the National Academy
    of Sciences 77:6144-6166.
Kaplanski, J., and Smelik, P. G., 1973, Analysis of the inhibition of
    ACTH release by hypothalamic implants of atropine, Acta Endocrinol
    73:651-659.
Kasper, S., Moises, H. W., and Beck, H., 1981, The anticholinergic
    biperiden in depressive disorders, Pharmakopsychiatrie 14:195-198.
Kato, Y., Chihara, K., Ohgo, S., and Imura, H., 1974, Effect of nico-
    tine on the secretion of growth hormone and prolactin in rats,
    Neuroendocrinology 16:237-242.
Krieger, H. P., and Krieger, D. T., 1970, Chemical stimulation of the
    brain: effect on adrenal corticoid release, Am. J. Physiol.
    218:1632-1641.
Krieger, D. T., and Krieger, H. P., 1967, Circadian pattern of plasma
    17-hydroxycorticosteroid. Alteration by anticholinergic agents,
    Science 155:1421-1422.
Krieger, D. T., Silverberg, A. I., Rizzo, F., and Krieger, H. P., 1968
    Abbolution of circadian periodicity of plasma 17-OHCS levels in
    the cat, Am. J. Physiol. 125(4):959-968.
Libertun, C., and McCann, S. M., 1973, Blockade of the release of
    gonadotropins and prolactin by subcutaneous or intraventricular
    injection of atropine in male and female rats, Endocrinology
    92(6):1714-1724.
Libertun, C., and McCann, S. M., 1974, Further evidence for cholin-
    ergic control of gonadotropin and prolactin secretion, Proc. Soc.
    Exp. Biol. Med. 147:498-504.
Mandell, A. J., and Knapp, S., 1971, The effects of chronic adminis-
    tration of some cholinergic and adrenergic drugs on the activity
    of choline acetyltransferase in the optic lobe of the chick brain
    Neuropharmacology 10:513-516.
Mendelson, W. G., Lantigua, R. A., Wyatt, R. J., Gillin, J. C., and
    Jacobs, L. S., 1981, Piperadine enhances sleep-related and
    insulin-induced growth hormone secretion: further evidence for a
    cholinergic secretory mechanism, J. Clin. Endocrinol. Metab.
    52:409-415.
Modestin, J. J., Hunger, J., and Schwartz, R. B., 1973a, Uber die
    depressogene wirkung von physostigmine, Arch. Psychiatr. Nervenkr.
    218:67.
Modestin, J. J., Schwartz, R. B., and Hunger, J., 1973b, Zur frage der
    beeinflussung schizophrener symptome physostigmine, Pharmakopsy-
    chiatrie 9:300-304.

Naumenko, E. V., 1968, Hypothalamic chemoreactive structures and the
    regulation of pituitary-adrenal function. Effects of local injec-
    tions of norepinephrine, carbacol and serotonin into the brain of
    guinea pigs with intact brains and after mesencephalic transection
    Brain Res. 11:1-10.
Neil, J. F., Himmelhoch, J. M., and Licata, S. M., 1976, Emergence of
    myasthenia gravis during treatment with lithium carbonate, Arch.
    Gen. Psychiatry 33:1090-1092.
Nurnberger, J., Gershon, E. S., Sitaram, N., Gillin, J. C., Brown, G.,
    Ebert, M., Gold, P., Jimerson, D., and Kessler, L., 1982a, Dextro-
    amphetamine and arecoline as pharmacogenetic probes in normals and
    remitted bipolar patients, Psychopharmacol. Bull. 17:80-82.
Nurnberger, J. I., Jimerson, D. C., Simmons, S., Tamminga, C., Nadi,
    N. S., and Gershon, E. S., 1982b, Responses to arecoline in
    normal twins and "well state" patients with affective disorder,
    Presented at the Society of Biological Society, 13th Annual
    Convention, Toronto.
Olds, J., 1958, Self-stimulation of the brain, Science 127:315-324.
Oppenheimer, G., Ebstein, R., and Belmaker, R., 1979, Effects of
    lithium on the physostigmine-induced behavioral syndrome and
    plasma cyclic GMP, J. Psychiatry Res. 14:133-138.
Ostrow, D. G., Halaris, A., Dysken, M. E., and Davis, J. M., 1980, Ion
    transport and neurotransmitter function in major affective dis-
    orders, Paper presented at the Society of Biological Psychiatry
    Annual Meeting, Boston.
Otsuka, K., 1966, Effects of atropine, eserine and tetramethylammonium
    on the adrenal 17-hydroxycorticosteroid secretion in anaesthetized
    dogs, Tohoku J. Exp. Med. 8:165-170.
Pestronk, A., and Drachman, D. B., 1980, Lith u reduces the number of
    acetylcholine receptors in skeletal muscle, Science 210:342-343.
Pradhan, S. N., and Kavat, K. A., 1972, Action and interaction of
    cholinergic agonists and antagonists on self-stimulation, Arch.
    Int. Pharmacodyn. Ther. 196:321-329.
Rausch, J., Janowsky, D. S., Risch, S. C., Huey, L. Y., and Swanson,
    G. W., 1982, Physostigmine effect on platelet serotonin uptake,
    in "Serotonin in Biological Psychiatry," B. Ho and E. Usdin,
    eds., Raven Press, New York.
Risch, S. C., Cohen, P. M., Janowsky, D. S., Kalin, N. H., Insel, T.
    R., and Murphy, D. L., 1981b, Physostigmine induction of depres-
    sive symptomatology in normal volunteer subjects, J. Psychiat.
    Res. 4:89-94.
Risch, S. C., Cohen, R. M., Janowsky, D. S., Kalin, N. H., and Murphy,
    D. L., 1980, Mood and behavioral effects of physostigmine on
    humans are accompanied by elevations in plasma beta-endorphin and
    cortisone, Science 209:1545-1546.
Risch, S. C., Janowsky, D. S., Judd, L. L., and Huey, L. Y., 1982c,
    Elevated plasma β-endorphin concentrations in depression and cho-
    linergically supersensitive release mechanisms, Psychopharmacol.
    Bull. 18(3):211-216.

Risch, S. C., Janowsky, D. S., Kalin, N. H., Cohen, R. M., Aloi, J. A. and Murphy, D. L., 1982a, Cholinergic β-endorphin hypersensitivity associated with depression, in "Biological Markers in Psychiatry and Neurology," I. Hanin and E. Usdin, eds., Pergamon Press, Oxford.

Risch, S. C., Janowsky, D. S., Siever, L. J., Judd, L. L., Rausch, J. L., Huey, L. Y., Beckman, K. A., Cohen, R. M., and Murphy, D. L., 1982b, Cholinomimetic-induced co-release of prolactin and beta-endorphin in man, Psychopharmacol. Bull. 18(4):21-25.

Risch, S. C., Kalin, N. H., and Janowsky, D. S., 1981a, Cholinergic challenges in affective illness, behavioral and neuroendocrine correlates, J. Clin. Psychopharm. 1:186-192.

Rowntree, D. W., Neven, S., and Wilson, A., 1950, The effects of di-isopropylfluorophosphonate in schizophrenia and manic depressive psychosis, J. Neurol. Neurosurg. Psychiatry 13:47-62.

Safer, D. J., and Allen, R. P., 1971, The central effects of scopola-mine in man, Biol. Psychiatry 3:347-356.

Samples, J., Janowsky, D. S., and Pechnick, R., and Judd, L. L., 1977, Lethal effects of physostigmine plus lithium in rats, Psychopharmacology 52:307-309.

Scheel-Krüger, J., 1971, Comparative studies of various amphetamine analogues demonstrating different interactions with the metabolism of catecholamines in brain, Eur. J. Pharmacol. 14:47-49.

Schildkraut, J. J., 1973, Norepinephrine metabolism in the pathophysi-ology and classification of depressive and manic disorders, in "Psychopathology and Pharmacology," J. Cole, A. Freedman and A. Friedhoff, eds., Johns Hopkins University Press, Baltimore.

Schildkraut, J. J., and Kety, S. S., 1967, Biogenic amines and emotion Science 156:21-30.

Shopsin, B., Janowsky, D. S., Davis, J. M., and Gershon, S., 1975, Rebound phenomena in mania patients following physostigmine, Neuropsychobiology 1:180-187.

Siever, L. J., Risch, S. C., and Murphy, D. L., 1981, Possible con-currence of cholinergic receptor hypersensitivity and adrenergic receptor hyposensitivity in affective disorders, Psychiatry Res. 5:108-109.

Singh, M. M., 1976, Dysphoric response to neuroleptic treatment in schizophrenia and its prognostic significance, Dis. Nerv. Sys. 37:191-196.

Singh, M. M., and Kay, S. R., 1979, Dysphoric response to neuroleptic treatment in schizophrenia: its relationship to autonomic arousal and prognosis, Biol. Psychiatry 14:277-292.

Singh, M. M., and Lal, H., 1982, Central cholinergic mechanisms, neuroleptic action and schizophrenia, in "Clinical Applications of Neuropharmacology," W. Essman and L. Valzelli, eds., pp. 337-389, Spectrum Publications, New York.

Sitaram, N.,1982, Pupillary changes following cholinomimetics, in "Biologic Changes in Psychiatry and Neurology," E. Usdin and I. Hanin, eds., Pergamon Press, New York.

Sitaram, N., Moore, A. M., Vanskiver, C., Blendy, J., Nurnberger, J. I., Gershon, E. S., and Gillin, J.C., 1981, Hypersensitive cholinergic functioning in primary illness, in "Cholinergic Mechanisms. Phylogenetic Aspects, Central and Peripheral Synapses and Clinical Significance," G. Pepeu and H. Ladinsky, eds., Plenum Press, New York.

Sitaram, N., Nurnberger, J., Gershon, E., and Gillin, J.C., 1980, Faster cholinergic REM sleep induction in euthymic patients with primary affective illness, Science 208:200-202.

Smith, J. A., 1980, Abuse of the antiParkinsonian drugs: A review of the literature, J. Clin. Psychiatry 41;351-354.

Subramanian, M. G., and Gala, R. R., 1976, The influence of cholinergic, adrenergic and serotonergic drugs on the afternoon surge of plasma prolactin in ovariectomized, estrogen-treated rats, Endocrinology 98:842-848.

Suzuki, T., Abe, K., and Hirose, T., 1975, Adrenal cortical secretion in response to pilocarpine in dogs with hypothalamic lesions, Neuroendocrinology 17(1):75-82.

Suzuki, T., Hirai, K., Yoshio, H., Kurouji, K-I, and Hirose, T., 1964, Effect of eserine and atropine on adrenocortical hormone secretion in unanesthetized dogs, J. Endocrinol. 31:81-82.

Tamminga, C., Smith, R. C., Change, S., Haraszti, J. S., and Davis, J. M., 1976, Depression associated with oral choline, Lancet II: 905.

Tissot, R., 1975, The common pathophysiology of monoaminergic psychoses: a new hypothesis, Neuropsychobiology 1:243-260.

Van Putten, T., and May, P. A., 1978, "Akinetic depression" in schizophrenia, Arch. Gen. Psychiatry 35:1101-1107.

Chapter 11

CHOLINERGIC NEUROPSYCHOPHARMACOLOGY
AND NEUROPATHOLOGY OF DEMENTIAS

Konrad C. Retz and Harbans Lal

Department of Pharmacology
Texas College of Osteopathic Medicine
Camp Bowie at Montgomery
Fort Worth, Texas 76107

---

1. INTRODUCTION

Currently it is estimated that more than five percent of the population above 65 years of age exhibit dementia and that the nursing home care for people so afflicted may exceed $6 billion per year (Katzman, 1976; Terry and Davies, 1980). Senile dementia has often

been accepted as a normal feature of "growing old." However, many
people retain good cognitive ability well into the eigth or ninth
decade in the absence of any other neurological symptoms. Presenile
dementia typically appears in people in their fifth decade and consists of a progressive deterioration of cognitive functions, especially recent memory. This latter form of dementia, presenile dementia of
the Alzheimer's type (SDAT) produces a neuropathology that is similar
to that of senile dementia including such features as: (a) neuritic
plaques with an extracellular core of amyloid; (b) neurofibrillary
tangles in the neuronal cell bodies; and (c) granulovacuolar degeneration especially in some hippocampal neurons (Constantinidis, 1978;
Selkoe et al., 1982). Because some genetic studies have indicated
that SDAT occurs as an autosomal dominant trait, it is possible that
SDAT and senile dementia may share some common genetic basis (Folstein
and Breitner, 1981; Heston et al., 1981).

The possibility of cholinergic system involvement in dementia has
been suggested by experimental, clinical and neuropathological studies.
Neuropsychopharmacological studies in animals have shown that cholinergic blockade tends to impair acquisition and retrieval in various
learning paradigms (see Spencer and Lal, Chapter 5). Correspondingly,
in clinical situations, antimuscarinic drugs have long been known to
produce deficits in recent memory (Longo, 1966; Drachman and Leavitt,
1976; Drachman, 1977, 1978a), which can be reduced by the administration of an acetylcholinesterase (AChE) inhibitor, physostigmine
(Drachman, 1977; Mewaldt and Ghoniem, 1979). Based on such insights,
drugs which increase central cholinergic activity have been investigated in patients with presenile and senile dementia. At the same
time, neuropathological studies have produced evidence which suggests
a relationship between cholinergic deficits in the brain and human,
as well as animal, aging and dementia. In this chapter, we review the
neuropharmacological and neuropathological data to evaluate the possible role of cholinergic mechanisms in dementia. Experimental data
have already been reviewed in Chapter 5 by Spencer and Lal.

2. NEUROPSYCHOPHARMACOLOGY OF DEMENTIA

2.1. Cholinergic Manipulations

It is feasible to enhance activity at cholinergic synapses by any
or all of the following approaches: (a) enhancing the rate of ACh
synthesis as a result of elevating levels of the precursor, choline;
(b) direct stimulation of postsynaptic muscarinic receptors; and (c)
inhibiting the hydrolytic catabolism of acetylcholine (ACh) by AChE
(Cooper et al., 1982). Moreover, it appears that rodents and nonhuman
primates exhibit subcellular changes in the CNS during senescence that
are similar to those seen in humans in at least the following aspects:
cortical atrophy; neuronal loss; cerebral microvascular histopathology; cerebral blood flow disorders; glial histopathology; and neuronal organelle histopathology (Miquel et al., 1983). These factors

have permitted extensive testing of the cholinergic hypothesis of memory dysfunction in both humans and experimental animals (see Bartus, et al., 1982; Spencer and Lal, this book).

2.1.1. Precursor Loading

Attempts to enhance muscarinic cholinergic activity by "precursor loading" with either lecithin or choline, the precursors to ACh, have been undertaken in both humans (see Bartus et al., 1982; Mohs et al., 1981; Goodnick and Gershon, 1983; Peters and Levin, 1982; Bajada, 1982; Johns et al., 1983; Thal et al., 1983) and experimental animals (Bartus, 1982; Bartus et al., 1983). The rationale for this approach is somewhat controversial (see Eckernas, 1977; Freeman et al., 1975; Wecker et al., 1978; Brunello et al., 1982; Flentge et al., 1981), although in vitro (Cohen and Wurtman, 1975; Haubrich et al., 1975; Hirsch and Wurtman, 1978) and in vivo (Jenden et al., 1982; Bartus and Dean, 1983; Haubrich et al., 1979) studies have shown that the rate of synthesis of ACh can indeed be increased under certain conditions. The therapeutic utility of this approach in patients with dementia requires that muscarinic neurons be present and capable of releasing sufficient amounts of ACh (Wurtman, 1983). Reviews describing 33 clinical studies have concluded that use of precursors alone is not able to produce consistent or significant improvement in cognitive function of either healthy elderly or SDAT patients (see Bartus et al. 1982; Mohs et al., 1981; Goodnick and Gershon, 1983). Although choline loading has been more successful in mice (Bartus, 1982) and monkeys (Bartus et al. 1983), the greatest improvement of memory in aged rats occurred when choline and piracetam, a nootropic, were coadministered (Bartus and Dean, 1981; Bartus et al., 1981). More recent clinical studies have shown that some aged and SDAT patients may have improved memory performance when either lecithin or choline is coadministered with physostigmine, an AChE inhibitor (Peters and Levin, 1982; Bajada, 1982; Thal et al., 1983). Nevertheless, at the present time, both clinical and animal studies suggest that the ACh precursor loading approach will not have great promise for management of dementias.

2.1.2. Mucarinic Agonists

A number of attempts to improve memory performance by stimulating muscarinic post-synaptic receptors have been made in humans (see Bartus et al., 1982; Goodnick and Gershon, 1983; Christie, 1982) and laboratory animals (see Bartus et al., 1982, 1983; Bartus and Dean, 1981; Bartus, 1982; Cherkin and Riege, 1983). This approach could be efficacious even in regions where cholinergic innervation is greatly diminished. In young adults, arecoline produced an improvement in cognitive ability that was decreased with elevation of dose (Davis et al., 1976, 1978; Risch et al., 1981). Arecoline has also been reported to increase cognitive ability in normal (Sitaram et al., 1978) and SDAT (Christie, 1982) patients. Arecoline and oxotremorine have been found to be capable of improving cognitive abilities in both monkeys

(Bartus, 1982; Bartus et al., 1981, 1982, 1983) and mice (Cherkin and
Riege, 1983). While the limited studies with arecoline and oxotremorine are supportive of a cholinergic hypothesis for cognition, short
half-lives and adverse effects in the autonomic nervous system limit
the clinical usefulness of these drugs in the management of CNS
diseases (Taylor, 1980).

2.1.3. Acetylcholinesterase Inhibitors

Elevation of synaptic ACh levels by inhibition of AChE has been
the cholinergic manipulation that has most reliably elevated cognitive
performance in both humans (see Bartus et al., 1982; Drachman, 1978b,
1981; Smith and Swash, 1980; Mohs et al., 1981; Ordy et al., 1981;
Goodnick and Gershon, 1983; Smith et al., 1982; Christie, 1982; Peters
and Levin, 1982; Bajada, 1982; Davis et al., 1982; Johns et al., 1983;
Meier-Ruge, 1983; Thal et al., 1983) and experimental animals (see
Bartus et al., 1982, 1983; Bartus, 1982; Bartus and Dean, 1981;
Cherkin and Riege, 1983). Physostigmine has been employed almost exclusively, although the longer acting 1,2,3,4-tetrahydro-5-aminoacri-
dine (THA) has been reported to be of some benefit in one of two
clinical studies (see Goodnick and Gershon, 1983), and shorter acting
edrophonium has been reported to increase memory in mice (see Cherkin
and Riege, 1983).

When surveying the studies using AChE inhibitors to improve cognition, the following conclusions become apparent: (a) in SDAT patients memory is improved slightly, but not restored to either that
of age-matched controls or young adults; (b) in general, cholinomimetics cause biphasic dose-effect responses -- improvement, followed
by impairment -- within a narrow therapeutic window; (c) cognitive
functions exhibit a differential sensitivity to cholinomimetics; and
(d) individuals exhibit great differences in sensitivity to cholinomimetics. As a result, it appears that even with increasing evidence
obtained from both behavioral and pathological studies in support of
the cholinergic hypothesis of memory, the use of cholinomimetic therapy alone is likely to have limited efficacy in the management of SDAT
and other dementias.

2.1.4. Cholinergic Interaction with Other Processes

The studies with cholinomimetics suggest that cognitive loss may
result from a specific cholinergic deficit acting in concert with
impairment of other physiological and biochemical processes. For
example, mice exhibit an age-dependent decrease in ACh release in
vitro, which can be reversed by 3,4-diaminopyridine, a treatment that
in vivo improves performance in the tight rope test (Gibson and
Peterson, 1983). Altered energy metabolism processes may be one such
underlying factor in the dementias. Although glucose utilization
appears to be well maintained in mice and adult humans during normal
senescence (Gibson and Peterson, 1982; Rapoport et al., 1983; Ferris

et al., 1983), the response to various insults can be decreased in senescense, e.g., oxotremorine enhancement of glucose uptake in rat visual cortex and altered cerebral ACh synthesis in hypoxic mice (Gibson and Peterson, 1982; Rapoport et al., 1983). Thus, it is significant that recent studies found that, when compared to normal elderly patients, demented elderly patients had a reduction in cerebral glucose metabolism correlated with cognitive impairment (Ferris et al., 1983).

2.2. Noncholinergic Manipulations and Dementia

2.2.1. Catecholaminergic and GABAergic Systems

Because the cholinergic deficits seen in SDAT may be superimposed upon more general metabolic deficits, it is instructive to consider the results of other pharmacological attempts to improve cognitive function in humans and laboratory animals. Many studies with CNS active amines and other neurotransmitters have been reported in humans (Ordy et al., 1981; Goodnick and Gershon, 1983; Bartus et al., 1983; Loew, 1980; Reisberg et al., 1983) with widespread consensus that the following agents administered alone are not capable of consistently producing a significant improvement of cognitive processes: (a) CNS stimulants -- methylphenidate, magnesium pemoline, dextroamphetamine; (b) catecholamine precursors -- L-DOPA; and (c) dopaminergic agonist -- bromocriptine. Similarly when monkeys were examined in an automated, computer controlled test of discrimination acquisition (Bartus et al., 1978), the following were found to produce insignificant effects: (a) dopamine precursor -- L-DOPA; (b) dopamine antagonist -- haloperidol; (c) beta-1 and -2 antagonist -- propranolol; (d) alpha-2 antagonist -- clonidine; and (e) GABA agonist -- muscimol (Bartus et al., 1983). The only exception to these findings, which are generally negative, has been observed in limited clinical studies (Ordy et al., 1981; Goodnick and Gershon, 1983), where the memory functions improved with pipradol.

2.2.2. Cerebral Vasodilation

A second group of drugs that has been examined in clinical studies is the vasodilators including the ergot alkaloids (Ordy et al., 1981; Goodnick and Gershon, 1983; Bartus and Dean, 1981; Loew, 1980; Branconnier, 1983). Again, the general consensus is that the following vasodilator agents, administered alone, do not produce reliably significant effects on cognitive performance: papaverine, cyclandelate, isoxsuprine, nylidrine, vitamin E, vincamine and cinnarizine. Naftidofuryl (nafronyl, PRAXILENE) a vasodilator that also elevates intracellular ATP levels, may be more beneficial (Goodnick and Gershon, 1983; Bartus and Dean, 1981; Branconnier, 1983). The most extensively studied ergot alkaloid, dihydroergotoxine (co-dergocrine mesylate, HYDERGINE), has many reported actions in addition to being a weaker vasodilator (see Ordy et al., 1981; Loew, 1980; Branconnier,

1983). Although this ergot has been no more reliable than other vasodilators in producing cognitive improvements, it has given more improvement in cognitive performance than has the prototypic vasodilator
papaverine (Goodnick and Gershon, 1983). Recent studies of vincamine
and dihydroergotoxine in aged monkeys also observed limited and unre-
liable improvements in cognitive function with these agents (Bartus
and Dean, 1981), similar to the results of the clinical studies.

     The lack of more encouraging findings with the cerebral vasodila-
tors is somewhat surprising in that cholinergic innervation of pial
and other cerebrovasculature has been found, which is apparently associated with processes of neurons containing vasoactive intestinal
peptide (Larson et al., 1976). Moreover, the ability of acetylcholine
to increase cerebral blood flow and the ability of vasoactive intestinal peptide to serve as a facilitatory modulator has been demonstrated
in in vitro and in vivo studies (Larsson et al., 1976; Heistad et al.,
1980; Krieger and Martin, 1981a,b).

2.2.3. Oxidative Cerebral Metabolism

     Another group of drugs includes those acting directly to improve
or enhance oxidative cerebral metabolism. Pyrithioxine, which is believed to enhance the uptake and consumption of glucose, has undergone
limited clinical trials (Reisberg et al., 1983). The nootropic agents
(Giurgia, 1976) -- piracetam, etiracetam, oxiracetam, pramiracetam --
are believed to directly stimulate the synthesis of ATP, and have been
examined in both clinical (Ordy et al., 1981; Goodnick and Gershon,
1983; Bartus and Dean, 1981; Loew, 1980; Branconnier, 1983) and experimental animal (Bartus and Dean, 1981; Bartus et al., 1983; Loew,
1980) studies. Although studies with piracetam administered alone may
be equivocal, piracetam has been shown to potentiate the effects of
precursor loading with choline in rats (Bartus and Dean, 1981; Bartus
et al., 1981). The newer agents, oxiracetam and pramiracetam, have
had limited studies which suggest that they may have greater efficacy
than piracetam (see Branconnier, 1983).

2.2.4. Lipofuscin Pigment

     A fourth approach has been to attempt to reverse the accumulation
of lipofuscin pigment, a concomitant event in mammalian aging (see Lal
and Nandy, 1979; Nandy, 1983). Centrophenoxine has been administered
for this purpose in both human (see Ordy et al., 1981; Bartus and
Dean, 1981; Branconnier, 1983) and animal (see Lal et al., 1973; Lal
and Nandy, 1979; Ordy et al., 1981; Bartus and Dean, 1981; Nandy,
1983, 1979; Ordy et al., 1981; Bartus and Dean, 1981; Nandy, 1983)
studies. The human studies have been limited, and like other pharmacological approaches, have produced inconsistent positive results.
Studies in aged monkeys (Bartus and Dean, 1981) and mice (Lal and
Nandy, 1979; Nandy, 1983) have been more encouraging suggesting a
further examination of the drug and the mechanisms underlying accumulation of lipofuscin pigment. However, it is not known if there is a

relationship between lipofuscin accumulation and cholinergic abnormalities.

2.2.5. Miscellaneous

     Finally, several approaches have been avocated because of their
potential effects on behavior or metabolic status in the aged. For
example, anticoagulant therapy has been examined in an effort to
reduce erythrocyte intravascular adhesion, and thereby improve cerebral blood flow (Bartus et al., 1983). Neuropeptide hormones -- ACTH
and component analogues, vasopressin and component analogues, oxyto-
cin, somatostatin -- have been examined because of their abilities to
alter behavior by inducing long-lasting biochemical events (Goodnick
and Gershon, 1983). The anticonvulsant, sodium valproate, has not
been examined in the aged or demented, but has been reported to affect
cognitive abilities in epileptic patients (see Reisberg et al., 1983).
Although all of these suggested approaches have had limited investigation, it is not certain that they are intended to address putative
deficits of either aging or dementia per se, or that they have any
relationship to brain cholinergic systems.

3.   NEUROPATHOLOGY OF DEMENTIA

     Recent pathological studies have shown that SDAT brains at
autopsy have a neuronal cell loss in the frontal and temporal cortices that is greater than that seen in age-matched controls. This
knowledge combined with the fact that two other neurodegenerative
diseases -- Parkinson's disease and Huntington's disease -- are known
to have regional neurotransmitter-specific deficits, has prompted the
search for the involvement of a similar neurochemical lesion in SDAT.
Some of the evidence to support such a specific cholinergic deficit
will now be presented.

3.1. Choline Acetyltransferase and Muscarinic Receptors in the Brain
      at Postmortem

     When the activity of the ACh biosynthetic enzyme, choline acetyl-
transferase (CAT), was measured in brains of patients who had died
with SDAT, there was a significant reduction in CAT activity in the
hippocampal formation and cerebral cortex relative to age-matched controls who had died of unrelated causes (Bowen et al., 1976; Davies and
Maloney, 1976; Perry et al., 1978; Davies, 1979; Davies et al., 1980).
Similarly, the activity of AChE in patients with SDAT was also reduced
in these two regions when compared to controls (Davies et al., 1980;
Perry et al., 1978; Davies, 1979; Pope et al., 1965; Bowen et al.,
1976). However, muscarinic cholinergic receptors were not decreased
in the cerebral cortex of SDAT patients (see Bartus et al., 1982).
When considering that CAT is now believed to be localized only in
cholinergic neurons, these findings suggested that SDAT patients could

have a neurologically significant loss of cholinergic neurons in the
cerebral cortex, However the loss of CAT activity seemed to be
greater than the degree of neuronal loss in the cerebral cortex, which
would suggest either the existence of a major extrinsic innervation
of cholinergic neurons to that structure, or the retrograde degeneration of efferents out of the cerebral cortex (see Coyle et al., 1983).

3.2. Loss of Cholinergic Innervation

Earlier studies of Shute and Lewis (1967) used a histochemical
stain for AChE to identify the cholinergic projections in the rat
brain. They concluded that large neuronal cell bodies in the basal
forebrain were the source of cortical cholinergic innervation. However, later studies demonstrated that non-cholinergic neurons could
stain for AChE (Butcher et al., 1975). Recent approaches using stereotaxic administration of excitatory amino acid neurotoxins (see
Coyle, 1982) to destroy neurons, but spare axons of passage, have
established that in the rat, the ventral globus pallidus is the source
of the cholinergic innervation to the cerebral cortex (Johnston et al.,
1979, 1981a, 1981b). Those lesions were able to reduce the activity
of CAT by up to 70 percent in the frontal cortex, while not affecting
neurochemical indices of cortical GABAergic function. The neuroanatomical boundaries of the magnocellular neurons include the ventral
and medial globus pallidus extending into the hypothalamus, the diagonal band of Broca, and the medial septal nucleus (Divac, 1976).
Studies in primates have shown that the location of these neurons
corresponds to the nucleus basalis of Meynert (Meynert, 1872; Gorry,
1963), that they are also cholinergic (McKinney et al., 1982), and
that they project primarily to the frontal, prefrontal and parietal
cortex (see Coyle et al., 1983). In primates, cholinergic neuronal
cell bodies in the medial septum and diagonal band of Broca innervate
the hippocampal formation and occipital cortex (see Coyle et al.,
1983). It is important to note that electrolytic lesions of the magnocellular neurons in rats can impair acquisition of active and passive avoidance conditioned responses (Lo Conte et al., 1982).

The neuroanatomical localization of the source of the major cholinergic innervation to the cortex, has prompted a greater interest
in the study of the nucleus basalis of Meynert in autopsy specimens
of patients with SDAT. Such studies have shown that cell densities
in that region are consistently decreased by as much as 75 percent in
number with no consistent alterations in adjacent regions (Whitehouse
et al., 1982). Furthermore, a study of neuritic plaques in the cerebral cortex of aged monkeys has established that the early plaques
were rich in AChE staining material, whereas the latter plaques had
much less AChE activity (Struble et al., 1982). Thus, it appears
that the functional decline in the innervation of the cerebral cortex
and/or the hippocampus by cholinergic neurons of the basal forebrain
could play a major role in the development of the cognitive deficit
in SDAT and senile dementia.

4.   CONCLUSIONS AND FUTURE DIRECTIONS

4.1. Current Status

It is certainly clear from behavioral, and pathological evidence as reviewed above and elsewhere (see Bartus et al., 1982; Spencer and Lal, Chapter 5; Coyle et al., 1983) that cholinergic deficits may play an important role in the pathogenesis of SDAT and other dementias. What is less certain are the following: (a) the nature and manner of cholinergic involvement; (b) if this involvement relates to changes in cholinergic sensitivity usually observed in senescence (see Lal and Carroll, 1979); and (c) whether or not the cholinergic deficit is the etiological agent or merely a concomitant occurrence. To address that issue, several neuropsychopharmacological agents have been employed in an effort to improve learning and memory in both experimental animals and humans. However, these approaches, utilizing both cholinergic and noncholinergic manipulations in the aged and demented, have failed to identify a single cholinomimetic agent that can restore learning and memory performance to that of normal adults. Instead, it appears that the most reliable and efficacious regimen is a concerted effort utilizing cholinomimetics combined with a nootropic agent to improve oxidative metabolism, which is necessary to maintain cholinergic function.

The neuropathological studies of dementia are less extensive than are the neuropsychopharmacological ones, but provide better evidence for the occurrence of cholinergic deficits in dementia. In particular, there seems to be a deficit in cholinergic projections from the magnocellular neurons in the nucleus basalis of Meynert to the cerebral cortex and from the medial septum and diagonal band of Broca to the hippocampal formation and occipital cortex. The potential importance of these deficits merits reiteration since electrolytic lesions of the magnocellular neurons in rats have been shown to impair acquisition of active and passive avoidance conditioned responses (Lo Conte et al., 1982).

4.2. Future Needs and Potential Approaches

Although cholinomimetic therapy alone has not yielded consistent significant improvement of cognitive function in either aged animals or demented patients, some of this inconsistency may result from not using a site-specific cholinergic agent, or from measurements of behaviors that do not specifically reflect recent memory. These concerns have already been stated by several investigators (see Drachman, 1978b, 1981, 1983; Ordy et al., 1981; Johns et al., 1983; Bartus et al., 1983; Sprott and Stavnes, 1975; Drachman et al., 1982; Corkin, 1982). One approach to this problem is the development of new cholinergic drugs which are more specific in interacting with neuronal processes underlying memory and learning. For clinical studies there must be a more selective description and assessment of presenile

dementia subsets from normal aged populations and dementias secondary
to other organic diseases (Drachman et al., 1982; Corkin, 1982;
Drachman, 1983). Studies in non-human primates have already benefited
from development of an automated, computer-controlled, self-paced
stimulus discrimination apparatus (see Bartus et al., 1978, 1983).
Studies in rodents have extensively used both passive and active
avoidance procedures to noxious stimulus, usually electrical shock
(see Sprott and Stavnes, 1975). By contrast, the T-maze problem --
which examines a more natural behavior and permits the measurement of
acquisition, retention, and reversal performance -- may see more use
in the future.

Because the rationale for correlation of cholinergic deficits
with cognitive deficits is very strong, one would expect to see the
development of animal models that permit examination of cognitive performance in the presence of varied degrees of cholinergic deficits.
In this regard, destruction of the nucleus basalis of Meynert by
excitatory amino acid neurotoxins, offers a potential primate and
rodent model of advanced states of dementias (see Coyle et al., 1983).
Ethycholine mustard aziridinium ion (AF64A), a recently characterized
toxin exhibiting a high degree of specificity for cholinergic neurons
(Mantione et al., 1981; Fisher and Hanin, 1980; Fisher et al., 1982),
may prove to be even more useful for this purpose.

Another development of interest is the recent report that genetic
manipulations may provide animal models exhibiting concurrent memory
deficits and cholinergic dysfunctions. For example, the New Zealand
Black (NZB) mouse was reported to possess deficits in learning of an
active avoidance task (Nandy et al., 1983), passive avoidance task
(Spencer and Lal, 1983) and abnormalities in cholinergic receptor
systems as well as decreased sensitivity to muscarinic drugs (Retz
et al., 1984).

Finally, although this review has focused upon the role of CNS
cholinergic status and pharmacological manipulations thereof in dementia, an open mind must be kept regarding the potential involvement of
other neurotransmitters, neuromodulators and homeostatic metabolic
processes. For example, recent animal studies have shown that
naloxone, an opiate antagonist, can improve learning and memory (see
Izquierdo, 1983), findings which are currently being examined in mul-
ticenter clinical trials.

REFERENCES

Bajada, S., 1982, A trial of choline chloride and physostigmine in
    Alzheimer's dementia, in "Alzheimer's Disease: A Report of
    Progress (Aging, Vol. 19)," S. Corkin. K. L. Davis, J. H.
    Growdon, E. Usdin and R. J. Wurtman, eds., pp. 427-432, Raven
    Press, New York.

Bartus, R. T., 1982, Effects of cholinergic agents on learning and memory in animal models of aging, in "Alzheimer's Disease: A Report of Progress (Aging, Vol. 19)," S. Corkin, K. L. Davis, J. H. Growdon, E. Usdin and R. J. Wurtman, eds., pp. 271-280, Raven Press, New York.

Bartus, R. T., and Dean, R. L., III, 1981, Age-related memory loss and drug therapy: Possible directions based on animal models, in "Brain Neurotransmitters and Receptors in Aging and Age-Related Disorders (Aging, Vol. 17)," S. J. Enna, T. Samorajski and B. Beer, eds., pp. 209-223, Raven Press, New York.

Bartus, R. T., and Dean, R. L., III, 1984, Cholinergic precursor therapy for geriatric cognition: Its past, its present, and a question of its future, in "Nutrition in Gerontology, (Aging, Vol. 26)," J. M. Ordy and D. Harman and R. B. Alfin-Slater, eds., Raven Press, New York.

Bartus, R. T., Dean, R. L., III, and Beer, B., 1983, An evaluation of drugs for improving memory in aged monkeys: Implications for clinical trials in humans, Psychopharmacol. Bull. 19:168-184.

Bartus, R. T., Dean, R. L., III, Beer, B., and Lippa, A. S., 1982, The cholinergic hypothesis of geriatric memory dysfunction, Science 217:408-417.

Bartus, R. T., Dean, R. L., III, Sherman, K. A., Friedman, E., and Beer, B., 1981, Profound effects of combining choline and piracetam on memory enhancement and cholinergic function in aged rats, Neurobiol. Aging 2:105-111.

Bartus, R. T., Fleming, D., and Johnson, H. R., 1978, Aging in the rhesus monkey: Debilitating effects on short-term memory, J. Gerontol. 33:858-871.

Bowen, D. M., Smith, C. B., White, P., and Davison, A. N., 1976, Neurotransmitter-related enzymes and indices of hypoxia in senile dementia and other abiotrophies, Brain 99:459-496.

Bowen, D. M., Smith, C. C. T., White, P., and Davison, A. N., 1976, Senile dementia and related abiotrophies: Biochemical studies on histologically evaluated human postmortem specimens, in "Neurobiology of Aging (Aging, Vol. 3)," R. D. Terry and S. Gershon, eds., pp. 361-378, Raven Press, New York.

Branconnier, R. J., 1983, The efficacy of the cerebral metabolic enhancers in the treatment of senile dementia, Psychopharmacol. Bull. 19:212-219.

Brunello, N., Cheney, D. L., and Costa E., 1982, Increase in exogenous choline fails to elevate the content or turnover rate of cortical, striatal or hippocampal acetylcholine, J. Neurochem. 38:1160-1163.

Butcher, L. L., Talbot, K., and Bilezikjian, L., 1975, Acetylcholinesterase neurons in dopamine-containing regions of the brain, J. Neural Transm. 37:127-153.

Cherkin, A., and Riege, W. H., 1983, Multimodal approach to pharmacotherapy of senile amnesias, in "Brain Aging: Neuropathology and Neuropharmacology (Aging, Vol. 21)," J. Cervos-Navarro and H.-I. Sarkander, eds., pp. 415-435, Raven Press, New York.

Christie, J. E., 1982, Physostigmine and arecoline infusions in
    Alzheimer's disease, in "Alzheimer's Disease: A Report of
    Progress (Aging, Vol. 19)," pp. 413-419, Raven Press, New York.
Cohen, E. L., and Wurtman, R. J., 1975, Brain acetylcholine: Increase
    after systemic choline administration, Life Sci. 16:1095-1102.
Constantinidis, J., 1978, Is Alzheimer's disease a major form of
    senile dementia? Clinical, anatomical, and genetic data, in
    Alzheimer's Disease: Senile Dementia and Related Disorders
    (Aging, Vol. 7)," R. Katzman, R. D. Terry and K. L. Bick eds.,
    pp. 15-25, Raven Press, New York.
Cooper, J. R., Bloom, F. E., and Roth, R. H., eds., 1982, "The
    Biochemical Basis of Neuropharmacology, 4th Ed.," pp. 77-108,
    Oxford University Press, New York.
Corkin, S., 1982, Some relationships between global amnesias and the
    memory impairments in Alzheimer's disease, in "Alzheimer's
    Disease: A Report of Progress (Aging, Vol. 19)," S. Corkin, K.
    L. Davis, J. Growdon, E. Usdin and R. J. Wurtman, eds.,
    pp. 149-164, Raven Press, New York.
Coyle, J. T., 1982, Excitatory amino acid neurotoxins, in "Handbook of
    Psychopharmacology, Vol. 15," L. I. Iversen, S. D. Iversen and S.
    H. Snyder, eds., pp. 237-269, Plenum, New York.
Coyle, J. T., Price, D. L., and DeLong, M. R., 1983, Alzheimer's
    disease: A disorder of cortical cholinergic innervation, Science
    219:1184-1190.
Davies, P., 1979, Neurotransmitter-related enzymes in senile dementia
    of the Alzheimer type, Brain Res. 171:319-327.
Davies, P., Katzman, R., and Terry, R. D., 1980, Reduced somatostatin-
    like immunoreactivity in cerebral cortex from cases of Alzheimer
    disease and Alzheimer senile dementia, Nature 288:279-280.
Davies, P., and Maloney, A. J. R., 1976, Selective loss of central
    cholinergic neurons in Alzheimer's disease, Lancet II 1403.
Davis, K. L., Hollister, L. E., Overall, J., Johnson, A., and Train,
    K., 1976, Physostigmine: Effects on cognition and affect in
    normal subjects, Psychopharmacologia 51:23-27.
Davis, K. L., Mohs, R. C., Davis, B. M., Levy, M. I., Horvath, T. B.,
    Rosenberg, G. S., Ross, A., Rothpearl, A., and Rosen, W., 1982,
    Cholinergic treatment in Alzheimer's disease: Implications for
    future research, in "Alzheimer's Disease: A Report of Progress
    (Aging, Vol. 19)," S. Corkin, K. L. Davis, J. H. Growdon, E. Usdin
    and R. J. Wurtman, eds., pp. 483-494, Raven Press, New York.
Davis, K. L., Mohs, R. C., Tinklenberg, J. R., Pfefferbaum, A.,
    Hollister, L. D., and Kopell, B. S., 1978, Physostigmine:
    Improvement of long-term memory processes in normal humans,
    Science 201:272-274.
Drachman, D. A., 1978b, Central cholinergic system and memory, in,
    "Psychopharmacology: A Generation of Progress," M. A. Lipton, A.
    DiMascio and K. F. Killam, eds., pp. 651-662, Raven Press, New
    York.

Drachman, D. A., 1983, How normal aging relates to dementia: A
    critique and classification, in "Aging of the Brain (Aging, Vol.
    22)," D. Samuel, S. Algeria, S. Gershon, V. E. Grimm and G.
    Toffano, eds., pp. 19-31, Raven Press, New York.
Drachman, D. A., 1977, Memory and cognitive function in man: Does the
    cholinergic system have a specific role? Neurology 27:783-790.
Drachman, D. A., 1978a, Memory, dementia and the cholinergic system,
    in "Alzheimer's Disease: Senile Dementia and Related Disorders
    (Aging, Vol. 7)," R. Katzman, R. D. Terry and K. L. Bick, eds.,
    pp. 141-148, Raven Press, New York.
Drachman, D. A., 1981, The cholinergic system, memory and aging, in
    "Brain Neurotransmitters and Receptors in Aging and Age-Related
    Disorders (Aging, Vol. 17)," S. J. Enna, T. Somarajski and B.
    Beer, eds., pp. 255-268, Raven Press, New York.
Drachman, D. A., Fleming, P., and Glosser, G., 1982, The multidimen-
    sional assessment for dementia scales, in "Alzheimer's Disease:
    A Report of Progress (Aging, Vol. 19)," S. Corkin, K. L. Davis,
    J. Growdon, E. Usdin and R. J. Wurtman, eds., pp. 109-118, Raven
    Press, New York.
Drachman, D. A., and Leavitt, J., 1976, Human memory and the cholin-
    ergic system. A relationship to aging? Arch. Neurol. 30:113-121.
Divac, I., 1976, Magnocellular nuclei of the basal forebrain project
    to neocortex, brain stem, and olfactory bulb. Review of some
    functional correlates, Brain Res. 93:385-398.
Eckernas, S., 1977, Plasma choline and cholinergic mechanisms in the
    brain. Methods, function and role in Huntington's chorea, Acta
    Physiol. Scand. Suppl. 449:1-62.
Ferris, S. H., De Leon, M. J., Wold, A. P., George, A. E., Reisberg,
    B., Brodie, J., Genter, C., Christman, D. R., and Fowler, J. S.,
    1983, Regional metabolism and cognitive deficits in aging and
    senile dementia, in "Aging of the Brain (Aging, Vol. 22)," D.
    Samuel, S. Algeria, S. Gershon, V. E. Grimm and G. Toffano, eds.,
    pp. 133-142 Raven Press, New York.
Fisher, A. and Hanin, I., 1980, Choline analogues as potential tools
    in developing selective animal models of central cholinergic hypo-
    function, Life Sci. 27:1615-1634.
Fisher, A., Mantione, C. R., Abraham, D. J., and Hanin, I., 1982,
    Long-term central cholinergic hypofunction induced in mice by
    ethylcholine aziridinium ion (AF64A) in vivo, J. Pharmacol. Exp.
    Ther. 222:140-145.
Flentge, F., Postrema, F., Medema, H. M., and Vandenberg, C. J., 1981,
    Acute choline administration in rat and mouse: No effect on dopa-
    mine metabolism in brain, Life Sci. 29:331-335.
Folstein, M. F., and Breitner, J. C., 1981, Language disorder predicts
    familial Alzheimer's disease, Johns Hopkins Med. J. 149:145-147.
Freeman, J. J., Choi, R. L., and Jenden, D. J., 1975, Plasma choline:
    Its turnover and exhange with brain choline, J. Neurochem.
    24:729-734.

Gibson, G. E., and Peterson, C., 1983, Amelioration of age-related deficits in acetylcholine release and behavior with 3, 4-diamino-pyridine, in "Aging of the Brain (Aging, Vol. 22)," D. Samuel, S. Algeria, S. Gershon, V. E. Grimm and G. Toffano, eds., pp. 337-348, Raven Press, New York.

Gibson, G. E., and Peterson, C., 1982, Biochemical and behavioral parallels in aging and hypoxia, in "The Aging Brain: Cellular and Molecular Mechanisms of Aging in the Nervous System (Aging, Vol. 20)," E. Giacobini, G. Filogano and A. Vernadakis, eds., pp. 107-122, Raven Press, New York.

Giurgia, C., 1976, Piracetam: Nootropic pharmacology of neurointe-grative activity, in "Current Developments in Psychopharmacology, Vol. 3," W. B. Essman and L. Valzelli, eds., pp. 222-273, Spectrum New York.

Goodnick, P. J., and Gershon, S., 1983, Chemotherapy of cognitive dis-orders, in "Aging of the Brain (Aging, Vol. 22)," D. Samuel, S. Algeria, S. Gershon, V. E. Grimm and G. Toffano, eds., pp. 349-361, Raven Press, New York.

Gorry, J. R., 1963, Studies on the comparative anatomy of the ganglion basale of Meynert, Acta Anat. (Basel) 55:51-104.

Haubrich, D. R., Gerber, N. H., and Pflueger, A. B., 1979, Choline availability and the synthesis of acetylcholine, in "Choline and Lecithin in Brain Disorders (Nutrition and the Brain, Vol. 5)," A. Barbeau, J. H. Growdon and R. J. Wurtman, eds., pp. 57-72, Raven Press, New York.

Haubrich, D. R., Wang, P. F. L., Clody, D. E., and Wedeking, P. W., 1975, Increase in rat brain acetylcholine induced by choline or deanol, Life Sci. 17:975-980.

Heistad, D. D., Marcus, M. L., Said, S. I., and Gross, P. M., 1980, Effect of acetylcholine and vasoactive intestinal peptide on cerebral blood flow, Am. J. Physiol. 239:473-480.

Heston, L. L., Mastri, A. R., Anderson B. E., and White, J., 1981, Dementia of the Alzheimer type, Arch. Gen. Psychiatry 38:1085-1090.

Hirsch, M. J., and Wurtman, R. J., 1978, Lecithin consumption increas-es acetylcholine concentrations in rat brain and adrenal gland, Science 202:223-225.

Izquierdo, I., 1983, Naloxone facilitation in memory, Trends in Pharmacol. 4:411.

Jenden, D. J., Weiler, M. H., and Gundersen, C. B., 1982, Choline availability and acetylcholine synthesis, in "Alzheimer's Disease: A Report of Progress in Research (Aging, Vol. 19)," S. Corkin, K. L. Davis, J. H. Growdon, E. Usdin and R. J. Wurtman, eds., pp. 315-326, Raven Press, New York.

Johns, C. A., Greenwald, B. S., Mohs, R. C., and Davis, K. L., 1983 The cholinergic treatment strategy in aging and senile dementia, Psychopharmacol. Bull. 19:185-197.

Johnston, M. V., McKinney, M., and Coyle, J. T., 1979, Evidence for a cholinergic projection to neocortex from neurons in basal fore-brain, Proc. Natl. Acad. Sci. USA 76:5392-5396.

Johnston, M. V., McKinney, M., and Coyle, J. T., 1981a, Neocortical cholinergic innervation: A description of extrinsic and intrinsic components in the rat, Exp. Brain Res. 43:159-172.

Johnston, M. V., Young, A. C., and Coyle, J. T., 1981b, Laminar distribution of cholinergic markers in neocortex: Effects of lesions, J. Neurosci. Res. 6:597-607.

Katzman, R., 1976, The prevalence and malignancy of Alzheimer disease. Arch. Neurol. 33:217-218.

Krieger, D. T., and Martin, J. B., 1981a, Brain peptides, N. Engl. J. Med. 304:876-885.

Krieger, D. T., and Martin, J. B., 1981b, Brain peptides, N. Engl. J. Med. 304:944-951.

Lal, H., and Carroll, P. T., 1979, Alterations in brain neurotransmitters related to senescence, in "Geriatric Psychopharmacology (Developments in Neurology, Vol. 3)," K. Nandy, ed., pp. 3-16, Elsevier/North Holland, New York.

Lal, H., and Nandy, K., 1979, Future drugs against senescence-related brain dysfunctions, in "New Frontiers in Psychotropic Drug Research," S. Fielding and R. C. Effland eds., pp. 51-74 Futura Publishing Co., Mount Kisco, New York.

Lal, H., Pogacar, S., Daly, P., and Puri, S., 1973, Behavioral and neuropathological manifestations of nutritionally-induced central nervous "aging" in the rat, in "Neurobiological Aspects of Maturation and Aging (Progress in Brain Research, Vol. 40)," D. H. Ford, ed., pp. 129-140, Elsevier Publishing Co., Amsterdam.

Larsson, L.-I., Edvinsson, L., Fahrenkrug, J., Hakanson, R., Owman, Ch., Schaffalitzky de Muckadell, O., and Sundler, F., 1976, Immunohistochemical localization of a vasodilatory polypeptide (VIP) in cerebrovascular nerves, Brain Res. 113:400-404.

Lo Conte, G., Bartolini, L., Casamenti, F., Marconcini-Pepeu, I., and Pepeu, G., 1982, Lesions of cholinergic forebrain nuclei: Changes in avoidance behavior and scopolamine actions, Pharmacol. Biochem. Behav. 17:933-937.

Loew, D. M., 1980, Pharmacologic approaches to the treatment of senile dementia, in "Aging of the Brain and Dementia (Aging, Vol. 13)," L. Amaducci, A. N. Davison and P. Antuono, eds., pp. 287-294, Raven Press, New York.

Longo, V. C., 1966, Behavioral and electroencephalographic effects of atropine and related compounds, Pharmacol. Rev. 18:965-996.

Mantione, C. R., Fisher, A., and Hanin, I., 1981, The AF64A-treated mouse: Possible model for central cholinergic hypofunction, Science 213:579-580.

McKinney, M., Struble, R. G., Coyle, J. T., and Price, D. L., 1982, Monkey nucleus basalis is enriched with choline acetyltransferase, Neuroscience 7:2363-2368.

Meier-Ruge, W., 1983, New prospects in neuropharmacology of senile dementia, in "Brain Aging: Neuropathology and Neuropharmacology (Aging, Vol. 21)," J. Cervos-Navarro and H.-I. Sarkander, eds., pp. 391-400, Raven Press, New York.

Mewaldt, P., Ghoneim, M. M., 1979, The effects and interactions of
    scopolamine, physostigmine and methamphetamine on human memory,
    Pharmacol. Biochem. Behav. 10:205-210.

Meynert, T., 1872, Vom Gehirn der Saugetiere, in "Handbuch der Lehre
    von den Geweben des Menschen und Thiere (Vol. 2)," S. Stricker,
    ed., pp. 694, Englemann, Leipzig.

Miquel, J., Johnson, J. E., Jr., and Cervos-Navarro, J., 1983, Compar-
    ison of CNS aging in Humans and experimental animals, in "Brain
    Aging: Neuropathology and Neuropharmacology (Aging, Vol. 21),"
    J. Cervos-Navarro and H.-I. Sarkander eds., pp. 231-258, Raven
    Press, New York.

Mohs, R. C., Davis. K. L., Rosenberg, G., Davis, B., Horvath, T.,
    Denigris, Y., Ross, A., Cummings, T., Decker, P., and Levy, M.,
    1981, Studies of cholinergic drug effects on cognition in normal
    subjects and patients with Alzheimer's disease, in "Brain Neuro-
    transmitters and Receptors in Aging and Age-Related Disorders
    (Aging, Vol. 17)," S. J. Enna, T. Samorajski and B. Beer, eds.,
    pp. 225-230, Raven Press, New York.

Nandy, K., 1983, Aging neurons and pharmacological agents, in "Brain
    Aging: Neuropathology and Neuropharmacology (Aging, Vol. 32),"
    J. Cervos-Navarro and H.-I. Sarkander, eds., pp. 401-413, Raven
    Press, New York.

Nandy, K., Lal, H., Bennett, M., and Bennett, D., 1983, Correlation
    between a learning disorder and elevated brain-reactive antibodies
    in aged C57BL/6 and young NZB mice, Life Sci. 33:1499-1503.

Ordy, J. M., Brizee, K. R., and Bartus, R. T., 1981, Neuropsycho-
    pharmacology: Drug modification of memory in relation to aging
    in human and nonhuman primate brain, in "Clinical Pharmacology
    and the Aged Patient (Aging, Vol. 16)," L. F. Jarvik, D. J.
    Greenblatt and D. Harman, eds., pp. 79-102, Raven Press, New York.

Perry, E. K., Tomlinson, B. E., Blessed, G., Bergman, K., Gibson, P.
    H., and Perry, R. H., 1978, Correlation of cholinergic abnormali-
    ties with senile plaques and mental test scores in senile demen-
    tia, Br. Med. J. 2:1457-1459.

Peters, B. H., and Levin, H. S., 1982, Chronic oral physostigmine
    and lecithin administration in memory disorders of aging, in
    "Alzheimer's Disease: A Report of Progress (Aging, Vol. 19),"
    S. Corkin, K. L. Davis, J. H. Growdon, E. Usdin and R. J.
    Wurtman, eds., pp. 421-426, Raven Press, New York.

Pope, A., Hess, H. H., and Lewin, H., 1965. Microchemical pathology
    of the cerebral cortex in pre-senile dementias, Trans. Amer.
    Neurol. Assoc. 89:15-16.

Rapoport, S. I., Duara, R., London, E. D., Margolin, R. A., Schmartz,
    M., Cutler, N. R., Partanen, M., and Shinowara, N. L., 1983,
    Glucose metabolism of the aging nervous system, in "Aging of the
    Brain (Aging, Vol. 22)," D. Samuel, S. Algeria, S. Gershon, V. E.
    Grimm and T. Toffano, eds., pp. 111-121, Raven Press, New York.

Reisberg, B., London, E., Ferris, S. H., Anand, R., and De Leon, M. J.
    1983, Novel pharmacologic approaches to the treatment of senile
    dementia of the Alzheimer's type (SDAT), Psychopharmacol Bull.
    19:220-225.

Retz, K. C., Spencer, D. G., Jr., Lasley, S. M., Lane, J. D., Frantz, N., and Lal, H., 1984, Cholinergic deficiencies in the NZB mouse: A potential animal model of presenile dementia? Fed. Proc. 43:624.

Risch, S. C., Cohen, R. M., Janowsky, D. S., Kalin, N. H., Sitaram, N. Gillin, J. C., and Murphy, D. L., 1981, Physostigmine induction of depressive symptomatology in normal human subjects, Psychiatry Res. 4:89-94.

Selkoe, D. J., Ihara, I., and Salazar, F. J., 1982, Alzheimer's disease: Insolubility of partially purified paired helical elements in sodium dodecyl sulfate and urea, Science 215:1243-1245.

Shute, C. C. D., and Lewis, P. R., 1967, The ascending cholinergic reticular system: Neocortical, olfactory and subcortical projections, Brain 90-497-520.

Sitaram, N., Weingartner, H., and Gillin, J. C., 1978, Human serial learning: Enhancement with arecoline and choline and impairment with scopolamine, Science 201:274-276.

Smith, C. M., Semple, S. A., and Swash, M., 1982, Effects of physostigmine on responses in memory tests in patients with Alzheimer's disease, in "Alzheimer's Disease: A Report of Progress (Aging, Vol. 19)," S. Corkin, K. L. Davis, J. H. Growdon, E. Usdin and R. J. Wurtman, eds., pp. 405-411, Raven Press, New York.

Smith, C. M., and Swash, M., 1980, Effects of cholinergic drugs in memory, in Alzheimer's disease, in "Aging of the Brain and Dementia (Aging, Vol. 13)," L. Amaducci, A. N. Davison and P. Antuono, eds., pp. 295-304, Raven Press, New York.

Spencer, D. G., Jr., and Lal, H., 1983, Specific behavioral impairments in associational tasks in mice with an autoimmune disorder, Soc. Neurosci. Abstr. 9:96.

Sprott, R. L., and Stavnes, K., 1975, Avoidance learning, behavior genetics, and aging: A critical review and comment on methodology Exp. Aging Res. 1:145-168.

Struble, R. G., Cork, L. C., Whitehouse, P. J., and Price, D. L., 1982 Cholinergic innervation in neuritic plaques, Science 216:413-415.

Taylor, P., 1980, Cholinergic agonists, in "Goodman and Gilman's The Pharmacological Basis of Therapeutics, 6th ed.," A. G. Gilman, L. S. Goodman and A. Gilman, eds., pp. 91-99, Macmillan, New York.

Terry, R. D., and Davies, P., 1980, Dementia of the Alzheimer type, Ann. Rev. Neurosci. 3:77-95.

Thal, L. J., Fuld, P. A., Masur, D. M., and Sharpless, N. S., 1983, Oral physostigmine and lecithin improve memory in Alzheimer's disease, Ann. Neurol. 13:491-496.

Wecker, L., Dettbarn, W.-D., and Schmidt, D. E., 1978, Choline administration: Modification of the central actions of atropine, Science 199:86-87.

Whitehouse, P. J., Price, D. L., Struble, R. G., Clark, A. W., Coyle, J. T., and DeLong, M. R., 1982, Alzheimer's disease and senile dementia: Loss of neurons in the basal forebrain, Science 215:1237-1239.

Wurtman, R. J., 1983, Choline availability and acetyl choline synthe-
     sis: Relation to Alzheimer's disease, in "Aging of the Brain
     (Aging, Vol. 22)," D. Samuel, S. Algeria, S. Gershon, V. E. Grimm
     and G. Toffano, eds., pp. 211-220, Raven Press, New York.

Chapter 12

CHOLINERGIC MECHANISMS, ADAPTIVE BRAIN PROCESSES AND PSYCHOPATHOLOGY
Commentary and A Blueprint for Research

Man Mohan Singh

Department of Psychiatry
Southern Illinois University
School of Medicine
P.O. Box 3926
Springfield, Illinois 62708, U.S.A.

---

1. INTRODUCTION

The data reviewed in this book implicate central cholinergic mechanisms in many processes in the train of events that convert sensory inputs into behavioral outputs or what may be broadly described

353

as "information processing." Included among these are: electrocortical arousal, REM sleep, attention, perception, input-output association formation, retrieval of past memories, motivation, mood, and behavioral outputs. This cuts a wide swathe in the realm of higher
brain functions.

One interpretation of such a broad sweep of cholinergic effects
may be that cholinergic neurons form part of many brain mechanisms
which serve different functions. Since one or more of those functions
are likely to be impaired in any psychopathological state, cholinergic
manipulations would tend to produce changes of relevance to many forms
of psychiatric illness, without necessarily indicating a specific or
fundamental role in the pathogenesis of any.

Another interpretation would be the opposite, that is, the central cholinergic mechanisms have a fundamental, possibly unique, function which can affect a variety of processes involved in brain behavior relations. As such, defects in cholinergic functions may be of
basic importance in the pathogenesis of a condition such as schizophrenia in which many higher brain functions are disturbed at once.

This chapter examines this question by attempting an analysis and
a synthesis of the information presented in the previous chapters. In
this context, it should be understood that the term "adaptive" has a
broader and a more restrictive connotation. The wider meaning applies
to all the processes such as optimal arousal, selective attention,
perceptual discrimination, and memory retrieval which lead to the
choice and execution of behaviors most successful in meeting environmental as well as internal demands of the organism. The narrower,
though not basically different, meaning relates to what ethologists
term "phenotypic adjustability," that is the facility with which old
behaviors can be changed and new behaviors formed in meeting varied
and changing demands of the environment. In this chapter, the term
adaptive function will refer to both these meanings but with greater
emphasis on the second type of usage. The brain may well be viewed
as an organ that frees behavior from the tyrannical and immediate control of sensory stimuli and thus permits flexibility and the formation
of newer, more successful behaviors in meeting the changing and complex demands of the environment.

2.   BRAIN ORGANIZATION

To understand the role of cholinergic pathways, one needs to have
some idea of the functional organization of the brain and where in
that organization these pathways fit. Figure 1 attempts to present a
very broad view of the brain organization based on important conceptual papers by a number of authors that deal with evolutionary brain
levels (MacLean, 1972, 1976; Isaacson, 1974), arousal mechanisms
(Routtenberg, 1968; Pribram and McGuiness, 1975; Vanderwolf and

Robinson, 1981), limbic system (Nauta and Domesick, 1981), basal
ganglia (Mettler, 1955; Hassler, 1978; Graybiel and Ragsdale, 1979),
frontal cortical areas (Nauta, 1971) and posterior cortical areas
(Mesulam and Geschwind, 1978; Mesulam et al., 1977). The only major
brain structure which has been left out is the cerebellum because,
although its role in the organization and coordination of motor
activity is well-known, the part it might play in the higher brain
processes has yet to be properly investigated.

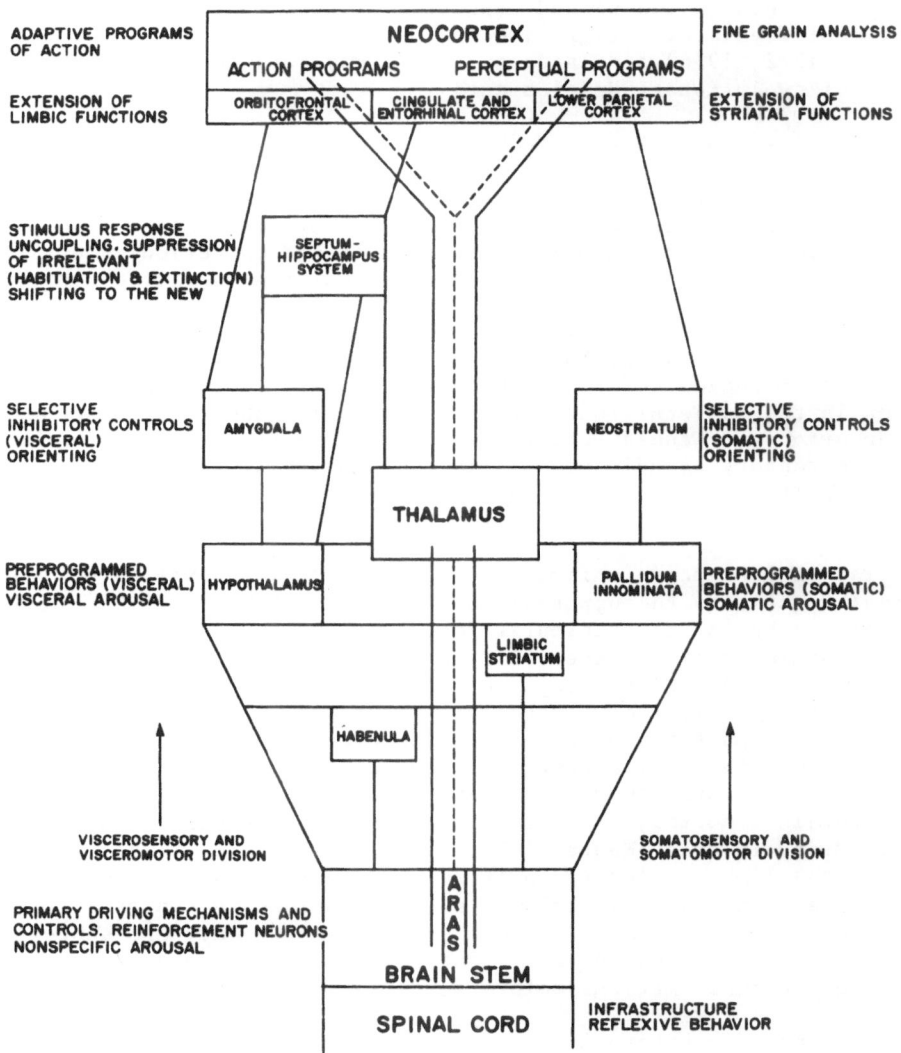

Fig. 1.   Levels of Brain Organization, Arousal, Attention, Stimulus-
          Response Processing and Adaptiveness.

The figure, which is not intended to be a comprehensive model of
the brain functions, emphasizes two basic organizational concepts.
The first recognizes the fact that the brain has two types of inputs
and outputs, namely, the somatic or exteroceptive reflecting the external milieu and visceral or interoceptive representing the internal
milieu. Apart from vertical interactions between various components
of each system, there is horizontal communication and integration between the two systems at successive levels including the brain stem,
diencephalon, subcortical limbic and striatal nuclei and the neocortex.
Related to this is the second concept, that is, the brain functions
at several levels of integration and adaptiveness which, according to
MacLean (1972, 1976) and Isaacson (1974) may represent different
stages of evolutionary development.

2.1. Cortical Input-Output Mechanisms

The exteroceptive inputs travel up to the brain stem via the
classical sensory pathways of the lemniscal system. After issuing
branches to the multisynaptic brain stem ascending reticular activating system (ARAS) and its thalamic extension, the so-called nonspecific thalamic nuclei, which together are involved in the regulation of
general cortical and behavioral activation or arousal (Magoun, 1958;
Lindsley, 1961; Hassler, 1978), these inputs form relays in the specific thalamic nuclei before reaching the primary sensory areas of the
cortex in the parietal, occipital and temporal lobes. As discussed
by Warburton and Wesnes (Chapters 1 and 8) the arrival of both the
specific sensory signals as well as the nonspecific activation signals
from ARAS at the cortex is probably needed for perception of, and attention to, stimuli.

The interoceptive information is carried via neural as well as
humoral signals to the hypothalamus, which is also the limbic extension of the brain stem reticular formation and serves what is termed
the autonomic or limbic arousal system (Routtenberg, 1968; Pribram and
McGuiness, 1975). With relays in the hypothalamus and/or the subcortical limbic nuclei, i.e., amygdala, septum and hippocampus, the interoceptive inputs reach the primary cortical areas of the limbic
system, i.e., the orbitofrontal cortex, which is connected with the
amygdala, the cingulate cortex, retrosplenial cortex, presubiculum
and entorhinal cortex, which receive hippocampal projections, and the
limbic midbrain area (Nauta, 1971; Nauta and Domesick, 1981). A good
part of the limbic information is relayed to the cortex through the
anterior and mediodorsal thalamic nuclei, so that in contrast to the
exteroceptive inputs which reach the cortex after only one subcortical
relay in the thalamus, the interoceptive inputs have a succession of
relays and transformations before reaching the cortex.

The specific exteroceptive information from the visual, auditory
and somatosensory cortices converges on to the inferior parietal
lobule which, in turn, connects with the somatic output mechanisms in

the frontal cortex and the subcortical striopallidal system, as well as the prefrontal cortex receiving limbic information from the amygdala and septal circuits and the cingulate and hippocampal gyri serving the hippocampal circuit (Petras, 1971; Nauta, 1971; Pribram and McGuiness, 1975; Nauta and Domesick, 1981). Exteroceptive signals from all modalities are also conveyed to the cingulate and parahippocampal gyri via the temporal neocortex (Nauta, 1971), so that more than any other limbic system, the hippocampal circuit seems to have a preferential relationship with the exteroceptive input systems. It is quite likely, therefore, that this circuit has a key role in the higher level input processing in the brain.

2.2. Striopallidal Circuit

Analogous to the exteroceptive sensory areas, the somatomator functions of the cortex are organized so that the precentral cortex serves as the specific motor area and, corresponding to the belt areas of the sensory cortex, the premotor cortex provides motor integrative functions. Forward of that is the so-called "frontal eye field" which has a strong connection with the inferior parietal lobule (see above) and is concerned with conjugate eye movements of the kind involved in paying attention to stimuli (Nauta, 1971). The rest of the frontal lobe, which has very close affinities with the limbic system (Nauta, 1971), seems to have a more general inhibitory control over behavioral outputs (Nauta, 1971; Pribram and McGuiness, 1975; Wilcott et al., 1976). The main subcortical input to the cortical motor or action program areas comes via the thalamus from the striopallidal system and cerebellum which are well-recognized for their role in somatomotor integration and control (Graybiel and Ragsdale, 1979).

The caudate-putamen or neostriatum receives inputs from the whole of the neocortex. Of the sensory areas, the parietal, especially the sensory motor, cortex provides particularly strong projections (Hassler, 1978; Graybiel and Ragsdale, 1979), and the putamen seems to be the main striatal component interposed between the inputs from the somatic sensory and somatic motor cortices (Künzle, 1977). The prefrontal cortex, with its strong limbic system affiliation, seems to project almost exclusively to the caudate in primates, so that the two components of the neostriatum may show some specialization of function (Goldman and Nauta, 1977). The nucleus accumbens-olfactory tubercle area, which is contiguous with the caudate-putamen and is designated limbic or ventral striatum (Heimer and Wilson, 1975), receives topographical projections from the allocortical formations of the limbic system, i.e., hippocampus, amygdala, and piriform cortex. The outputs from the neostriatum and limbic striatum are directed respectively to the pallidum and substantia innominata or ventral pallidum, which represent the output ends of the striopallidal chains (Heimer and Wilson, 1975; Hassler, 1978; Graybiel and Ragsdale, 1979). A large portion of the pallidal projection goes through the VA-VL complex of the thalamus to the neocortex, particularly the motor and

premotor cortex and the parietal lobe, thus completing the cortico-
striato-pallido-thalamo-cortical circuit concerned with somatomotor
or action programs (Hassler, 1978). The projections from the
substantia innominata also spread to most or all of the neocortex,
providing a pathway for limbic influence over the functional state of
the cortex as a whole (Nauta and Domesick, 1981; Robinson, Chapter 2,
this book).

A second circuit connecting the neocortex with the striopallidal
system involves the intralaminar thalamic nuclei, especially the
center median nucleus which has a massive size in primates. The intralaminar thalamic nuclei, mainly the center median and parafascicular nuclei, form parts of the so-called nonspecific or diffuse thalamic projection system (Jasper, 1949) which has a widespread influence
on cortical activation and represents a thalamic counterpart and/or
extension of the mesencephalic reticular system of Moruzzi and Magoun
(1949). While the latter seems to have some direct connections with
the cortex (Starzl and Magoun, 1951), the nonspecific thalamic system
seems to have its diffuse cortical effects through the striopallidal
neuronal chains (Hassler, 1978), thus implicating the striopallidal
system in the control of cortical and behavioral arousal and attention.
Besides the nonspecific sensory inputs travelling up through the
neuronal chains of the brain stem reticular formation, the center
median - parafascicular complex of the intralaminar, or what Hassler
(1978) terms the truncothalamic, nuclei receive inputs from the neocortex, principally the motor cortex (Graybiel and Ragsdale, 1979).
The truncothalamic nuclei project to the striatum or the outer segment
of the pallidum from where the impulses meet in the outer and inner
segments of the pallidum. From there, some projections go back to the
truncothalamic nuclei, thus forming a closed loop, while others are
diffusely transmitted to the cortex through the VA-VL thalamic complex
(Hassler, 1978), thus completing the cortico-thalamo-strio-pallido-
thalamo-cortical circuit.

On the basis of experiments involving stimulation, at various
intensities and frequencies, of parts of the striatum, pallidum, and
truncothalamic nuclei in freely moving animals as well as other types
of preparations, Hassler (1978) has concluded that the striopallidal
neuronal chain forms an integral part of the nonspecific thalamo-cortical activating system, which he calls the truncothalamic system to
avoid the term nonspecific. This system, he believes is involved in
the somatic and emotional aspects of arousal and attention such as
turning towards an object or an event in the contralateral field and
suppression of activities other than those attracting attention. In
this, the role of the pallidum is essentially excitatory so that its
stimulation produces turning of eyes, head and the rest of the body to
the opposite side along with signs of alertness and vigilance such as
dilatation of the palpebral fissure and the pupils. The role of the
striatum is to exercise inhibitory control over these processes on the
basis of information received from the neocortex and other sources.

The interconnections between the inferior parietal lobule, the strio-pallido-thalamic nuclei and the frontal eye fields may be particularly important in these functions because activity in all these areas is related to attentional behaviors, and their damage can produce contra-lateral inattention and sensory neglect (Nauta, 1971; Ungerstedt and Pycock, 1974; Mesulam et al., 1977; Mesulam and Geschwind, 1978). Other structures which can be implicated in the attentional processes carry limbic information (see below) and are also closely connected with this circuitry.

Besides the cortical and thalamic connections outlined above, the neostriatum and limbic striatum receive important afferents from the dopaminergic neurons of the substantia nigra and the serotonergic neu-rons of the raphe nuclei in the midbrain. These neurons, along with the more caudally situated norepinephric neurons of the locus ceruleus and the reticular formation, are phylogenetically ancient systems which seem to modulate basic adaptive neural and hormonal processes concerned with arousal, locomotion, thermal regulation, defense and reproduction (Dahlström, 1969). Arising from very small discrete areas, all in the brain stem, these neurons have widespread distribu-tion and influence in the somatic as well as visceral domains, sug-gesting a general drive-control or drive-modulation role for them (Olds, 1976).

Of the three monoaminergic systems, the dopaminergic seems to have a preferential relationship with the somatic output systems rep-resented by the striopallidal complex and the frontal cortex and may be regarded as a primary driving mechanism for the somatic output system. This is suggested not only by the fact that most of the nigral dopaminergic projections are aimed at the neostriatum and limbic striatum, while others terminate in the frontal and limbic cor-tices (Graybiel and Ragsdale, 1979), but also by the observation that the effects of dopaminergic activation are similar to those produced by pallidal stimulation i.e., attentional fixation on and repetition of stereotyped motor patterns (Randrup and Munkvad, 1968; Ellinwood et al., 1973; Matthysse, 1977; Hassler, 1978; Singh and Lal, 1982). However, the main input into the substantia nigra is from the limbic structures, reaching it directly and, more importantly, through the limbic striatum and habenula (Graybiel and Ragsdale, 1979; Nauta and Domesick, 1981). This input reaches the zona compacta, the source of nigrostriatal pathway, directly, as well as indirectly through the zona reticulata which connects with the zona compacta as part of the strionigral loop in which the afferent limb is the nigrostriatal path-way from the zona compacta, while the efferent limb is the striatal projection to the zona reticulata (Scheel-Krüger, Chapter 4). This means that the striopallidal complex, through its drive neurons, is under limbic control and thus responsive to influences such as motiva-tion, mood, and affect. Furthermore, through the zona reticulata pro-jections to the mediodorsal as well as the VA-VL thalamic nuclei, this influence may serve to modulate the whole striopallidal connection with the cortex. Of particular interest may be the zona reticulata

access to the frontal eyefields through the mediodorsal thalamic
nucleus (Akert, 1964), because through this channel limbic mechanisms
may be able to direct the attentional functions of the striopallidal
system.

The limbic influence over the striopallidal system is exerted
through connections other than those with the substantia nigra. Most
prominent among these are direct and indirect projections from the
septal-hippocampal system. As summarized in an elegant review by
Nauta and Domesick (1981), direct hippocampal projections reach the
anteroventral part of the striatum, while indirect projections reach
the mediodorsal striatum through the cingulate cortex and the whole
of the striatum through a conduction route that travels over the
dorsum of the thalamus through the habenular complex and reaches the
midbrain raphe nuclei, which then send serotonergic projections to the
corpus striatum. Considering that a good part of the input to the
limbic striatum, and thence to the nigral complex, also represents the
hippocampal outflow, it can be appreciated the that septal-hippocampal
system has a great deal to do with the functioning of the striopallidal system. However, direct and indirect projections to the latter
also come from the amygdala.

An important aspect of these limbic-striatal connections is that
they largely flow from the limbic system to the striatum suggesting
that the striopallidal system is under limbic regulation. According
to Isaacson (1974), this control is essentially of an inhibitory
nature, which is consistent with MacLean's (1972, 1976) triune brain
model whereby the limbic system ("paleomammalian brain") is viewed as
a later evolutionary development which served to increase the adaptiveness of the organism by providing inhibitory control over the
tendency of the phylogenetically older striopallidal complex ("the
reptilian brain" or R-complex) to emit preprogrammed, stereotyped
behaviors.

It should be noted that the dopaminergic system, through its
nigrostriatal and mesolimbic divisions, affects both the somatomotor
striopallidal complex as well as the visceral influence on that
through the limbic striatum (Graybiel and Ragsdale, 1979). In addition, it sends fiber projections to the amygdala as well as to the
limbic system-affiliated frontal, cingulate and entorhinal cortices.
The serotonergic fiber system originating in the mesencephalic raphe
nuclei reflects the limbic-striopallidal association even more because
its striopallidal projection is matched by a widespread projection,
through the medial forebrain bundle, to all the subcortical as well
as cortical components of the limbic system (Andén et al., 1966;
Ungerstedt, 1971; Nauta and Domesick, 1981). However, the norepinephric system, which originates in the lower brain stem, projects
through the medial forebrain bundle largely to the limbic system
structures where its distribution corresponds to that of the serotonergic system (Fuxe, 1965; Ungerstedt, 1971). The brain self-stimulation studies suggest that the norepinephrine neurons may serve as the

drive mechanism for reward or pleasure within the limbic system (Olds, 1976). One might, therefore, conceptualize these as the primary drive neurons for the motive functions of the limbic system, while the dopamine neurons serve to drive the purposive, instrumental behavior functions of the striopallidal system and the serotonergic neurons perform some general, possibly inhibitory functions, common to both the systems.

From this outline, it can be seen that the striopallidal system is interposed as a subcortical loop between the somatosensory and somatomotor mechanisms of the neocortex on the one hand and between the limbic and neocortical mechanisms on the other. In view of the very broad range of cortical and limbic information it receives and the extensiveness of the output it provides to the cortical motor as well as to the sensory systems, its function is likely to be of a general rather than a discrete nature. The traditional view has been that basal ganglia regulate essentially the mechanical and geometric aspect of movements begun by the motor cortex. This belies the phenomenal amount of input coming into this system from the sensory cortex, its subjection to the limbic control and its involvement in the reticulo-thalamo-cortical arousal mechanisms. On anatomical grounds alone, one would have to suspect that the striopallidal system is involved in the activation, sensory-motor integration and motivational regulation of programmed behavior. Therefore, it might be more plausible to view it as a system involved in the initiation, monitoring and modification of behavior in terms of somatosensory feedback as well as information concerning the motivational and emotional significance of the action and its consequences. Such indeed is the emerging concept (Kornhuber, 1971; DeLong, 1972; Matthysse, 1974; Villablanca and Marcus, 1975; Teuber, 1976; Cools and Van den Bercken, 1977; Hassler, 1978). Based on evolutionary considerations and the results of studies such as those involving electrical stimulation of basal ganglia or chemical activation of the dopaminergic or cholinergic mechanisms of this system, it has been suggested that the primitive functions of the midbrain-basal ganglia complex, (the so-called "R-complex"), which is derived from its reptilian past, is to emit and attend to species-typical preprogrammed behaviors or primary automatisms (MacLean, 1972, 1976; Isaacson, 1974; Hassler, 1978), whereas the later development of the limbic ("paleomammalian") and cortical ("neomammalian") superimpositions have provided it the capability for developing, emitting and modifying secondary automatisms or programmed behaviors acquired through intentional action and learning (Isaacson, 1974; Hassler, 1978). In neurophysiological and neuropsychological terms, Pribram and McGuiness (1975) have suggested that the basal ganglia-centered mechanisms are concerned with vigilant readiness ("what is to be done?") or activation of perceptual expectancies and motor readiness signaling intention to act, i.e., processes such as those believed to be reflected in the contingent negative variation in brain electrical activity (Tecce, 1972). In biochemical and pharmacological terms, the activation of automatic behaviors and the

resultant attentional fixation or perseveration may be a consequence
of dopaminergic activity (Randrup and Munkvad, 1970; Ellinwood et al.,
1973; Matthysse, 1977), while cholinergic and possibly serotonergic
systems may be involved in mechanisms which introduce variability and
adaptive flexibility in the behavioral operations (Cools and Van den
Bercken, 1977; Van den Bercken and Cools, 1979; Pribram and McGuiness,
1975).

2.3. Limbic Circuits

These concepts recognize that the somatic output system centered
on the striopallidal complex is under limbic regulation, which is suggested by the neuroanatomical fact of predominantly one way projections from the limbic system to the extrapyramidal system. However,
within the limbic organization, developmentally, anatomically and
functionally, two systems or circuits can be differentiated - one
centered on the amygdala complex and the other on the hippocampal
formation. Of these, the amygdala system may be considered as the
visceral counterpart of the striopallidal somatic output system. This
is suggested not only by its role in visceromotor arousal, orienting
or attention, agonistic and affiliative behaviors, active and passive
avoidance, sexual activity and feeding activities (Kaada, 1972;
Pribram and McGuiness, 1975; Kling and Steklis, 1976), but also by the
fact that it shares with the striopallidal complex its embryological
development (Humphrey, 1972) and the dopaminergic input from substantia nigra (Ungerstedt, 1971; Stevens, 1973; Emson et al., 1979). On
the other hand, the hippocampus, which does not have a close embryological link with the striopallidal complex and receives few if any
dopaminergic fibers, may be part of the circuitry concerned mainly
with input processing and perceptual control of goal-directed behavior
through some form of coordination of the basal ganglia and amygdala
circuits on the one hand and of the posterior (input) and anterior
(output) parts of the cortex on the other (Pribram and McGuiness,
1975; Pribram and Isaacson, 1975).

Funneling information upstream, downstream and between the two
limbic systems, and also providing the command neurons for drives and
visceral activity, is a continuum of gray matter intermingled in the
fibers of the medial forebrain bundle which extends from the limbic
zones of the midbrain tegmentum, including the origins of the three
monoaminergic systems (i.e., serotonergic, norepinephric, and dopaminergic), to the septal area on the cortical end (Nauta and Domesick,
1981). In its arrangement as a mixture of gray and white matter, and
also as a repository of command neurons for motivational drive mechanisms (e.g., Gloor, 1972) this continuum resembles the brain stem reticular formation and may be considered as the limbic extension of the
reticular activating system, much as the truncothalamic nuclei seem
to be the striopallidal or somatic extension. Included in this continuum, from the cortical end to the brain stem, are the septum,
limbic striatum, substantia innominata, preoptic area, hypothalamus
and the limbic midbrain areas, which include the ventral tegmental

area (dopaminergic), raphe nuclei (serotonergic), interpeduncular nucleus (cholinergic) and locus ceruleus (norepinephric). In addition, the habenular complex, despite its distance from the above structures, may be included in the continuum, because it shares with them the characteristic of providing an intermediate station for the reciprocal limbic forebrain-midbrain circuit (Nauta and Domesick, 1981).

2.4. Cortical Connections of Limbic Circuits

On the cortical end, the amygdala receives exteroceptive inputs in a topographically organized fashion through anterior portions of the superior, middle and inferior temporal gyri and the mediolateral aspects of the temporal pole (Herzog and Van Hoesen, 1976; Turner et al., 1980). This information remains modality-specific to a surprising degree because each sensory system (i.e., vision, audition, taste) seems to terminate on a specific part of the amygdala complex (Turner et al., 1980). In addition to these sensory inputs, which are one or two steps removed from the primary sensory areas, the amygdala receives olfactory information more directly through the paleocortical piriform cortex (Lammers, 1972). The amygdala thus serves as an integrative center for the two types of exteroceptive input and a major connecting link between them and the central visceral mechanisms of the preoptic-hypothalamic continuum (Herzog and Van Hoesen, 1976), through which the affective relationships of the sensory inflow can be elaborated and expressed. The cortical efferents from the amygdala reach the orbitofrontal cortex via a subcortical conduction route, the ventral amygdalofugal pathway, that passes through the preoptic-hypothalamic area on its way to the magnocellular portion of the mediodorsal thalamus, which in turn projects to the orbitofrontal cortex (Lammers, 1972; Nauta and Domesick, 1981). The latter is reciprocally connected to the inferior temporal cortex which sends afferents to the amygdala. Another source of frontal input to the amygdala circuits arises as a widespread topographic projection from the frontal convexity to the temporal gyri which provide afferents to the amygdala complex (Whitlock and Nauta, 1956; Pandya and Kuypers, 1969; Nauta, 1971). This provides the anatomical basis for the two reciprocally-acting amygdala-centered systems that have been distinguished, namely, a visceroautonomic inhibitory pathway with the orbitofrontal cortex at the rostral pole and a visceroautonomic facilitatory pathway in which the dorsolateral frontal cortex represents the cortical end (Pribram and McGuiness, 1975).

The cortical connections of the hippocampus are significantly different from those of the amygdala. Information from the visual, auditory and somatic cortical fields reaches the hippocampal formation through two interconnected routes, the inferior parietal lobule and the rostral half of the temporal neocortex, both of which are the convergence zones for inputs from the three sensory association areas Pandya and Kuypers, 1969; Nauta, 1971; Petras, 1971; Van Hoesen and Pandya, 1975; Van Hoesen et al., 1975). This information seems to be

much more processed or supramodal than that reaching the amygdala
(Mesulam et al., 1977; Turner et al., 1980), and connects with the
hippocampal or Papez's circuit on both its input and output sides,
represented respectively by the juxtahippocampal cortex (entorhinal
area and parahippocampal gyrus) and the cingulate gyrus. The circuit
is in the form of a closed loop in which hippocampal projections in
the fornix reach the anterior thalamic nucleus directly as well as
indirectly through the mammillary body and the mammillothalamic tract;
the anterior thalamic nucleus then projects via the fasciculus cinguli
to the cingulate gyrus, retrosplenial cortex and presubiculum, and the
circuit is finally completed by the presubiculum projection to the
entorhinal cortex, from which begins the perforant pathway to the hippocampus (Nauta and Domesick, 1981). Thus, in its thalamic connection
also, the hippocampal circuit remains distinct from the amygdala
circuit. This distinction is further evident in the hippocampal relations with the frontal cortex where most of the fibers for the cingulate and parahippocampal gyri originate from the dorsal convexity
cortex, especially in an area of the principal sulcus which lies
fairly close to the frontal eye field. These areas receive strong
projections from the inferior parietal lobule and rostral temporal
cortex, which have close connections with the hippocampal circuit
(Nauta, 1971; Petras, 1971; Mesulam et al., 1977). These connections
may be of great interest for the anatomy of attention, because attentional failure and sensory neglect can result from ablations of many
of the areas, especially the cingulate cortex, inferior parietal
lobule and the frontal eye field, involved in this network (Mesulam
et al., 1977). One might well surmise from these connections that the
hippocampal circuit has a significant role in the mechanisms of perceptual attention. In this context, it may be interesting to note
that the cingulate cortex - the recipient of the hippocampal outputs -
sends few if any projections to the central limbic structures such as
the hypothalamus, septum and amygdala (Domesick, 1969, 1972) which
provide the visceroautonomic outflow and are implicated in the visceral aspects of arousal and attention (see below). Its projections
go mainly to the parietal and temporal sensory association areas of
the neocortex, the frontal neocortex and various nuclei of the thalamus (Isaacson, 1974). This would implicate it mainly in the somatosensory and somatomotor components of attention where its role might
be to indicate the emotional and motivational significance of exteroceptive inputs.

2.5. Subcortical Connections of Limbic Circuits

The subcortical connections of the amygdala circuit seem to be
weighted towards the structures that provide viceroautonomic outflow,
while those of the hippocampal system seem to have a particular relationship to the structures which provide limbic input to the extrapyramidal system and the neocortex.

Numerous fibers that form into a dorsal pathway (the stria terminalis) and a ventral pathway (the ventral amygdalofugal system)

establish reciprocal connections between various parts of the amygdala
complex and the ergotopic (sympathetic) as well as trophotropic (parasympathetic) parts of the preoptic area and the hypothalamus, from
where originate the visceroautonomic outflow to the autonomic neurons
of the brain stem and the spinal cord (Lammers, 1972; Kaada, 1972;
Kuypers and Maisky, 1975; Saper et al., 1976). The medial group of
amygdala nuclei may have a preferential relationship with the medial
sympathetic zone of the hypothalamus while the lateral group may be
connected mainly to the lateral parasympathetic zone of the hypothalamus (Koikegami, 1963, 1964; Egger and Flynn, 1967). In addition to
these, the amygdala has been shown to establish a direct reciprocal
connection with a number of midbrain nuclei concerned with visceral
inputs and outputs (Nauta and Domesick, 1981). Through these connections, the amygdala, and the frontal neocortical areas with which it
is connected, can modulate the visceral processes initiated by the
diencephalic command neurons of the hypothalamus and the visceromotor
nuclei (Kaada, 1972; Gloor, 1972).

Another set of connections would permit the amygdala to influence
the extrapyramidal system. These are the projections via both the
fiber systems of the amygdala to the limbic striatum and substantia
innominata which, as described before, connect with and influence various parts of the striopallidal system (Nauta and Domesick, 1981).
Thus the amygdala circuits are in a position to simultaneously affect
the subcortical visceral as well as somatic output mechanisms - an
anatomical arrangement well-suited for a pivotal role in the control
of behavioral arousal and orienting which these circuits are believed
to have (Pribram and McGuiness, 1975). In a review of the relevant
lesioning and neurophysiological studies in monkeys, Pribram and
McGuiness (1975) noted that amygdalectomy results in a failure of behavioral habituation leading to repetitious locomotor orienting reaction, an effect also produced by an orbitofrontal lesion. At the same
time, the phasic heart rate responses accompanying attentional processes are lost but there is a tonic elevation of heart rate. The
electrodermal responses during orienting are also reduced in most
subjects. Corresponding to this, the resection of the dorsolateral
frontal cortex produces a loss of visceroautonomic components of
orienting. The overall picture from an amygdalectomy is that of a
persistent and nonspecific defense reaction similar to that produced
by the stimulation of the so-called defense region of the hypothalamus.
Therefore, it may be concluded that a dual fronto-amygdala system is
crucially important for specific control and attentional direction of
the arousal generated in the hypothalamus and also possibly in the
striopallidal circuits. It may be noted in this context that the role
of amygdala-centered mechanisms in fight-flight or agonistic behavior,
as well as the related affiliative behavior, is well-documented
(Kaada, 1972; Kling and Steklis, 1976). The destruction of the amygdala, orbitofrontal cortex or the temporal pole in monkeys results in
social isolation, avoidance and loss of affiliative behaviors. The
overall behavioral effect of amygdala seems to be excitatory
(Isaacson, 1974).

The principal subcortical connections of the hippocampal formation involve the septum on the afferent end and various structures
connected with the extrapyramidal system and the neocortex on the
efferent end.

Standing at the head of the septal-diencephalic-midbrain continuum of the central limbic structures, the septal area occupies a significant position as the cross-roads of extensive neural traffic from
almost all the subcortical as well as cortical constituents of the
limbic system in its widest sense (Isaacson, 1974). It is thus able
to funnel both upstream as well as downstream limbic information into
the hippocampal system, with which, mainly through the so-called precommissural fornix, it establishes two-way connections. Its close
link to the hippocampus is suggested not only by the extensiveness of
these connections but also by the fact that many of the functional
consequences of a septal lesion are similar to those that follow a
hippocampectomy (Isaacson, 1974). Through its intimate downstream
connections with various parts of the hypothalamus, it may be conceived as an intermediary between the hippocampus and the hypothalamus, although many direct connections are also to be found between the
latter structures. However, it is remarkable that, in contrast to
almost every other part of the limbic system, the hippocampus, when
stimulated produces few if any autonomic effects (Kaada, 1951). This
may mean that the hypothalamus is mostly afferent to the hippocampus,
or that the relationship between the two concerns functions other than
the visceroautonomic outflow from the hypothalamus.

The subcortical extrapyramidal connections of the hippocampal
system follow two different conduction lines. The first, by way of
precommissural fornix, is to the limbic striatum and substantia innominata (Heimer and Wilson, 1975), where they are joined by projections from the amygdala, so that through this route, the basal ganglia
system may be thought of as being under a dual limbic control
(Graybiel and Ragsdale, 1979). These connections would permit the
hippocampal system to influence virtually the whole of the dopaminergic system. However, since there is no direct dopaminergic innervation of the hippocampus, any feedback by the dopamine system is likely
to be indirect through the septum – limbic striatum – innominata continuum. The second conduction line leads to the serotonergic raphe
nuclei in the midbrain via the stria medullaris, which connects the
septum (as well as the lateral preoptic-hypothalamic region) with the
habenula, and the fasciculus retroflexus, which connects the habenula
with the interpeduncular nucleus and the raphe nuclei; the raphe
nuclei then send projections to the basal ganalia and almost all the
limbic structures including the hippocampal formation (Herkenham and
Nauta, 1977, 1979; Hillarp et al., 1966; Nauta and Domesick, 1981).
Thus, the hippocampal circuit is able to affect the activity of the
neurons of origin for both the monoaminergic projections i.e., dopaminergic and serotonergic, for the striopallidal network. At the
same time, as mentioned before, the hippocampus establishes direct

subcortical connections with the striatum, and also reaches it from
the cortical end through a cingulate projection (Nauta and Domesick,
1981). This means that the hippocampal circuit, through its subcortical and cortical projections, has a bipolar link with the striopallidal system.

Through its influence on the dopaminergic and the serotonergic
systems, the hippocampal circuit is also in a position to affect the
amygdala circuit, which receives strong projections from these systems.
Further interactions with the amygdala circuit are likely in the
septum - limbic striatum - innominata continuum, which receives dual
limbic cortical projections, as well as at the frontal neocortical
level. Very few direct fiber connections between the hippocampus and
amygdala seem to exist.

Through the septum - limbic striatum - innominata continuum, the
hippocampal system, like the amygdala system, establishes a route to
the neocortex of a most encompassing nature, because large neurons in
these structures, especially the substantia innominata, seem to send
a widespread projection to the neocortex. From the diffuseness of
this projection, it is reasonable to assume that the influence of
this pathway is of a general rather than a specific character.

Anatomically, therefore, the hippocampus-centered circuit is
distinguished by the following characteristics: (1) on the cortical
end, it relates predominately to the areas which serve integrative,
and possibly attention-control, function in the exteroceptive input
system, while on the subcortical end, it sends multichannel but largely unreciprocated projections into the striopallidal circuit, and also
a very diffuse projection into the neocortex; (b) unlike the other two
major subcortical systems, it receives no dopaminergic input, except
indirectly throught the septal connection; and (c) its limbic character is indicated mainly by the fact that it has many connections with
the central limbic structures of the septal - hypothalamic - mesencephalic continuum, but in terms of visceroautonomic outflow it seems
to have little impact, so that its role may be conceived as mainly
providing limbic system input and control in the exteroceptive aspects
of the brain organization. In addition, as will be discussed in the
next section, this circuit may have a pivotal role in the cholinergic
mechanisms of the brain.

To highlight the functional significance of this anatomical arrangement, it may be stated, as a simplified generalization, that the
hippocampal circuit seems to be essentially inhibitory on the behavioral output end but facilitatory in terms of input processing. This
is suggested by the behavioral and perceptual consequences of experimental hippocampal destruction as well as by the relationships between
the electrical activity of the hippocampus and various stages of information processing.

Based on the literature reviewed by Isaacson (1974), the results of bilateral hippocampal destruction in animals may be summarized as follows: hyperactivity and poor habituation in an open field situation; decreased distractibility or poor orienting to novel stimuli during performance of well-learned or predominant behavioral acts in a situation; poor performance in situations requiring withholding of responses such as passive avoidance and differential reinforcement of low rate or DRL tasks; perseveratory behavior in tasks such as spontaneous alternation where normal animals alternate their visits to the arms of a Y or T maze, and various learning situations where the animal has to change responses, strategies or perceptual hypotheses to obtain reinforcement or avoid punishment; and poor discrimination performance in tasks involving successive discrimination, shift from one type of perceptual hypothesis to another, replacement of a previously learned response with a new one (discrimination reversal), the choice of a correct response from two possible responses, and the detection of a positive or rewarded cue from several negative or unrewarded cues.

In terms of the brain electrical activity, a rhythmical or synchronized, 4 to 8 Hz theta wave pattern in the hippocampus accompanies the desynchronized, low voltage fast activity, i.e., activation pattern, in the neocortex when a state of arousal is produced by sensory stimulation or electrical stimulation of the brain stem or limbic arousal mechanisms (Green and Arduini, 1954; Torü, 1961; Anchel and Lindsley, 1972). The behavioral correlate of this is believed to be orienting toward and attending to stimuli in the environment (Bennett, 1970). With intended or overt voluntary action, suggesting possibly an engagement of the motor programs relevant to the prevailing motivation and environmental incentives, the rhythmical theta continues (Dalton and Black, 1968; Vanderwolf, 1969, 1971). The theta power apparently shows an increase when the contingent negative variation in the brain electrical activity, signifying an expectant attention or a motor readiness signal, gives way to a sharp positivity indicating the start of the intended response (Grandstaff and Pribram, 1972). However, any alteration in ongoing behavioral sequence is attended with an increase in the hippocampal electrical frequencies (Kamp et al., 1971), while the arrest of ongoing behavior is associated with a desynchronization of electrical activities in the hippocampus (Bennett and Gottfried, 1970). The response of hippocampal neurons to a stimulus presentation is slow to develop and lasts well beyond the time required for sensory processing in the specific as well as the association areas of the cortex suggesting that the hippocampus deals with something other than the specific aspects of sensory input (Vinogradova, 1970). Habituation of this response occurs with repeated stimulus presentation but dishabituation occurs with any change in stimulus configuration.

Thus, it seems clear that the hippocampal circuit is involved in input processing as well as inhibitory control of behavior. However, it is probably not concerned with sensory discrimination or perception

as such because not only has the sensory information lost its specificity by the time it reaches the hippocampus but animals with hippocampal lesions are still capable of sensory discrimination (Isaacson,
1974; Pribram and Isaacson, 1975). Neither does it seem to be a general inhibitor of responses because hippocampectomized animals still
have the capability to inhibit responses in certain situations, e.g.,
passive avoidance learned before the lesion, go - no go alternation
and object reversal (Wishart and Mogenson, 1970; Mahut, 1971; Olton,
1972; Pribram and Isaacson, 1975). The indistractibility of the
lesioned animals also is evident mainly while performing well-established behaviors (Isaacson, 1974) and it is reflected more in somatomotor performance than perception because perceptual distractibility
is still demonstrable (Douglas and Pribram, 1969).

The role of the hippocampus-centered circuit in input processing
and attention as well as control of responses may be concerned essentially with circumstances where incoming external and internal information signals the need for a modification or change in the strategum
or behavior in use. According to a proposal elaborated by Pribram and
his collaborators (Douglas and Pribram, 1966; Pribram, 1971; Pribram
and McGuiness, 1975; Pribram and Isaacson, 1975), the hippocampus is
part of a mechanism that recognizes an error, mismatch, uncertainty
or new development in a situation and then sets into motion neural
processes which can devise a new plan of action. This, it would ac-
complish by inhibiting ongoing or habitual behavior and facilitating
attention to new or supplementary information. The hippocampal circuit thus provides added flexibility or adaptiveness to the organism.

Based on the work of Macadar et al. (1974) and others, Pribram
and McGuiness (1975) have proposed that the hippocampal circuit
remains under tonic inhibition, indicated by the rhythmical theta,
through the activity of catecholaminergic mechanisms when the organism
is engaged in orienting or voluntary behavior for which the catecholaminergic inputs to the amygdala and basal ganglia circuit provide
the driving force. However, when a signal requiring change in behavior comes down to the brain stem reticular system from the cortex, the
serotonergic mechanisms act to decrease this inhibition on the hippocampus, producing a desynchronization of hippocampal electrical activity and a mobilization of the hippocampal circuit, which disengages
the input and output control mechanisms of the amygdala and the basal
ganglia circuits, thereby interrupting an ongoing behavioral program,
and thus permits the cortical circuits to devise a modified or a new
program of action.

Pribram and McGuiness (1975) have indeed proposed a comprehensive
model which considers not only the functional relations between the
amygdala-, the basal ganglia-, and the hippocampus-centered circuits
but also the role played by the brain stem monoaminergic projections
to these structures. This model, which has been explained in parts in
the foregoing outline, seems to fit the anatomical arrangement of the

connections between these circuits quite nicely and has few serious competitors as a framework for considering information processing in the brain. In essence, it states that, corresponding to the functions of the three cortical-subcortical circuits, three types of attention can be defined. The first consists of an orienting reaction to stimuli and is controlled by the amygdala circuit, while the second, controlled by the striopallidal circuit, involves vigilant readiness to respond. Both are energized by the catecholaminergic neurons and control attentional-intentional behavior as long as the stimulus-response coupling can take place within a fairly stable and certain environment in which, so to speak, the rules of the game do not change. However, with the appearance of any uncertainty, change or perturbation, arising from new external or internal information, including presumably that related to memories, motivations and the consequences of behavior, a third type of attentional process becomes necessary, in which the hippocampal circuit has a crucial role. This process would involve suspension of the ongoing program of action and attending to the new data so that a new strategy or solution can be developed by the cortical mechanisms. This function is thought to be released by the serotonergic inhibition of the inhibitory control exercised on the hippocampal mechanisms by the catecholamine neurons. When the behavior is completely automatic and thus does not involve the attention-intention processes, none of the three cortical-subcortical circuits is needed, while during any defensive action (fighting or fleeing), both the orienting and the action readiness mechanisms are believed to be involved simultaneously.

The role of the brain cholinergic pathways is not spelled out in this fomulation. However, as will be discussed in the next section, the cholinergic neurons may have a crucial part in the hippocampal circuit functions.

3.   CHOLINERGIC MECHANISMS AND THE HIPPOCAMPAL CIRCUIT

Apart from the cholinergic neurons in the striatum, where they have an essentially local function (see above), most of the neurons of the central cholinergic mechanisms seem to belong to the limbic system (Robinson, Chapter 2). Much like the monoaminergic systems of the brain stem, these neurons provide widespread projections from a small locus of origin, which, perhaps significantly, is situated in the limbic extension of the brain stem reticular formation. Characteristically, they have large, easily recognized, cell bodies which are to be found in the limbic core in a continuum of structures including, from the rostral end, septum, nucleus of the diagonal band of Broca, lateral preoptic area and substantia innominata.

Within the framework of the brain organization outlined above, the cholinergic projections from these structures may be conceptualized as comprising two pathways. One of these, corresponding to the

ventral tegmental pathway of Shute and Lewis (1967, 1975), seems to be
part of the reticulocortical projection system concerned with arousal
and attention. It consists of the cholinergic fibers arising in the
magnocellular neurons of the substantia innominata and lateral preoptic area and reaching all parts of the neocortex as well as portions
(mostly the lateral nuclei) of the amygdala (Robinson, Chapter 2).
In an essentially serial arrangement, the brain stem monoaminergic
projections, reaching the innominata-preoptic area through the septal-
limbic striatal connections, or possibly directly, are afferent to
this cholinergic pathway. The second cholinergic projection corresponds to the "cholinergic limbic system" of Shute and Lewis (1967,
1975) and is part of the septal-hippocampal circuit, which seems to
be arranged so as to form a loop that connects with the first, i.e.,
the reticulocortical, projection system at the point of intersection
between the brain stem monoaminergic pathways and the cortical cholinergic radiation. The fibers of this pathway originate in the cholinergic neurons located in the medial septum and the adjacent nucleus
of the diagonal band and form the septal radiation to the hippocampus,
thus occupying an afferent position with respect to the latter
(Robinson, Chapter 2). As discussed earlier, the hippocampal output,
which is believed to be mediated by glutaminergic neurons (Walaas and
Fonnum, 1980), goes to the limbic striatum-substantia innominata continuum, thus completing one part of the cholinergic limbic loop.
Another part is constituted by the hippocampal return to the septal-
nucleus of the diagonal band area, which in turn is connected with the
limbic striatum-substantia innominata continuum. Yet another part
consists of the hippocampal projection to the habenula, from where a
cholinergic pathway (which also contains cholinergic fibers from the
septum) goes to the interpeduncular nucleus, and the loop is completed
by the interpeduncular projection to the raphe nuclei, which provide
the serotonergic neurons for the septal-nucleus of the diagonal band
area as well as the limbic striatum-substantia innominata complex
(Robinson, Chapter 2; Nauta and Domesick 1981). Thus, through three
different routes, the cholinergic neurons of the septal-hippocampal
system could affect all the brain stem monoaminergic pathways and the
core limbic structures situated at the junction of the brain stem
reticular system pathways (i.e., monoaminergic neurons) and the cholinergic cortical projection on the one hand, and the limbic circuits
and the striopallidal circuit on the other. Furthermore, since the
cholinergic output from the substantia innominata-lateral preoptic
area goes not only to the cortex but also to the amygdala (which sends
a return projection thus completing another loop), the hippocampal
outputs could affect the amygdala circuit operations at the same time.

    Such an anatomical arrangement, if correct, would seem to place
the cholinergic system in an important, if not crucial, position in
relation to the hypothesized role of the hippocampal circuit (see
above) in disengaging stimulus-response connections and providing inhibition of behavioral output while facilitating input processing in
situations such as those requiring new solutions to problems. The

notable similarity of the effects of the hippocampal lesions with
those produced by central cholinergic blockade lends support to this
position (Douglas, 1972, 1975). At the same time, this arrangement
suggests a conceptual model that could explain the apparent paradox
of behavioral suppression coupled with cortical arousal produced by
cholinergic stimulation (Karczmar, 1975, 1979; Hingtgen and Aprison,
1976; Wauquier and Clincke, Chapter 3). The model might also clarify
the situation created by the experimental data which suggest cholinergic involvement in a large number of functions and which can be
interpreted to support hypotheses which assign mainly input-control,
memory, or output-control functions to the brain cholinergic
mechanisms.

     To examine and expand these statements, some of the pertinent
data should be considered. A good starting point for this would be
the behavioral and cortical arousal. As discussed in reviews by
Karczmar (1979) and Warburton and Wesnes (Chapter 1), there is ample
evidence to suggest that cortical desynchronization accompanied by
local acetylcholine release is produced by a pharmacological increase
of central cholinergic activity, intraventricular instillation of
cholinomimetics, as well as a local injection of cholinergic agents
in the brain stem reticular formation or its limbic extension. The
involvement of a cholinergic mechanism in cortical activation produced
by direct reticular stimulation or sensory input is also well supported by the experimental data. This evidence, when considered with the
results of cholinergic and anticholinergic effects on information
processing in animals and humans, suggests to Warburton and Wesnes
(Chapters 1 and 8) that the central cholinergic mechanisms serve
selective attention in input processing.

     However, amphetamine-induced behavioral and cortical arousal,
which is due to catecholaminergic stimulation and produces an attentional fixation and behavioral stereotypies (Randrup and Munkvad,
1970; Ellinwood et al., 1973; Matthysse, 1977), is also attended with
acetylcholine release from the cortex (Robinson, Chapter 2). According to the evidence reviewed by Robinson, this acetylcholine release
is probably due to the amphetamine action on norepinephrine neurons.
Corresponding changes in the hippocampus consist of electrical synchronization and the production of rhythmical theta suggesting, as
proposed by Pribram and McGuiness (1975), a (direct or indirect) tonic
inhibitory action of the catecholaminergic neurons on this system
(Vanderwolf and Robinson, 1981). This type of electrical activity in
the hippocampus, besides being produced by amphetamines, seems to
accompany all voluntary movements, and is not affected by cholinergic
blockade (Vanderwolf and Robinson, 1981). Therefore, one might conclude that under such circumstances the so-called limbic cholinergic
system, as part of the hippocampal circuit, is disengaged or suppressed, while the cortical cholinergic mechanism is active and functions in series with the brain stem catecholaminergic pathways which,
through their actions on the amygdala and the striopallidal circuits

produce orienting and behavioral arousal. In terms of the Pribram and McGuiness (1975) model, the input and output or the stimulus and response mechanisms are engaged or linked together and the organism is involved in carrying out attentional-intentional action programs. Clearly, under these circumstances, the brain cholinergic systems cannot be viewed as of a piece or serving only the input processing functions.

Quite a different constellation of phenomena occur when the behaving organism changes or stops ongoing behavior, or when stimulation of all the cholinergic systems in the brain takes place as a result of a systemic administration of a centrally active cholinergic agent such as physostigmine. As was mentioned earlier, the hippocampal frequencies increase with any change in behavioral sequence (Kamp et al., 1971) and become irregular or desynchronized when there is an arrest of ongoing behavior (Bennett and Gottfried, 1970). According to the evidence reviewed by Vanderwolf and Robinson (1981), these types of electrical phenomena in the hippocampus involve cholinergic activity and are blocked by an atropinic, and that their characteristic behavioral correlate is an alert immobile state. A similar state, termed Alert Non-Mobile Behavior, has been described by Karczmar (1977), as a characteristic effect of cholinergic drugs. There is cortical desynchronization and the animal is alert and seemingly attentive but shows an arrest of motor activity. This means that when both the limbic and the cortical cholinergic systems are active, there is an inhibition of the output mechanisms but a facilitation of input processing, because an arrest of ongoing behavior would necessarily interrupt or suspend the action-generated inputs and thus permit "undivided" attention to other types - internal or external - of information. In terms of the model presented earlier, these events could be appropriately characterized as a process of disengaging the stimulus-response connections or loosening the links between the orienting and response set mechanisms needed for carrying out a behavioral program. Such a process would not only be helpful or adaptive in situations requiring a change of strategy but may be necessary to terminate a behavior once its goal has been achieved.

A logical location for this disconnection to take place would be at the point of intersection in the limbic core between the limbic, the striopallidal and the brain stem reticular or drive mechanisms (see above). The importance of the hippocampal circuit in this function was discussed earlier. What can be added to that proposal here is that the integrity of the septal-hippocampal cholinergic mechanisms may be crucial for such a role of the hippocampal circuit.

A large body of data on the effects of central cholinergic blockade on attention, learning and goal-directed behavior would seem to support this view, because these effects are remarkably similar to those produced by bilateral hippocampectomy (Douglas, 1972). Included among such effects are: increased locomotor activity; enhanced shuttle-box learning and two-way active avoidance but poor one-way

active avoidance and passive avoidance; loss of spontaneous alternation; deficient successive discrimination; poor maze learning; and
deficits in habituation (Douglas 1972, 1975; Hingtgen and Aprison,
1976). Accompanying these behavioral effects, there is the expected
loss of acetylcholine-related electrical responses of the hippocampus. Also, related undoubtedly to interference with the cortical cholinergic system, there is a change in the electrical activity of the
cortex which, depending upon the dose of the anticholinergic agent,
is characterized by the loss of desynchronization related to alert
immobile behavior and the appearance of excessive amounts of high
voltage slow waves along with low voltage fast activity in the resting state (Singh and Kay, Chapter 9). Both the excessive motor activity and the appearance of low voltage fast rhythms in the resting
electrocortical activity may be an indication of the released catecholaminergic mechanisms, because amphetamine intensifies the atropine-induced hyperactivity, leading to constant movement and continuous low voltage fast activity (Vanderwolf, 1975; Schallert et al.,
1980). The latter also suggests that, besides the cholinergic mechanism of cortical arousal, there is also an arousal mechanism related
to the catecholaminergic systems which continues to function in atropinized subjects (Vanderwolf and Robinson, 1981).

In the Pribram and McGuiness (1975) schema, serotonergic projections from the raphe nuclei are thought to be responsible for releasing the hippocampal circuit from tonic catecholaminergic inhibitory
control. The same mechanisms should apply for bringing the septo-hippocampal cholinergic mechanism into play. There is some evidence to
support this. The electrical stimulation of the median raphe nucleus
in the rat produces a fear-like behavioral freezing accompanied by
neocortical desynchronization and a theta rhythm in the hippocampus
(Graeff et al., 1980). A similar response can be produced by a conditioned stimulus indicating inescapable foot shock. The hippocampal
theta in such a situation can be blocked by an anticholinergic agent.
However, a serotonin antagonist is not effective, suggesting that the
serotonin neurons are probably not acting directly on the hippocampal
cholinergic neurons.

By way of a summary, it might be said that two cholinergic projection systems - one to the neocortex and the other to the hippocampus - arise in the limbic core or reticular formation. They seem to
function in two modes. In one mode, the cortical system is active but
the hippocampal system is silent, the stimuli are bonded to the responses, and the organism is engaged in orienting and the goal-directed actions facilitated by the activity of catecholaminergic drive
neurons. The input mechanisms in this situation may be thought of as
being open to all forms of information but expectedly dominated by
the action-generated inputs. In the second mode, both the cholinergic
systems are active and, largely through the operation of the hippocampal circuit, the action programs, and therefore the action-generated inputs, are suspended or held at bay when other forms of information derived from external inputs, memories and motivational stimuli

can be preferentially attended to so as to devise new plans and
strategies. Such an operational mechanism would give the organism
added flexibility and adaptiveness. Also, it would create the framework in which the purely mental processes described as thinking and
reasoning in human language could take place effectively (Pribram and
McGuiness, 1975).

A brief mention should also be made of the striatal cholinergic
neurons at this point. According to observations reported by Cools
and Van den Bercken (1977) and Van den Bercken and Cools (1979), cholinergic stimulation in the neostriatum increases variability in motor
activity. If this is correct, then the function of the striatal cho-
liergic system may also be viewed as providing increased flexibility
in behavior.

Between the three systems, the cholinergic neurons could obviously be involved in a large number of brain functions. It is not surprising, therefore, that cholinergic and anticholinergic effects have
been found in a wide array of functions concerned with both the input
and the output processing. However, a common thread does seem to
emerge from the varied phenomena in which the cholinergic neurons seem
to play a part, that is, these neurons seem to be part of the brain
mechanisms which give flexibility and improved adaptiveness to the
organism.

4.   BEHAVIORAL CONTROL, ADAPTIVENESS AND CHOLINERGIC MECHANISMS

Having outlined a functional anatomical brain model, and the
place the cholinergic systems seem to occupy in that model, an analysis and integration of various hypotheses of central cholinergic functions can now be attempted.

4.1. Input Processing and Selective Attention

Based on a historical review of the literature, Warburton and
Wesnes (Chapter 1) have made a strong case for the notion that the
brain cholinergic mechanisms have their main role in input processing
by mediating selective attention to stimuli of relevance.

Supporting this hypothesis are experiments in which anticholinergic drugs impair performance in stimulus discrimination tasks where
the "correct," significant," or "relevant" stimulus or cue has to be
distinguished from others and responded to in order to obtain a reward
or avoid punishment. Physiological range cholinergic stimulation can
counteract this impairment and may improve performance in normal
individuals. Thus, in learnig to perform tasks requiring discrimination of stimuli, anticholinergics appreciably retard task acquisition
in animals, particularly when a relevant stimulus has to be distinguished from several irrelevant stimuli or when multiple relevant cues

are involved (e.g., Whitehouse, 1967). Once the tasks have been learned, the administration of an anticholinergic before repeat trials increases the number of errors in performance, but this time more so when a single right cue has to be picked out from the background of irrelevant stimuli than when multiple cues are available to point to the correct (i.e., reinforced) response (e.g., Warburton and Heise, 1972; Warburton, 1974; Heise, 1975). On the other hand, experiments suggesting increased cholinergic function in the cortex in response to a stimulus-rich environment as well as an association between problem-solving ability and the genetically-determined cholinergic function of the cortex may be regarded as the other side of the same coin.

In humans, cholinolytics have also been found to cause distracti-bility and impaired performance in tasks requiring detection of fig-ures embedded in a larger design (Callaway and Band, 1958), certain numeral sequences appearing randomly among rapidly presented series of digits (Wesnes and Warburton, 1983), or colors while dealing with distracting meanings of words (Callaway and Band, 1958). Experiments by Warburton and Wesnes (Chapters 1 and 9) found that nicotine, which besides stimulating nicotinic receptors for acetylcholine can cause a release of acetylcholine at the cortex, can not only counteract this impairment but improve performance beyond that seen in controls.

Another type of evidence which, Warburton and Wesnes believe, supports their thesis, and also suggests the mechanism involved is electrophysiological. Muscarinic as well as nicotinic activity in the brain leads to cortical desynchronization, which is generally related to a state of alertness and attention. During discrimination tasks, the efficiency of performance seems to be related to the electroen-cephalographic frequency so that increased frequencies, suggesting electrocortical arousal, correlate with improved signal detections (Groll, 1966; O'Hanlon and Beatty, 1977). Also, acetylcholine facil-itates sensory evoked potentials at the cortex, and both the effi-ciency and direction of attention to stimuli seem related to the size of the evoked potentials (Schwent and Hillyard, 1975). In their stud-ies with nicotine, Warburton and Wesnes found that along with improved signal detection, there was a decreased latency of the later compo-nents of the evoked potentials, which are thought to be related to the attention-intention processes.

While arguing for the input-processing hypothesis of cholinergic function, Warburton and Wesnes have taken a position against the long-held view that cholinergic mechanisms mediate suppression of behavior-al outputs in circumstances such as non-reward or punishment. Their reasoning is that under anticholinergic treatment, the animals do not seem to show so much a perseverative repetition of responses which go unreinforced and are, therefore, incorrect, but that due to an appar-ently poor stimulus control of behavior, the animals appear to show too much random behavior. In other words, the cholinergic systems may be considered to improve control over behavior through stimulus selec-tion rather than through response selection.

In considering this hypothesis, it should be pointed out that the pharmacological experiments with cholinergics and anticholinergics on which it is based would necessarily involve all the cholinergic systems of the brain. This means that the individual would be in a mode of operation in which both the cortical as well as the septal-hippocampal cholinergic systems are simultaneously active or blocked. In nature, where the two systems can probably act separately, this situation would represent only one of the several possible operational combinations.

Further, it should be noted that the electrocortical arousal associated with cortical cholinergic activity may occur in situations, such as amphetamine-induced behavioral arousal, where the attentional process becomes less adaptive due to distractibility on the one hand and a tendency towards attentional fixation, related probably to behavioral stereotypy, on the other. In the case of attentional fixation, one might even talk of the organism becoming over-selective, and the adaptational problem arises because of difficulty in shifting attention from a useless task to one which may be more significant at the time. Also, as discussed earlier, for cortical arousal, the cholinergic mechanism is not the only one available, because another mechanism related to the catecholamine systems is also involved.

As such, the specific cholinergic influence on input processing and selective attention which is of adaptive importance may be related not so much to the cholinergic electrocortical effects but to what the septal-hippocampal cholinergic system adds to that process. Warburton and Wesnes (Chapter 1) have reviewed the data which suggest that this might be the case.

However, in discussing the role of the septal-hippocampal cholinergic system, one is talking more about what the hippocampal circuit contributes to the behavior than about what the brain cholinergic mechanisms as a whole do. Therefore, the question to be asked is how does the hippocampal circuit, of which the septal-hippocampal cholinergic pathway is a part, facilitate selective attention?

From the functional-anatomical standpoint, the close relationship between the hippocampal circuit and the sensory processing areas of the neocortex discussed earlier would support the idea that this circuit, and therefore, the cholinergic system, is involved in input processing. However, this circuit also has strong connections with the extrapyramidal output control mechanisms, and from the available evidence, the behavioral function of the hippocampal circuit seems to be essentially inhibitory. What purpose does this serve in selective attention and input processing? Also, one must ask the question as to what specific adaptive purpose does the unique cholinergic effect of an Alert Non-Mobile Behavior have? In this context, it should be noted that there is much evidence to suggest that cholinergic activity reduces the behavioral activation and repetitiousness induced by dopaminergic activity (Singh and Lal, 1982).

Based on the earlier analysis, the most plausible answer to these questions would seem to be that by providing inhibitory control over behavior, the hippocampal circuit can, when needed, free up the input-processing mechanisms from the constraints exercised by the action-generated inputs. Thus disengaged from the response control, the input mechanisms can more effectively deal with other information and lead to the development of newer, possibly more effective, stimulus-reponse connections. Such a mechanism would be of obvious value in circumstances where new information has to be attended to, conflicting or competing demands have to be met, or the perceptuo-motor plan or strategy in use has to be revised to meet the internally and externally determined goals. Also, in situations which involve mainly internal manipulations of information and stimulus-response associations, as in human functions of thinking and reasoning, keeping the response mechanisms in check would be a necessary part of the process. Much effort, leading to the familiar mental fatigue, would be involved in this because the natural tendency of a living organism to react to stimuli has to be kept in active restraint until such time that a somatomotor response is necessary or called for (Pribram and McGuiness, 1975). It is, therefore, a special type of attentional process which requires effort and in which both input facilitation and output inhibition may be involved.

In any type of discrimination task, in fact, withholding of response to the irrelevant and unrewarded stimuli may be thought of as the crucial ingredient in learning to respond only to the relevant and rewarded stimulus. The more the irrelevant or competing stimuli, and the more ambiguous, uncertain and complex the situation, the more important would be the mechanism which can facilitate this. Therefore, an argument could be made that the facilitation of discriminative performance by the cholinergic mechanisms in general, and the hippocampal circuit in particular, may depend as much on the response suppression as on the input-facilitation.

It would seem, therefore, that the brain cholinergic mechanisms may be involved on both the input and output sides of the behavioral chain and should not be viewed purely as the input-selection or the output-control mechanisms.

There is no reason to expect the hippocampal or other cholinergic systems to be involved in all forms of behavioral suppression. As mentioned earlier, both the amygdala and the striopallidal systems have mechanisms for inhibiting behavior. These may or may not be dependent on the cholinergic system activity. Similarly, it would probably be wrong to assume that the cholinergic systems are important at every stage, and in all forms, of stimulus processing and the attention-intention process. The discrimination studies in which cholinergic effects have been demonstrated are essentially concerned with the process by which specific stimuli become significant to the organism and take on cue functions in goal-directed behavior. This may be

a relatively late stage in sensory processing in which limbic information conveyed by the cholinergic mechanisms (and other limbic systems)
would be of obvious importance. Such a process would no doubt involve
the sensory integration or association areas of the cortex with which
hippocampal and other limbic mechanisms establish close contacts.
However, actual sensory differentiation may be an earlier stage process taking place in the modality-specific cortices or the contiguous
belt areas. In this, the cholinergic mechanisms may be of little
significance, or the cortical cholinergic system may be involved while
the septal-hippocampal system is not. Thus, the two major components
of the cholinergic system may have different roles in input processing.
Likewise, in terms of attentional functions, cholinergic activity may
be important only in certain types of attentional process. Orienting
to new stimuli, with accompanying phasic acceleration of heart rate,
vigilant readiness for input categorization tasks, in which there is
a tonic deceleration of heart rate, and the concentration involved in
reasoning to decide on a response, when the heart rate shows a tonic
increase, are apparently three different attention-intention processes
(Pribram and McGuiness, 1975). Which of these most involves one or
more of the cholinergic systems is not known at this point.

     Therefore, the issue of whether the cholinergic function is
mainly on the input side or the output side may not be the important
question in trying to understand what the cholinergic systems contribute to the brain's mission. One might do much better to ask: What
are the circumstances or the adaptational contexts in which one or
more of the cholinergic pathways, and the circuits including them,
come into play? When do their input and output control functions,
separately and together, become important in the initiation, execution, modification and termination of goal-directed activity? How do
the different cholinergic systems interact with each other, and with
other neurotransmitter systems, and as such, what part do they play
in the operations of the major cortical-subcortical circuits? Rather
than talk about a general behavioral-suppression or input-selection
function for the cholinergic mechanisms, we probably need to define
the context-related, specific input-output functions, in which these
mechanisms, individually or combined, become especially important in
the organism-environment interactions.

4.2. Memory

     Facilitation of retrieval of information from memory stores, ac-
cording to Spencer and Lal (Chapter 5), is the best unifying concept
for describing the central cholinergic functions.

     Their arguments are based on the same sorts of behavioral pharma-
cological studies as considered by Warburton and Wesnes. The animals
learn various types of stimulus-response associations to obtain rewards or avoid punishment; the efficiency with which they acquire the
task provides a measure of acquisition, while the degree to which the

initial training is reflected in repeat performance later provides a measure of memory process of one kind or another. Cholinergic and anticholinergic drugs are given before, during or after learning and repeat testing to study their effects on acquisition, input and output aspects of performance, memory formation, consolidation of memory and the retrieval of the past memories.

Like Warburton and Wesnes, Spencer and Lal have taken the position that the cholinergic mechanisms are not primarily concerned with response suppression. Therefore, much of what was said above could be repeated here.

However, they also disagree with Warburton and Wesnes in some respects. In the studies reviewed by them, which were concerned mainly with anticholinergic effects on tasks involving relatively simple stimulus discriminations, cholinergic blockade was generally found to impair acquisition performance, indicating difficulty in selecting relevant (reinforced) from the irrelevant stimuli. Nevertheless, they argued that this was not necessarily due to deficits in attention or sensory discrimination but could be explained as one of the consequences of memory retrieval impairment which was more clearly demonstrable in the repeat tests designed to measure recall. Decreased stimulus sensitivity, suggesting a sensory discrimination difficulty, was observed in some instances but did not seem to be the main factor responsible for impaired performance.

Considering the nature of these studies, in which the animal essentially learns that certain quite ordinary stimuli are "significant" due to the related motivational states produced by the rewards and punishments, one wonders if attention, stimulus selection, memory formation and retrieval can really be distinguished as separate processes purely on the basis of behavioral analysis. Let us take the studies which have shown that acquisition impairment by cholinolytics is much greater when the animal has to distinguish a relevant signal from many irrele nt ones or when it has to learn a multi-cued task. The most plausible explanation would be that the cholinergic mechanisms are important for selective attention. However, could it not be that the difficulty occurs due to a failure to "recall" the many unsuccessful stimulus-response combinations in this situation?

For making these distinctions, behavioral analysis probably has to be combined with other forms of analysis, such as biochemical, neurophysiological, and iontophoretic. As an illustration, the work of Matthies et al., (1975) might be cited. Using a shock-motivated brightness discrimination procedure, they found through the iontophoretic method that the sensitivity of cortical neurons to acetylcholine increased considerably with successful conditioning. Then to test the role of the hippocampal cholinergic system, they instilled an anticholinergic into the dorsal hippocampus immediately before and after acquisition. This caused a considerable delay in extinction of behavior which occurred in controls within three days. As the next step, they measured various pools of acetylcholine in the hippocampus during and, at various points, after the acquisition. There was a sequence of changes, starting with a 500 percent increase in free acetylcholine during acquisition, which corresponded to what might be described as the life history of the memory trace. This would clearly suggest that the hippocampus has a role in memory formation. However, in another series of tests, the rats learned shock-motivated position discrimination. Unlike the brightness discrimination, this behavior did not show any extinction three days after acquisition, and the corresponding acetylcholine parameters were totally different in that no changes occurred in the acetylcholine fractions during or after the learning procedures. This suggests that there might not be a uniform role for cholinergic mechanisms in memory functions. Rather, it might be a function determined by the part these systems play in a particular type of motivated behavior.

Since memories are records of stimulus-response association which have proven significant due to certain motivational consequences, all the limbic systems which contribute to motivated behaviors are to be expected to participate in memory functions. This would include the cholinergic mechanisms, especially those in the hippocampus. However, as such, these systems may not be unique. Other limbic systems, which contribute to the function of translating the organism's internal states and needs into behavior, might be expected to contribute to the memory processes. Evidence supports this. Thus severe impairment in monkeys occurs after a combined but not by separate removal of the amygdala and hippocampus, suggesting that the two main limbic circuits collaborate in the memory functions (Mishkin, 1978).

The important question, therefore, may not be whether the cholinergic mechanisms take part in the formation and recall of memories, but what are the existential circumstances or states - internal or external - in which cholinergic systems, such as those in the hippocampal circuit, become particularly important? Thus, if the broader attention-intention model of Pribram and McGuiness (1975) were correct, retrieval would fit in nicely as a necessary component of the hypothesized hippocampal circuit function of monitoring the onging behavior in terms of preset goals and the memory of what has gone before, and then triggering a series of changes on the input and output side that lead to stimulus-response disconnection and the formation of a new behavioral program or strategy. However, retrieval would not be the only or a unique function of the cholinergic mechanisms.

4.3. Aggression and Fear

Evidence reviewed by Bell and Brown (Chapter 6) strongly suggests that a cholinergic mechanism, probably one centered on the acetylcholine-rich basolateral amygdala, mediates certain forms of aggression, particularly those associated with a strong, usually negative, affect,

such as pain and irritability. It should be recalled at this point
that the amygdala receives cholinergic input from the same source
that provides the cortical projection, so that the two, the cortical
and the amygdala cholinergic mechanisms, may be thought of as being
linked.

On the face of it, the cholinergic mediation of the excitatory
behavior of aggression would seem inconsistent with the idea that cholinergic activity generally leads to behavioral inhibition. On closer
analysis, however, this inconsistency seems more apparent than real.
The electrical or cholinergic stimulation of the so-called aggression
area of the amygdala complex leads to a defensive-reaction characterized by heightened arousal, orienting behavior and a defensive posture
but seldom an attack behavior (Kaada, 1972); the same area serves the
escape-avoidance behavior (Grossman, 1972). The attack neurons, as
Bell and Brown have discussed, are in the hypothalamus and other parts
of the limbic and brain stem core, and on these, the amygdala circuit
seems to exercise a dual modulatory control in which the cholinergic
and norepinephric mechanisms may have opposing functions, while the
serotonin effects may be, in some ways, synergistic to the acetylcholine effects (Kaada, 1972; Karli et al., 1972). Thus, consistent with
their anatomical link with the cortical cholinergic projections, the
contribution of the cholinergic neurons of the amygdala circuit may
be to increase arousal and attention while providing selective restraint on the lower level attack mechanisms in circumstances where
behavioral choices for survival have to be quickly made. The cholinergic mechanisms of the septal-hippocampal system are also concerned
with aggressive behavior and may make a particular contribution to the
perceptual evaluation of the threatening situation (Rodgers and Brown,
1976).

Stimulation in areas of amygdala which are different from the
defense zones, and where serotonergic endings seem to be concentrated,
lead to a reaction of fearful withdrawal characterized by signs of
arousal, restless looking around, loss of sphincter control and withdrawal from the situation (Kaada, 1972; Hall, 1972). Electrical stimulation at the origin of the serotonergic fibers in the midbrain also
produces a fear-like behavioral freezing in the rat which is accompanied by a cholinergic theta activity in the hippocampus (Graeff
et al., 1980). Thus in another type of a situation, the cholinergic
mechanisms seem to be involved, along with the serotonergic mechanisms, in producing a combination of arousal, attention and behavioral
restraint. Also, as in a defense reaction, the activity of the amygdala and the hippocampal circuits is coordinated. In this context,
it may be mentioned that the two limbic systems, by virtue of their
somewhat different relations with the neocortex may influence the
sensory channels differently. Thus, the amygdala circuit, due to its
preferential relation with the frontal cortex which, according to
Pribram (1960, 1967), produces chunking of all the information, may
tend to reduce sampling of new alternatives in a situation. The hippocampal circuit, on the other hand, may permit a greater sampling of

novel alternatives in a situation because of its preferential relationship with the posterior cortex which is believed to allow greater
freedom for the sensory channels to remain separate (Pribram, 1960,
1967). The effects of the posterior cortical lesions, in many
respects, resemble the effects of the hippocampal lesions.

In relation to aggression, one other observation highlighted by
Bell and Brown should be mentioned. Unlike the muscarinic cholinergic
activity, the nicotinic cholinergic activity seems to have a generally
anti-aggression effect. This suggests a possible antagonism between
the two types of cholinergic receptors in aggression. It also raises
the larger issue, which future studies must address, that similar differences between the muscarinic and nicotinic effects might occur in
other behaviors in which cholinergic mechanisms have been implicated.

4.4. Stress

Stress as a reaction to conflicts, hard or impossible to solve
problems, and inescapable difficulties, represents situations marked
by great uncertainty. Cholinergic, especially hippocampal, mechanisms
should be of considerable adaptive significance in such circumstances. The experiment with inescapable shock reported by Karczmar and
Richardson (Chapter 7) seems to suggest that. After a period of pur-
poseless hyperactivity, stereotypic acts and undirected aggression,
the animals gave up and became immobile. At the height of this
stress, the acetylcholine content of the midbrain-diencephalon was
significantly elevated, suggesting perhaps that the mesodiencephalic
cholinergic mechanisms were called into play but could not operate
because no solution to the problem existed. After the inescapable
shock test, the stressed animals performed better than controls, suggesting possibly the enhanced activity of the cholinergic mechanisms
primed by the stressful experience.

The immobility seen in this experiment would be an example of the
Pavlovian transmarginal inhibition, which is a generalized inhibitory
state that supervenes in unresolvable conflict situations. Douglas
(1972, 1975) believes this form of nonspecific inhibition to be an
immature or primitive function of the hippocampus which can appear in
adulthood under some circumstances. The mature function of the hippocampus is selective inhibition which would be expected to operate in
normal circumstances provided the problem is solvable. The maturation
of the hippocampal function seems to be a genetically-determined process which, according to Douglas (1975), takes about a month to complete in rats and 3.5 to 4 years in humans. Pure-bred strains of rats
with delayed hippocampal maturation are known. However, stress or
cortisol injections during the maturation can also apparently retard
the appearance of functions thought to be due to a mature hippocampal
mechanism.

Isaacson (1974) has also noted the similarities between the behavioral effects of frustration and the hippocampal lesions. The

hippocampal lesions tend to lower the threshold for frustration-
induced effects in many animals, thus suggesting once again the importance of the hippocampal circuit in dealing with circumstances marked
by uncertainty, ambiguity and frustration.

5.   CHOLINERGIC MECHANISMS AD PSYCHOPATHOLOGY

5.1. Schizophrenia

    Of all the disease states considered in this book, the cholin-
ergic processes may prove to be of the greatest relevance for the
pathogenesis of schizophrenia. Evidence reviewed by Karczmar and
Richardson (Chapter 7), Warburton and Wesnes (Chapter 8) and Singh and
Kay (Chapter 9), suggests that many of the phenomena due to cholinergic deficits are also characteristic of one or more forms of schizophrenia. Included among these are difficulty in sustaining attention
or concentration, impairment of selective attention and cognitive processing, poor perceptual discrimination and problem-solving, hallucinatory behavior, disorganization of thinking, electroencephalographic
abnormalities characterized by excessive amounts of delta, theta and
fast beta but decreased amounts of alpha and slow beta frequencies,
abnormalities of evoked potentials, a tendency towards stereotyped
repetitiousness of behavior and a relative failure of behavioral
habituation.

    Perhaps the most fundamental feature that is common between the
cholinergic deficiency syndrome, especially one produced by hippocampal lesions, and schizphrenia, is the loss of flexibility in behavior
and decreased ability to deal with the new, or what Shakow (1971,
1977) has described as neophobia. The state of perceptual distractibility combined with behavioral indistractibility which follows bilateral hippocampectomy (Douglas and Pribram, 1969) seems also to be
remarkably like the combination of increased activity in the posterior
or input parts and decreased activity in the frontal or output parts
of the cortex, which cerebrography has shown to be characteristic of
chronic nonparanoid schizophrenics (Ingvar and Franzén, 1974, Franzén
and Ingvar, 1975).

    In humans, anticholinergic drugs produce a psychosis which resem-
bles the schizophrenic psychosis in many ways, and is often misdiag-
nosed as such. But this psychosis is also characterized by an altered
state of awareness, a delirious or confusional aspect, which is typically not associated with schizophrenia, so that anticholinergic psychosis may be considered questionable as a model for schizophrenia.
However, the condition produced by bilateral hippocampectomy in monkeys does not seem to have this delirious aspect – at least to the
extent one can make this judgement from observation of animal behavior.
In all other respects, the picture is highly reminiscent of a schizophrenic disorder (Singh and Kay, 1982). Could it be that the altered

state of awareness in anticholinergic psychosis results from the fact that, in addition to the interruption of the hippocampal cholinergic system, the cortical cholinergic system is also blocked in this situation? If that were the case - an issue which only further research could resolve - one would have an interesting possibility to consider, that is, it is perphaps the septal-hippocampal cholinergic system which is of main relevance to the pathogenesis of schizophrenia, but that the disruption of the cortical cholinergic system can add a confusional element to the clinical picture of psychosis. This raises the wider issue of the limitations of a purely pharmacological model of mental illness, and suggests the need for building models that combine pharmacological with neuroanatomical and other types of information.

Pharmacological studies in normal and schizophrenic individuals overall seem to support the possibility of a cholinergic involvement in schizophrenia (Singh and Kay, Chapter 9). Thus, there is fairly good evidence that, besides producing schizophrenia-like symptoms, the anticholinergic drugs exacerbate schizophrenia and, perhaps most significantly, counteract the antipsychotic activity of neuroleptics, which are believed to exercise their therapeutic effect by blocking the catecholaminergic, especially dopaminergic, transmission. These observations are understandable in terms of the relationships between the catecholaminergic and cholinergic pathways outlined earlier, and further support the idea that an impairment of the hippocampal circuit function may be a significant factor in the pathogenesis of schizophrenia (Singh and Kay, 1982). Apropos this, it should be noted that the effects of complete hippocampectomy in animals are not improved by cholinergic stimulation, because the cholinergic neurons are afferent in the hippocampal circuit (Douglas, 1975), but are improved somewhat by a neuroleptic, because the catecholaminergic systems are on the receiving end, and are probably released from an inhibitory control by the removal of the hippocampus (Isaacson, 1972). However, if hippocampectomy is not complete in an adult animal, the behavioral consequences can be reversed by cholinergic stimulation (Douglas, 1975). This may provide an explanation for the observation that the countertherapeutic anticholinergic effect is least evident in the poor prognosis or nuclear type of schizophrenics, in whom hippocampal impairment, if any, would be expected to be most marked, but is quite marked in the acute, good prognosis, schizophreniform, or catatonic types of cases, in whom any hippocampal impairment would presumably be partial.

Also consistent with this model are the results of treatment trials with cholinergic agents. Some therapeutic effect seems to occur in patients of the type in whom cholinolytics have the most adverse effect. However, little therapeutic effect is seen in the poor prognosis, nuclear nonparanoid schizophrenics. On the contrary, these patients may be highly resistant to muscarinic effects, although nicotinic effects may be preserved. This suggests a severe deficiency and hyporeactivity of the muscarinic cholinergic mechanisms. These are also the cases marked by a combination of increased blood flow and reactivity in the posterior cortex and decreased blood flow and reactivity in the frontal cortex.

A third group of patients, belonging to the paranoid subtype of schizophrenia, may be different yet. Anticholinergics, when combined with neuroleptics, have little countertherapeutic effect in these patients. However, they might be particularly sensitive to both cholinergic and anticholinergic psychotogens, thus raising the possibility of overly sensitive cholinergic mechanisms (Chapter 9, Section 8.3), similar to those suspected in depression (see below).

The possibility of three different psychobiological types of schizophrenia in terms of cholinergic processes might be the most important conceptual suggestion from the reviews of the literature. It not only emphasizes the heterogeneity of schizophrenia and the pitfalls of formulating any unitary pharmacological hypothesis for this syndrome, but points to an array of future investigative possibilities. Elsewhere, a consideration of psychophysiological, neurophysiological and pharmacological data suggested a similar tripartite division of schizophrenia (Singh, 1981; Singh and Kay, 1982; Singh and Lal, 1982). The findings of these reviews are summarized at the end of Chapter 9.

Whether or not the cholinergic mechanisms prove to be of a primary etiological significance for any type of schizophrenia, it seems clear that studies based on manipulations of various cholinergic systems could provide valuable insights into the neurobiological basis of schizophrenic psychopathology.

5.1. Affective Disorders

Janowsky et al. (Chapter 10) have reviewed a body of clinical and experimental data which seem to implicate the central cholinergic mechanisms in affective disorders. They have hypothesized that depression may be due to a relative cholinergic excess, and mania due to a relative cholinergic deficit, in the brain.

The main points in favor are that cholinergic stimulation with an anticholinesterase seems to worsen a depressed mood, reduces manicky behavior and mood, and reverses methylphenidate-induced exacerbation of mania, while anticholinergic drug use sometime results in euphoria. From behavioral, neurophysiological and neuroendocrine data, there is also an emerging suggestion of cholinergic supersensitivity in depression which, according to recent findings (Nurnberger et al., 1983), may be a genetically-determined correlate of vulnerability to affective disorder. This may prove to be the most interesting observation presented by Janowsky et al.

There are several points against the cholinergic hypothesis of manic-depressive illness as formulated by these authors. Thus, nicotine which, as reported by Warburton and Wesnes (Chapters 1 and 8), releases acetylcholine at the cortex, has an obvious reinforcing character and is not a dysphoriant. On the other hand, anticholinergic drugs are not effective antidepressants. Even more critical is the fact that increasing cholinergic blockade, though possibly euphoriant in early stages, leads to a clinical picture of schizophreniform psychosis, not mania. Nor is there is any evidence to suggest a decreased cholinergic sensitivity or reactivity in manic patients. Indeed, data on the effects of organophosphates (Singh and Kay, Chapter 9) suggest that these patients react much as normals do to cholinergic stimulation.

However, from the involvement of the cholinergic pathways in the limbic systems which seem to be concerned with signalling, and coping with, states of uncertainty, conflict and danger, it is not difficult to see that cholinergic activity might be associated with a feeling of distress. The hypothesized effort involved in the hippocampal function of restraining motor outputs while the situation creating uncertainty or conflict is being attended to and resolved may also contribute to this negative affect. Therefore, when cholinergic mechanisms are pharmacologically activated, the brain should be expected to respond as if the organism is facing an uncertain or threatening situation. This does not necessarily mean that cholinergic activity leads to dysphoric mood because, except in an inescapable impasse, the mobilization of adaptive mechanisms including cholinergic neurons should lead to the resolution of a problem and, therefore, a positive mood. As such, the association between depression and cholinergic transmission may be explained thus: the characteristic ideas of hopelessness and impending doom trigger the cholinergic mechanisms, but since there is no resolution, the cholinergic mechanisms continue to be activated leading possibly to receptor supersensitivity in the same manner as the chronic organophosphate exposure is believed to do (Chapter 9, Section 4). The critical question then is not whether cholinergic mechanisms produce depression but why the adaptive circuits they are involved in are unsuccessful in resolving the perceived impasse in the depressed patients, especially since there is usually no external obstacle? What blocks the effective operation of these circuits?

In this conceptual scheme, an explanation may also be found for the previously suggested (Chapter 9, Section 8.3) possibility of cholinergic sensitivity in paranoid schizophrenics – a condition also associated with a persistent perception of threat – and the proposed relationship between this condition and manic-depressive illness (Taylor and Abrams, 1974).

5.3. Dementia

Corresponding to the issue of a specific role for cholinergic

mechanisms in memory discussed earlier, there is a "cholinergic hypothesis" of dementia which proposes that the typical impairment of
memory in this condition may be due to the loss of cholinergic
functions. The review on this subject by Retz and Lal (Chapter 11),
and other recent reviews (Bartus et al., 1982), suggest that in
Alzheimer's dementia there is a loss of cholinergic markers and of
cholinergic neurons which is significantly greater than that associated with normal aging. However, the decrease in muscarinic receptor
density does not seem too much higher. Many other neurotransmitter
systems also show corresponding declines with advancing age as well
as dementia, and there is no evidence to suggest a selective loss of
the cholinergic system. There is some evidence to suggest that the
degree of cognitive decline in dementia correlates with the decrease
in cholinergic markers as well as the neuropathological markers. However, the main approach available to elucidate the pathogenesis of
memory loss in dementia is pharmacological, involving tests with various neurotransmitter precursors and agonists. The results of these
tests seem to show that cholinergic agonists, especially when combined
with agents which can increase oxidative metabolism in the brain, can
produce small but measurable improvement in the short term memory of
dementing individuals. Manipulations of other neurotransmitters, and
also of a variety of neurohormones, are generally without any reliable
effect on memory in such cases. Thus, there is some support for the
idea that memory impairment in dementia may be related to the loss of
cholinergic function. However, the therapeutic value of cholinergic
agents is quite limited.

6.   CONCLUDING REMARKS

Introspectively, the preparation of this essay has been exhaust-
ing work, requiring a great deal of mental effort accompanied by a
roller-coaster of emotions, because it involved reconciling many conflicting viewpoints, searching for a new synthesis of a vast amount
of information, and finding a way to express the synthesis in clear
scientific language within the framework of a reasonably organized
whole. This has brought home in a personal way the enormous importance to human adaptiveness of the brain mechanisms which can make
such a process possible. The study of cholinergic functions seems to
offer great promise for understanding the nature and operations of
such mechanisms in normal humans as well as in those who suffer from
major adaptive dysfunctions seen in conditions such as schizophrenia,
manic-depressive illness and Alzheimer's disease.

Building on the current knowledge, future research must develop
sufficient refinement to make functional distinctions between different cholinergic pathways and the neuronal circuits which incorporate
them, because it is quite likely that they serve different adaptive
processes. This will not be accomplished merely by studying the behavioral effects of generalized pharmacological stimulation or interruption of cholinergic transmission in the brain. How to do it might

be a tall order, but it seems that an interactive study of different
neurotransmitter systems and the use of a combination of pharmacological and other research methods, such as sterotaxic lesions, biochemical assays and neurophysiological measurements, might prove to be
very fruitful in this respect.

The functional differentiation between the muscarinic and nicotinic cholinergic systems will also have to be elaborated because already there is some evidence to suggest that the two might serve different and even opposite adaptive purposes.

The investigative effort so far has been focused on defining the
role of central cholinergic activity in individual functions related
to input or output processing by the brain, and then attempting to
find which of these functions, such as stimulus sensitivity, arousal,
perceptual attention, memory, response suppression, etc., is the primary service of this activity. Many theories of cholinergic function
have, therefore, arisen. As the reviews in this book have shown,
there is some validity to each view. But what seems to be missing is
the recognition that different cholinergic effects may be part of a
pattern which has adaptive significance in terms of certain external
and internal conditions. Only through an ethologically-oriented integrative approach, especially one which takes into account the anatomical arrangement of various neuronal systems, might it be possible
to fully appreciate the purpose served by the cholinergic neurons in
various adaptive mechanisms of the brain.

If adaptiveness means setting aside or forgetting the percepts,
plans, and actions which are unnecessary or ineffective, and learning,
remembering and trying new solutions, then the circuits in which cholinergic neurons, especially those of the limbic system, participate
may be of strategic importance in the brain organization. Their apparent ability to at once enhance input processing and restrain outputs, and possibly produce a stimulus-response disengagement, suggests
that this may be so.

These are important issues to tackle for understanding the
brain's adaptive mechanisms and how those mechanisms become impaired
in psychopathology. The loss of selective attention, disturbance of
arousal, inflexibility and stereotypy of behavior and neophobia are
characteristic features of schizophrenic disorders. The study of cholinergic effects in these areas may well produce a fundamental understanding of schizophrenic pathology. Beyond that, there is a heuristic possibility of being able to recognize and define certain psychobiological subgroupings of this syndrome in terms of cholinergic functions and dysfunctions. Yet, it may be that the cholinergic mechanisms are of no primary etiological significance for schizophrenia.

The study of cholinergic functions in relation to depression,
and possibly paranoid schizophrenia, may prove to be of interest in a

different way. Through this, it may be possible to define the conditions - perceived threat, conflict or impasse - which trigger the cholinergic mechanisms, and therby engage the circuits which can facilitate the resolution of those conditions. More importantly, it should
give us an understanding of the mechanisms that produce new solutions
and execute the plans to resolve or exit from a demanding and distressing situation, for these mechanisms are clearly not functioning well
in disorders such as depression.

    At the same time, the role cholinergic mechanisms might have in
forming and recalling memories is being elaborated by studies in animals as well as in demented humans.

ACKNOWLEDGEMENT

    I am pleased to acknowledge the assistance provided by Barbara
Mason.

REFERENCES

Akert, K., 1964, Comparative anatomy of frontal cortex and thalamo-
    frontal connections, in "The Frontal Granular Cortex and
    Behavior," J.M. Warren and K. Akert, eds., pp. 372-396, McGraw
    Hill, New York.
Anchel, H., and Lindsley, D. B., 1972, Differentiation of two reticu-
    lohypothalamic systems regulating hippocampal activity, Electro-
    encephalogr. Clin. Neurophysiol. 32:209-226.
Andén, N.-E., Dahlström, A., Fuxe, K., Larson, K., Olson, L., and
    Ungerstedt, U., 1966, Ascending monoamine neurons to the telen-
    cephalon and diencephalon, Acta Physiol. Scand. 67:313-326.
Bartus, R. T., Dean, III, R. L., Beer, B., and Lippa, A. S., 1982, The
    cholinergic hypothesis of geriatric memory dysfunction, Science
    217:408-417.
Bennett, T. L., 1970, Hippocampal EEG correlates of behavior,
    Electroencephalogr. Clin. Neurophysiol. 28:17-23.
Bennett, T. L., and Gottfried, J., 1970, Hippocampal theta activity
    and response inhibition, Electroencephalogr. Clin. Neurophysiol.
    29:196-200.
Callaway, E., and Band, I., 1958, Some psychopharmacological effects
    of atropine, Arch. Neurol. Psychiatry 79:91-102.
Cools, A. R., and Van den Bercken, J. H. L., 1977, Cerebral organiza-
    tion of behavior and the neostriatal function, in "Psychobiology
    of Striatum," A. R. Cools, A. H. M. Lohman, and J. H. L. Van den
    Bercken, eds., pp. 119-140, North Holland Publishing Company,
    Amsterdam.
Dahlström, A., 1969, Fluorescence histochemistry of monoamines in the
    central nervous system, in "Basic Mechanisms of the Epilepsies,"
    H. H. Jasper, A. A. Ward, and A. Pope, eds., pp. 212-217, Little
    Brown, Boston.

Dalton, A., and Black, A. H., 1968, Hippocampal electrical activity during the operant conditioning of movement and refraining from movement, Comm. Behav. Biol. 2:267-273.

DeLong, M., 1972, Activity of basal ganglia neurons during movement, Brain Res. 40:127-135.

Domesick, V. B., 1969, Projections from the cingulate cortex in the rat, Brain Res. 12:296-320.

Domesick, V. B., 1972, Thalamic relationships of the medial cortex in the rat, Brain Behav. Evol. 6:457-483.

Douglas, R. J., 1972, Pavlovian conditioning and the brain, in "Inhibition and Learning," R. Boakes and M. Halliday, eds., pp. 529-553, Academic Press, London.

Douglas, R. J., 1975, The development of hippocampal function: Implication for theory and therapy, in "The Hippocampus, Vol. 2," R. L. Isaacson, and K. H. Pribram, eds., pp. 327-361. Plenum Press, New York.

Douglas, R. J., and Pribram, K. H., 1969, Distraction and habituation in monkeys with limbic lesions, J. Comp. Physiol. Psychol. 69:473-480.

Douglas, R. J., and Pribram, K. H., 1966, Learning and limbic lesions, Neurophychologia 4:197-220.

Egger, M. D., and Flynn, J. P., 1967, Further studies on the effects of amygdaloid stimulation and ablation on hypothalamically-elicited attack behavior in cats, Prog. Brain Res. 27:165-182.

Ellinwood, Jr., E. H., Sudilovsky, A., and Nelson, L. M., 1973, Evolving behavior in the clinical and experimental amphetamine (model) psychoses, Am. J. Psychiatry 130:1088-1093.

Emson, P. C., Björklund, O., Lindvall, O., and Paxinos, G., 1979, Contributions of different afferent pathways to the catecholamine and 5-hydroxytryptamine innervation of the amygdala: A neurochemical and histochemical study, Neuroscience 4:1347-1357.

Franzén, G., and Ingvar, D. H., 1975, Absence of activation in frontal structures during psychological testing of chronic schizophrenics, J. Neurol. Neurosurg. Psychiatry 38:1027-1032.

Fuxe, K., 1965, The distribution of monoamine terminals in the central nervous system, Acta Physiol. Scand. 64 (Suppl. 247):38-85.

Gloor, P., 1972, Temporal lobe epilepsy: Its possible contribution to the understanding of the significance of the amygdala and of its interactions with neocortical-temporal mechanisms, in "The Neurobiology of the Amygdala, "B. E. Eleftheriou, ed., pp. 423-457, Plenum Press, New York.

Goldman, P. S., and Nauta, W. J. H., 1977, An intricately patterned prefronto-caudate projection in the rhesus monkey, J. Comp. Neurol. 171:369-386.

Graeff, F. G., Quintero, S., and Gray, J. A., 1980, Median raphe stimulation, hippocampal theta rhythm and threat-induced behavioral inhibition, Physiol. Behav. 25:253-261.

Grandstaff, N. W., and Pribram, K. H., 1972, Habituation: Electrical changes in the visual system, Neuropsychologia 10:125-132.

Graybiel, A. M., and Ragsdale, C. W., 1979, Fiber connections of the basal ganglia, Prog. Brain. Res. 51:239-283.

Green, J. F., and Arduini, A., 1954, Hippocampal electrical activity in arousal, J. Neurophysiol. 17:533-557.

Groll, E., 1966, Central nervous system and peripheral activation variables during vigilance performance, Z. Exp. Angew. Psychol. 13:248-264.

Grossman, S. P., 1972, The role of the amygdala in escape-avoidance behaviors, in "The Neurobiology of the Amygdala," B. E. Eleftheriou, ed., pp. 537-551, Plenum Press, New York.

Hall, E., 1972, Some aspects of the structural organization of the amygdala, in "The Neurobiology of the Amygdala," B. E. Eleftheriou, ed., pp. 95-121, Plenum Press, New York.

Hassler, R., 1978, Striatal control of locomotion, intentional actions and of integrating and perceptive activity, J. Neurol. Sci. 36:187-224.

Heimer, L., and Wilson, R. D., 1975, The subcortical projections of the allocortex: Similarities in the neural associations of the hippocampus, the piriform cortex, and the neocortex, in "Golgi Centennial Symposium," M. Santini, ed., pp. 177-193, Raven Press, New York.

Heise, G. A., 1975, Discrete trial analysis of drug action, Fed. Proc. 34:1898-1903.

Herkenham, M., and Nauta, W. J. H., 1977, Afferent connections of the habenular nuclei in the rat: A horseradish peroxidase study, with a note on the fiber-of-passage problem, J. Comp. Neurol. 173:123-146.

Herkenham, M., and Nauta, W. J. H., 1979, Efferent connections of the habenular nuclei in the rat, J. Comp. Neurol. 187:19-48.

Herzog, A. G., and Van Hoesen, G. W., 1976, Temporal neocortical afferent connections to the amygdala in the rhesus monkey, Brain Res. 115:57-69.

Hillarp, N.-Å, Fuxe, K., and Dahlström, A., 1966, Demonstration and mapping of central neurons containing dopamine, noradrenaline, and 5-hydroxytryptamine and their reactions to psychopharmaca, Pharmacol. Rev. 18:(No. 1, Part 1):727-741.

Hingtgen, J. N., and Aprison, M. H., 1976, Behavioral and environmental aspects of the cholinergic system, in "Biology of Cholinergic Function," A. M. Goldberg, and I. Hanin, eds., pp. 515-566, Raven Press, New York.

Humphrey, T., 1972, The development of the human amygdala complex, in "The Neurobiology of the Amygdala," B. E. Eleftheriou, ed., pp. 21-80, Plenum Press, New York.

Ingvar, D. H., and Franzén, G., 1974, Abnormalities of cerebral blood flow distribution in patients with chronic schizophrenia, Acta Psychiatr. Scand. 50:425-462.

Isaacson, R. L., 1972, Neural systems of the limbic brain and behavioral inhibition, in "Inhibition and Learning," R. A. Boakes and M. S. Halliday, eds., pp. 41-71, Academic Press, New York.

Isaacson, R. L., 1974, "The Limbic System," Plenum Press, New York.

Jasper, H. H., 1949, Diffuse projection systems - The integrative action of the thalamic reticular system, Electroencephalogr. Clin. Neurophysiol. 1:405-420.

Kaada, B. R., 1972, Stimulation and regional ablation of the amygdaloid complex with reference to functional representations, in "The Neurobiology of the Amygdala," B. E. Eleftheriou, ed., pp. 205-281, Plenum Press, New York.

Kaada, B. R., 1951, Somato-motor, autonomic and electrocorticographic responses to electrical stimulation of "rhinencephalic" and other structures in primates, cat and dog: A study of responses from the limbic, subcallosal, orbito-insular, piriform and temporal cortex, hippocampus fornix and amygdala, Acta Physiol. Scand. 24 (Suppl. 83):1-285.

Kamp, A., Lopes DaSilva, F. H., and Storm Van Leeuwen, W., 1971, Hippocampal frequency shifts in different behavioral situations, Brain Res. 31:287-294.

Karczmar, A. G., 1975, Cholinergic influences on behavior, in "Cholinergic Mechanisms," P. G. Waser, ed., pp. 501-529, Raven Press, New York.

Karczmar, A. G., 1977, Exploitable aspects of central cholinergic function, particularly with respect to the EEG, motor, analgesic and mental functions, in "Cholinergic Mechanisms and Psychopharmacology," D. J. Jenden, ed., pp. 679-708, Plenum Press, New York.

Karczmar, A. G., 1979, Brain acetylcholine and animal electrophysiology, in "Brain Acetylcholine and Neuropsychiatric Disease," K. L. Davis, and P. A. Berger, eds., pp. 265-310, Plenum Publishing Corp., New York.

Karli, P., Vergnes, M., Eclancher, F., Schmitt, P., and Chaurand, J. P. 1972, Role of the amygdala on the control of "mouse-killing" behavior in the rat, in "The Neurobiology of the Amygdala," B. E. Eleftheriou, ed., pp. 553-580, Plenum Press, New York.

Kling, A., and Steklis, H. D., 1976, A neural substrate for affiliative behavior in nonhuman primates, Brain Behav. Evol. 13:216-238.

Koikegami, H., 1963, Amygdala and other related limbic structures: Experimental studies on the anatomy and function. I. Anatomical researches with same neurophysiological observations, Acta Med. Biolog. (Niigata), 10:161-277.

Koikegami, H., 1964, Amygdala and other related limbic structures: Experimental studies on the anatomy and function. II. Functional experiments, Acta Med. Biolog. (Niigata) 12:73-266.

Kornhuber, H. H., 1971, Motor functions of cerebellum and basal ganglia: The cerebellocortical saccadic (ballistic) clock, the cerebellonuclear hold regulator, and the basal ganglia ramp (the voluntary speed smooth movement) generator, Kybernetik 8:157-162.

Künzle, H., 1977, Projections from the primary somatosensory cortex to basal ganglia and thalamus in the monkey, Exp. Brain Res. 30:481-492.

Kuypers, H. G. J. M., and Maisky, V. A., 1975, Retrograde transport of horseradish peroxidase from spinal cord to brain stem cell groups in the rat, Neurosci. Lett. 1:9-14.

Lammers, H. L., The neural connections of the amygdaloid complex in
    mammals, 1972, in "The Neurobiology of the Amygdala," B. E.
    Eleftheriou, ed., pp. 123-144, Plenum Press, New York.
Lindsley, D. B., 1961, The reticular activating system and perceptual
    integration, in "Electrical Stimulation of the Brain," D. E.
    Sheer, ed., University of Texas Press, Austin.
Magoun, H. W., 1958, "The Waking Brain," Charles Thomas, Springfield.
Macadar, A. W., Chalupa, L. M., and Lindsley, D. B., 1974, Differen-
    tiation of brain stem loci which affect hippocampal and neocorti-
    cal electrical activity, Exp. Neurol. 43:499-514.
Mahut, H., 1971, Spatial and object reversal learning in monkeys with
    partial temporal lobe ablations, Neuropsychologia 9:409-424.
Matthies, H., Ott, T., and Kammerer, E., 1975, Cholinergic influences
    on learning, in "Cholinergic Mechanisms," P. G. Waser, ed.,
    pp. 493-499, Raven Press, New York.
Matthysse, S., 1974, Schizophrenia: Relationship to dopamine trans-
    mission, motor control and feature extraction, in "The Neuro-
    sciences: Third Study Program," T. O. Schmitt, and T. G. Worden,
    eds., pp. 733-737, MIT Press, Cambridge.
Matthysse, S., 1977, The biology of attention, Schizophr. Bull.
    3(3):370-372.
Mesulam, M.-M., and Geschwind, N., 1978, On the possible role of
    neocortex and its limbic connections in the process of attention
    and schizophrenia: Clinical cases of inattention in man and
    experimental anatomy in monkey, J. Psychiatr. Res. 14:249-259.
Mesulam, M.-M., Van Hoesen, G. W., Pandya, D. N., and Geschwind, N.,
    1977, Limbic and sensory connections of the inferior parietal
    lobule (Area PG) in the rhesus monkey: A study with a new method
    for horseradish peroxidase histochemistry, Brain Res. 136:393-414.
Mettler, F. A., 1955, Perceptual capacity, functions of the corpus
    striatum and schizophrenia, Psychiatr. Q. 29:89-111.
Mishkin, M., 1978, Memory in monkeys severely impaired by combined
    but not by separate removal of amygdala and hippocampus, Nature
    273:297-298.
Moruzzi, G., and Magoun, H. W., 1949, Brain stem reticular formation
    and activation of the EEG, Electroencephalogr. Clin. Neurophysiol.
    1:455-473.
MacLean, P. D., 1972, Cerebral evolution and emotional processes: new
    findings on the striatal complex, Ann. N.Y. Acad. Sci.
    193:137-139.
MacLean, P. D., 1976, Sensory and perceptive factors in emotional
    functions of the triune brain, in "Biological Foundations of
    Psychiatry, Vol. 1." R. G. Grenell and S. Gabay, eds.,
    pp. 177-198, Raven Press, New York.
Nauta, W. J. H., 1971, The problem of the frontal lobe: A reinterpre-
    tation, J. Psychiatr. Res. 8:167-187.
Nauta, W. J. H., and Domesick, V. B., 1981, Ramifications of the
    limbic system, in "Psychiatry and the Biology of the Human
    Brain," S. Matthysse, ed., pp. 165-188, Elsevier North Holland,
    Amsterdam.

Nurnberger, Jr., J., Sitaram, N., Gershon, E. S., and Christian
    Gillin, J., 1983, A twin study of cholinergic REM induction,
    Biol. Psychiatry 18:1161-1165.
O'Hanlon, J. F., and Beatty, F., 1977, Concurrence of electroencepha-
    lographic and performance changes during a simulated radar watch
    and some implications for the arousal theory of vigilance, in
    "Vigilance Theory: Operational Performance and Physiological
    Correlates," G. Mackie, ed., pp. 189-201., Plenum Press, London.
Olds, J., 1976, Reward and drive neurons: 1975, in "Brain-Stimulation
    Reward," A. Wauquier and E. T. Rolls, eds., pp. 1-27, North
    Holland Publishing Company, Amsterdam.
Olton, D. S., 1972, Behavioral and neuroanatomical differentiation of
    response suppression and response-shift mechanisms in the rat, J.
    Comp. Physiol. Psychol. 78:450-456.
Pandya, D. N., and Kuypers, H. G. J. M., 1969, Cortico-cortical con
    nections in the rhesus monkey, Brain Res. 13:13-36.
Petras, J. M., 1971, Connections of the parietal lobe, J. Psychiatr.,
    Res. 8:189-201.
Pribram, K. H., 1971, Languages of the Brain Experimental Paradoxes
    and Principles in "Neuropsychology," Prentice Hall, Englewood
    Cliffs. Pribram, K. H., 1967, Memory and the organization of
    attention, in "Brain Function," D. B. Lindsley and A. A.
    Lumsdaine, eds., University of California Press, Berkeley.
Pribram, K. H., 1960, The intrinsic systems of the forebrain, in
    "Handbook of Physiology, Neurophysiology II," J. Field, H. W.
    Magoun and V. E. Hall, eds., American Physiological Society,
    Washington, D.C.
Pribram, K. H., and Isaacson, R. L., 1975, Summary, in "The Hippocam-
    pus," R. L. Isaacson and K. H. Pribram, eds., pp. 429-441, Plenum
    Press, New York.
Pribram, K. H., and McGuiness, D., 1975, Arousal, activation and
    effort in the control of attention, Psychol. Rev. 82:116-149.
Randrup, A., and Munkvad, I., 1968, Behavioral stereotypies induced by
    pharmacological agents, Pharmacopsychiatry 1:18-26.
Randrup, A., and Munkvad, I., 1970, Biochemical anatomical and psycho-
    logical investigations of stereotyped behavior induced by ampheta-
    mines, in "Amphetamines and Related Compounds," E. Costa and S.
    Garratini, eds., pp. 695-713, Raven Press, New York.
Rodgers, R. J., and Brown, K., 1976, Amygdaloid function in the
    central cholinergic mediation of shock-induced aggression in the
    rat, Aggress. Behav. 2:131-152.
Routtenberg, A., 1968, The two-arousal hypothesis: Reticular forma-
    tion and limbic system, Psychol. Rev. 75:51-80.
Saper, C. B., Loewy, A. D., Swanson, L. W., and Cowan, W. M., 1976,
    Direct hypothalamo-autonomic connections, Brain Res. 177:305-312.
Schallert, T., DeRyck, M., and Teitelbaum, P., 1980, Atropine stereo-
    typy as a behavioral trap: A movement subsystem and electroence-
    phalographic analysis, J. Comp. Physiol. Psychol. 94:1-24.
Schwent, V. L., and Hillyard, S. A., 1975, Evoked potential correlates
    of selective attention with multichannel auditory inputs, Electro-
    enceph. Clin. Neurophysiol. 38:131-138.

Shakow, D., 1971, Some observations on the psychology (and some fewer
    in the biology) of schizophrenia, J. Nerv. Ment. Dis. 153:300-316.
Shakow, D., 1977, "Schizophrenia, Selected Papers. Psychology Issues
    10, No. 2," International Universities Press, New York.
Shute, C. C. D., and Lewis, P. R., 1967, The ascending cholinergic
    reticular systems: Neocortical, olfactory and subcortical projec-
    tions, Brain 90:497-520.
Shute, C. C. D., and Lewis, P. R., 1975, Cholinergic pathways 1. His-
    tochemical localization, Pharmacol. Ther. 1:79-87.
Singh, M. M., 1981, Cholinergic mechanisms and the psychobiology of
    schizophrenia, in "Biological Psychiatry 1981," C. Perris, G.
    Struwe and B. Jansson, eds., pp. 793-800, Elsevier/North Holland,
    Amsterdam.
Singh, M. M., and Kay, S. R., 1982, Towards a psychobiological model
    of schizophrenia: A clinical neuroscientist's view, in "Psycho-
    biology of Schizophrenia," M. Namba and H. Kaiya, eds.,
    pp. 93-107, Pergamon Press, Oxford.
Singh, M. M., and Lal, H., 1982, Central cholinergic mechanisms,
    neuroleptic action and schizophrenia, in "Neuropharmacology:
    Clinical Applications," W. B. Essman and L. Valzelli, eds.,
    pp. 337-389, Spectrum Publications, New York.
Starzl, T. E., and Magoun, H. W., 1951, Organization of the diffuse
    thalamic projection system, J. Neurophysiol 14:133-146.
Stevens, J. R., 1973, An anatomy of schizophrenia?, Arch. Gen.
    Psychiatry 29:177-189.
Taylor, M., and Abrams, R., 1974, Manic-depressive illness and para-
    noid schizophrenia: A phenomenological, family and treatment-
    response study, Arch. Gen. Psychiatry 31:640-642.
Tecce, J. J., 1972, Contingent negative variation (CNV) and psycho-
    logical processes in man, Psychol. Bull. 77:73-108.
Teuber, H. L., 1976, Complex functions of basal ganglia, in "The Basal
    Ganglia," M. D. Yahr, ed., pp. 151-168, Raven Press, New York.
Torü, S., 1961, Two types of pattern of hippocampal electrical activ-
    ity induced by stimulation of hypothalamus and surrounding parts
    of rabbit's brain, Jpn. J. Physiol. 11:147-157.
Turner, B. H., Mishkin, M., and Knapp, M., 1980, Organization of the
    amygdalopetal projections from modality-specific cortical asso-
    ciation areas in the monkey, J. Comp. Neurol. 191-515-543.
Ungerstedt, U., 1971, Stereotaxic mapping of the monoamine pathways in
    the rat brain, Acta Physiol. Scand. 197 (suppl. 367):1-48.
Ungerstedt, U., and Pycock, C., 1974, Functional correlates of dopa-
    mine neurotransmission, Bull. Schweiz. Akad. Med. Wiss. 30:44-55.
Van den Bercken, J. H. L., and Cools, A. R., 1979, Role of the neo-
    striatum in the initiation, continuation and termination of
    behavior, Appl. Neurophysiol. 42:106-108.
Vanderwolf, C. H., 1969, Hippocampal electrical activity and voluntary
    movement in the rat, Electroencephalogr. Clin. Neurophysiol.
    26:407-418.
Vanderwolf, C. H., 1971, Limbic-diencephalic mechanisms of voluntary
    movement, Psychol. Rev. 78:83-113.

Vanderwolf, C. H., and Robinson, T. E., 1981, Reticulo-cortical activity and behavior: A critique of the arousal theory and a new synthesis, Behav. Brain Sciences 4:459-514.

Van Hoesen, G. W., and Pandya, D. N., 1975, Some connections of the entorhinal (area 28) and the perirhinal (area 35) cortices of the rhesus monkey. I. Temporal lobe afferents, Brain Res. 95:1-24.

Van Hoesen, G. W., Pandya, D. N., and Butters, N., 1975, Some connections of the entorhinal (area 28) and perirhinal (area 35) cortices of the rhesus monkey. II. Frontal lobe afferents, Brain Res. 95:25-38.

Villablanca, J. R., and Marcus, R. J., 1975, Effects of caudate nucleus removal in cats. Comparison with effects of frontal cortex ablation, UCLA Forum Med. Science 18:273-311.

Vinogradova, O., 1970, Registration of information and the limbic system, in "Short-term Changes in Neural activity and Behavior," G. Horn and R. H. Hinde, eds., Cambridge University Press, Cambridge.

Warburton, D. M., 1974, The effect of scopolamine on a two-cue discrimination, Q. J. Exp. Psychol. 26:395-404.

Warburton, D. M., and Heise, G. A., 1972, The effects of scopolamine on double alternation in rats, J. Comp. Physiol. Psychol. 81-523-532.

Wesnes, K., and Warburton, D. M., 1983, Effects of scopolamine on stimulus sensitivity and response bias in a visual vigilance task, Neuropsychobiology 9:154-157.

Whitehouse, J. M., 1967, Cholinergic mechanisms in discrimination learning as a function of stimuli, J. Comp. Physiol. Psychol. 63:448-451.

Whitlock, D. G., and Nauta, W. J. H., 1956, Subcortical projections from the temporal neocortex in macaca mulatta, J. Comp. Neurol. 106:183-212.

Wilcott, R. C., Sabol, B. A., and Yurcheshen, R. P., 1976, Frontal cortex and response suppression in the rat, Brain Behav. Evol. 13:116-124.

Walaas, I., and Fonnum, F., 1980, Biochemical evidence for glutamate as a transmitter in hippocampal efferents to the rat brain, Neuroscience 5(10):1691-1698.

Wishart, T. B., and Mogenson, G. J., 1970, Effects of lesions of the hippocampus and septum before and after passive avoidance training, Physiol. Behav. 5:31-34.

INDEX

Acetylcholine (ACh)
  and cortical desynchronization,
      17, 22–23, 196, 227–229
  and dopamine interactions,
      106–131
    in depression, 106
    in Huntington's disease, 106
    in mania, 106
    in Parkinsonism, 106–108
    in schizophrenia, 106–109, 252
    in tardive dyskinesia, 106
  as neurotransmitter in the
      brain, 17–18
  release from the cortex, 17, 64,
      196–197, 229
  and sensory inputs, 18, 196,
      227–229
  turnover, 38, 40–41, 44, 194
Acetylcholinesterase (AChE)
  activity in the brain and
      behavior, 6–8
  cortical-subcortical ratio and
      behavior, 7–8
  containing neurons in the brain,
      18, 37–51, 116, 124, 195
  in schizophrenic brain, 286–287
  in dementias, 341
Active avoidance, 148–150
  cholinergic effects on, 148–150
  antimuscarinic effects on,
      149–150, 374
Adaptive behavior, 2–11, 200–206,
      249, 354, 369, 373,
      375–384
  and acetylcholine, 2–11,
      200–206, 249, 373, 375–384
  and brain acetylcholinesterase,
      6–8

Adaptive behavior (continued)
  and brain cholinesterase, 6–8
  definition of, 354
  and hippocampal circuit, 369,
      373, 377–379
Aggression, 161–183, 206, 365,
      381–383
  and amygdala, 49, 166–167,
      170–174, 365, 381–383
  brain model of, 174–176, 381–383
  and caudate nucleus, 170, 174
  and cholinergic circuits, 174,
      381–383
  defensive, shock-induced (SIDF),
      164–167, 174–177, 206
  and dopamine mechanism, 179–180,
      182
  fear induced, 162–163, 206
  and hippocampus, 166, 170, 382
  in humans, 180–182
  and hypothalamus, 165, 167,
      170–171
  instrumental, 163
  inter-male, 162
  irritable, 163, 170–171, 179–182
  isolation-induced, 169–170, 178
  maternal, 163
  and midbrain tegmentum, 168–170,
      174–175
  and muscarinic blockade, 165–171
  and muscarinic stimulation, 49,
      165–171
  and neurotransmitter interac-
      tions, 179, 206, 382
  and nicotine stimulation,
      176–182, 383
  and norepinephrine mechanism,
      179, 382

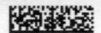